P9-EMR-804

* * * * * *

ALLERGY-FREE GARDENING

* * * * * *

ALLERGY-FREE

The Revolutionary Guide to Healthy Landscaping

GARDENING

Thomas Leo Ogren

Ten Speed Press
Berkeley Toronto

Ten Speed Press
PO Box 7123
Berkeley, California 94707
www.tenspeed.com

Distributed in Australia by Simon and Schuster Australia, in Canada by Ten Speed Press Canada, in New Zealand by Southern Publishers Group, in South Africa by Real Books, in Southeast Asia by Berkeley Books, and in the United Kingdom and Europe by Airlift Book Company.

Cover Design by Mary Rose O'Leary
Book Design by Jeffery Edward Puda
Original Illustrations by Paquerette
Photography by Tom Ogren, Frank Mullin, Shelby Stover, and J. Frank Schmidt and Son Company

Library of Congress Cataloging-in-Publication Data on file with the publisher.
ISBN 1-58008-166-5 (paper)
ISBN 1-58008-200-9 (cloth)

First printing, 2000
Printed in the United States of America

1 2 3 4 5 6 7 8 9 10 — 05 04 03 02 01 00

Dedication

*　*　*　*　*　*　*　*　*　*　*　*

I would like to dedicate this book to Dr. Thomas Myers, my grandfather, and to Katherine Scott, my great friend. Both of these wonderful people have long since passed on to the great garden above. More than any others, when I was a small boy, they encouraged me to love Nature and especially gardening.

"The female of the species is less deadly than the male."
—with apologies to Kipling

Contents

List of Illustrations

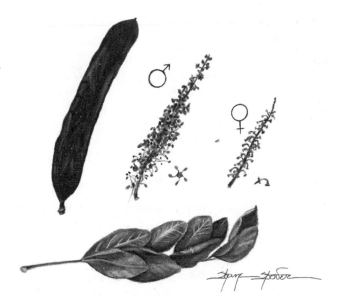

Acknowledgments

I would especially like to thank Dr. David Stadtner, M.D., of Stockton, California, for his advice and strong support. Dr. Stadtner (an allergist and a good one) told me that Hippocrates advised his medical students to learn all they could about the flora (plants) of the area in which they planned to practice, so that they would better understand the needs of their patients. It was good advice back then and is just as good today.

The first time I ever talked to Dr. Stadtner, as I was telling him about all the amazing things I was discovering, he said to me, "The more you look, the more you'll find. That's true in allergy study and in all of science for that matter."

I would also like to thank my fellow writer, Vicki Leon, author of the *Uppity Women Series*, for her vigorous encouragement of this project since I told her about my ideas many years ago. I also want to thank my wonderful wife, Yvonne, for her steady help and encouragement, and for the loss of thousands of hours of possible quality time we might well have spent together had I not been researching plants and allergy. No writer could have a more understanding or supportive wife.

Likewise, my four children, Sarah, Hildur, Naomi, and Josh have also tolerated me as I worked long into the night doing this labor of love. Sarah and Hildur are fine writers in their own right. They acted as my first agents and had the good sense to send this book to Ten Speed Press.

My first editor at Ten Speed, Heather Garnos, is certainly due thanks for *discovering* me. The editor who actually put this book together, Jason Rath, is owed much gratitude for all his hard work, his sense of humor, and his keen insight. Thanks, too, to Lorena Jones for getting this book finalized.

Ten Speed Publisher Kirsty Melville has long been interested in publishing a book on the subject, and was always a pleasure to work with.

My sister Rachel Clark, one of the first to steer me towards plant-allergy research, has long been a staunch believer in the ultimate importance of this work. My sister Mary Rose O'Leary, a very talented commercial artist, designed and created the simply marvelous book cover.

My brothers, Paul and David, always thought I was headed in the right direction here, and Paul especially contributed greatly to the manuscript with his many ideas and extensive help in collecting data.

My sister Liz and her husband, Dr. Dan Krieger, were always supportive, and also roamed around the state with me helping to chase down just the right photographs.

Many of the photographs in this book are from two talented friends, Frank Mullin and Shelby Stover. Shelby also taught me how to use a camera. The drawing of carob tree in the book is from the award-winning young artist, Shane Stover.

Thanks are also due to J. Frank Schmidt and Son Company for use of some of their fine photos of female maple trees.

I was also quite lucky to have over seventy incredible line drawings from the multi-talented young Cajun artist, Paquerette. Her incredible art work dresses up many a page in *Allergy-Free Gardening*.

Likewise, I am indebted to the USDA for permission to use line drawings from their wonderful 1949 Yearbook, *Trees*, drawn by the talented Miss Leta Hughey, of the U.S. Forest Service, and by Sidney H. Horn, of Ames, Iowa. Thanks also to David Nowak of the USDA Forest Service, Northwestern Research Station.

Special thanks are also in order for my enthusiastic literary agent, Sheree Bykofsky; to Joann Woy for her unusually thorough copyediting; to Barbara King for her careful job of proofreading; to Jane Bethard-Tracy for her help with the photos and invaluable editorial assistance; and to Jeff Puda, the creative book designer.

Special thanks are also due to the brilliant allergist and writer, Doris Rapp, M.D., for her early consideration and advice.

At the University of California, Davis, I was greatly assisted in plant hunting by Dr. Warren Roberts, the director of the UC Davis Arboretum. Also at UC Davis I was given much cheerful help going through the wonderful greenhouse collections by the greenhouse supervisor, Tim Metcalf, and his able assistant, Ernesto Sandoval.

At the Seattle Arboretum I was given good advice by Randall Hitchin, John, David, Jade, and Lou. The Seattle Arboretum staff is extremely knowledgeable and does a fabulous job at keeping the entire grounds looking lush. At the Los Angeles Arboretum I was given good advice by botanist David Lofgren.

At Cal Poly University, San Luis Obispo, my graduate committee, doctors Gene Offerman, Dale Smith, and Glen Casey, all encouraged and helped me to follow through with the project. Botany professor Dr. Lee Parker gave me all his data from four years of daily pollen collections, samples collected from the top of the Fisher Science Building at Cal Poly.

I owe a special debt of gratitude to Dr. Walter H. Lewis, professor of biology at Washington University, St. Louis, senior botanist at the Missouri Botanical Gardens, and lead author of the seminal work, *Airborne and Allergenic Pollen of North America*, John Hopkins University Press. Professor Lewis contributed valuable editing, and the wonderful photographs of individual pollen grains used in the text. Of the thousands of publications I've read on pollen and allergy, no single author has impressed or influenced me as greatly as Walter H. Lewis. Walter Lewis's remarkable wife, microbiologist, professor, and writer, Memory Elvin Lewis, also helped proof this book, and I am indebted to her for both her valuable suggestions and her warm, generous friendship.

My parents, two remarkable people, Bud and Paula Ogren, were always enthusiastic and pushed, prodded, and bugged me to get it all down on paper. They also very graciously volunteered to proofread the entire text—believe me, no easy task. I warned them before they started that when they were done they might know more about allergy and horticulture than they ever intended to know.

My father actually did proof every single word and comma in this text and without a doubt the entire book is far more readable, easier to understand, and much better constructed because of his numerous intelligent contributions.

To all of these wonderful people, thank you all so much. I could never have finished the book without your help.

Thomas Leo Ogren

Foreword

David A. Stadtner, M.D.

V ery rarely do we come across an idea that is both exceptionally good and revolutionary in its scope; the book *Allergy-Free Gardening* by Thomas Leo Ogren is such an idea.

I am eighty years old now and have been a practicing allergist for more than fifty years. In the past I often advised people to avoid the "toxic" highly allergenic shrubs and trees, but my knowledge of botany was limited. I only knew that certain plants were notorious for causing symptoms. When I started to practice in Stockton, California, I had the university botanist drive around town with me and point out the flora.

Today, allergies themselves are given short shrift in American medical schools, and perhaps in Europe as well. Students preparing for a medical career will receive only one or two lectures on the subject during a four-year course of intense study.

At one time, allergists were required to learn a great deal of botany, but I think those days have gone the way of the kindly family doctor. I recall that Hippocrates advised his students to study the winds and ecology of an area in which they planned to practice. It was good advice then and equally important today.

In Stockton, we are tortured by the pollen of walnuts, pecans, and olives. People who live close to our cherry and almond orchards sometimes develop severe asthma from the pollen. There are many more trees, shrubs, and ground covers that cause allergies in our area, but few of us are aware of the actual culprits. This book is a great leap forward because it combines allergy study and horticulture.

Detecting allergies is often difficult for the average person, because many reactions are not immediate. There are two kinds of allergy in regard to time. Most people have their allergy attack start within thirty minutes of exposure or sooner. This is often called "immediate." There are also those who do not have any symptoms at all until hours later, usually six to eight hours. This delay makes it hard to know what kind of pollen it is that has affected you.

There are many interesting stories in the study of allergy. The story of the castor bean is one. Early in World War II, the defense industry needed castor oil as a lubricant. Many farmers planted huge fields of castor beans. Nothing happened the first year, but starting in the second, the farmers and their close neighbors began to have severe allergic reactions to the pollen, some nearly catastrophic. Today, remains of those castor beans grow here and there in many American cities, still causing frequent cases of asthma.

Before this book, if you wanted to plant a landscape with allergy-free plants, you had few places to turn for advice. Some landscapers knew that fruitless mulberries and olive trees caused allergy, but that was about it. Several things especially make this work so valuable. The allergy scale in the book, assigning all plants a simple 1 to 10 allergy rating, is a marvelous idea. All plants, just like all people, are not created equal. Certain trees, for example, may cause allergy, but not to many people. Other trees or shrubs will cause almost no allergy, some will cause none at all, and some will cause a great deal of suffering. Ogren's allergy scale addresses this problem head on.

Another fine idea in this book is the reasoning about the dioecious species of plants. Dioecious (separate-sexed) plants cause far more than their share of allergies, because the male plants usually produce so much airborne pollen. These species, which include many common plants such as willows, ash, and maples, are often described as the worst allergy offenders. What the author figured out here is that the flip side is also true. If the males are the worst, then the females are the best! This is a simple idea, perhaps, but up until now no one had really addressed it.

The author has done an immense amount of work gathering information on allergenic and non-allergenic plants. Allergies cause a huge amount of pain and suffering. There are many medical treatments for allergies, and none of them is perfect. All of them have side effects.

The very best treatment for allergy is to avoid the offending substance. When the state or city park department plants trees for shade, they can end up causing immense suffering because of their poor choice of trees. Homeowners, too, unknowingly make poor choices and cause themselves years of allergy as they surround their houses with allergy-causing trees, shrubs, and lawns.

Allergy-Free Gardening is a well-written and greatly needed book. The science on which it has been developed is sound, and the book should withstand the test of time. It is my hope that the subject will become very popular. If the recommendations are followed, we will reduce dramatically the high costs that plant allergies impose on the susceptible individual and on our society. The author has made a valuable contribution to our good health, and now it is up to us to put the information to work.

Allergy-Free Gardening should be on the shelf of every serious gardener. All allergy specialists would be wise to own a copy, and certainly the book should be in the library of every nursery and municipal park department. Perhaps most important of all, this text should be required reading for every college student of landscape design or horticulture.

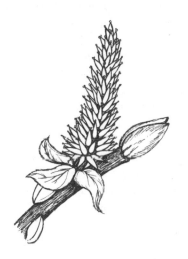

Introduction

"Gardening," said Sir Francis Bacon, "is the purest of human pleasures."

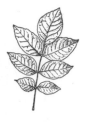

We create our landscapes and gardens to give us pleasure, to soothe our weary nerves, to reconnect us to Mother Nature, to entertain us, sometimes to feed us, and always to beautify our surroundings. Our gardens show our friends and neighbors that we know and appreciate fine trees, shrubs, vines, annuals, and perennials. "Gardening," said Sir Francis Bacon, "is the purest of human pleasures." But as anyone who has allergies knows all too well, hay fever, rashes, and asthma are far from pleasurable. The concept—the soul—of this book is simply that through research, common sense, and knowledge, we can create fabulous landscapes and gardens that will not make us, our children, or our neighbors sick. As gardeners, we can control what we plant and dramatically limit allergens in our own yards. This book was written with the serious gardener always in mind. It is intended to be a useful tool for making informed choices and a handy reference that you can take to the nursery with you.

When you buy trees and shrubs, check the plant tags and compare the scientific name, and cultivar name if given, with the allergy ranking in this text. All the plants here are listed in alphabetical order by their scientific names, and they have also been cross-referenced by their common names.

(**Please note**: Nursery tags, as yet, do not give the sex of separate-sexed plants, thus it is crucial to know the exact cultivar name and then to compare it to the listing in this text.)

Over a decade ago, I decided to research gardening and allergy so that I could create an allergy-free garden in my own yard. My wife, Yvonne, has long had both hay fever and asthma and I was, after all, a horticulturist. I soon found that there was very little written for the layman on the subject.

I talked to every nurseryman, horticulture professor, and landscape designer I could find who would listen to my questions. I visited local and university libraries. I got on the Internet and searched. I pored over dusty old texts of allergy study and botany. I read books on pollen and on the numerous flowering systems of the plant kingdom. For more than a dozen years I clipped every newspaper and magazine article remotely connected to allergy. I conducted allergy tests using pollen of plants I had not found documented but that I suspected of being allergenic. We especially conducted sniff tests, in which myself and others sniffed individual flowers and then gauged the response or lack of response. I also did many scratch tests on myself and willing others. We simply made a light scratch on the arm, not so deeply as to draw any blood, rubbed in pollen, and evaluated the results: a slight itching, a little redness and itch, on up through the worst, which was when the scratched-in pollen caused a red and raised itchy welt. Interestingly, itchiness is one of the biggest indicators of allergy, whether itchy skin, nose, eyes, or ears. Pollen can make you itch!

On occasion I did another type of allergy test in which subjects simply held pollen or flowers suspected of causing them allergy. First we would measure their pulse rate before holding the sample and then re-measure the pulse when holding the substance. Often a pollen found to be allergenic would raise the pulse rate considerably. This test can be reliable if done right but is not as easy as the sniff or scratch test.

A word of warning here: Please! All would-be self-allergists, some of this self-testing is not particularly safe. On several occasions subjects had severe reactions. The best way is to go to an allergist and have them test you.

The more I looked, the more I found. The more I found, the more excited I became about the chance to get a handle on this problem. I decided that what was needed was a good, easy-to-understand book, exactly the sort of book I myself had been trying to find.

In the last few years, other books on the subject of allergy-free gardening have appeared, written mainly for gardeners. Much of the material in these books is good, and they all assert that beautiful, showy, highly colored flowers cause few allergies. And this is true, to a point. However, there are many, many exceptions. A *Catalpa* tree, for example, has large, nicely colored, insect pollinated flowers—but it still causes quite a bit of allergy. And there are dozens of other examples.

It is easy to oversimplify the subject. All trees and shrubs, flowers, ground covers, houseplants, grasses, and whatnot simply cannot be divided into two groups—good plants and bad plants. Almost any plant could cause someone some degree of allergy, somewhere.

Pollen is the main culprit in allergies (although molds are certainly important too; see page 154), and all the flowering plants, except separate-sexed females, have pollen. The real question is, How much of an allergy threat does this particular plant pose in the garden or landscape? There are hundreds of thousands of different kinds of plants with multitudes of different flowering systems. They are not simply all good or all bad.

These same books list ash, maple, poplar, and willow as trees and shrubs to avoid planting. Here they have completely missed the boat! All of these species have separate-sexed trees or shrubs—and no, I repeat, no—female-only plant ever sheds *any* pollen. These lists of what to avoid contain fine plants that I have ranked as totally allergy-free shrubs and trees.

Ogren Plant-Allergy Scale (OPALS™)

Because many useful plants do not fall neatly into a "good" or "bad" category relative to allergy, a rating system for plants and allergy has been devised here, using a large set of criteria of allergen-related factors applied to each particular plant. This index rates plants on a 1 to 10 scale, with 1 being the best, most allergy-free selections, and 10 being the worst.

OPALS was built chiefly by asking two questions: First, "What do plants that are known to cause very little or no allergy have in common?" And second, "What do plants that are known to cause allergies have in common?" The system is not perfect, but it is based on solid, scientific principles. OPALS is also a first of a kind, because there has never been a plant-allergy scale in existence before it.

In this system, annuals are compared to other annuals, perennials to perennials, shrubs to shrubs, and trees to trees. Obviously, a small perennial with a rating of 7 will not cause as much allergy as a large tree with the same rating. OPALS takes into account all plant-related allergies including inhalant pollen allergy, odor allergy, reactions to contact with the leaves, stems, sap, roots, bulbs, and so forth. The greatest weight is given to direct inhalant pollen allergies, especially to those that may easily provoke asthma.

There are very many very good plants whose pollen will not cause hay fever or asthma, but which, at the same time, may be quite capable of causing rash or itching. These plants often rate fairly well, 4s and 5s commonly. They are usually not a problem if the gardener is aware that they can cause contact allergy, and thus watches out for these reactions.

Poisonous properties are also considered in OPALS, but this is not usually a heavily weighted factor. If a plant has highly poisonous pollen, this is always taken into account. Many plants are quite poisonous when eaten, but do not otherwise present much potential for allergy. No highly poisonous plants, however, are ever given a rating of 1.

Using this system, is it possible not only to rate individual plants, but also entire landscapes.

One positive sign for the future is that the United States Department of Agriculture (USDA) Urban Forestry Effects Model is now going to include an allergy component—something it was unable to do before—based on the rating system in this book. By multiplying actual species' biomass by each species' allergy rating, a numerical rank can be given to each city studied.

Discussed in this text are thousands of plants, including all the most important horticultural plants used in the United States. Additionally, a great many plants from other countries are included, ones not necessarily used in the United States, but species with high allergenic potential. If a tree, shrub, perennial, biennial, annual, houseplant, or herb poses a serious allergy risk to many, and is commonly used in gardening, it is probably in this book.

Avoidance is the key in allergy relief. Avoid being exposed. The fewer allergenic plants in the garden, the less chance of exposure. Allergy develops from repeated exposure, often from daily exposure. The plants closest to where we work, go to school, or live are those most capable of creating this overexposure.

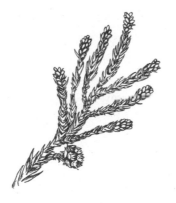

I

What Is Allergy-Free Gardening?

Camellia japonica
TINGLEY

Allergy on the Increase

Just because you don't have allergies now, doesn't mean you never will.

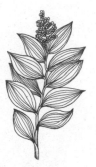

Naysayers will no doubt criticize this work by saying that we can do little to limit allergenic pollen in our yards and neighborhoods, that most serious allergies are caused by airborne weed pollen, like ragweed, that blow in on us from more rural areas no matter what we do with our own landscapes. In fact, however, landscaped urban areas produce their own heavy pollen loads.

Several years ago, in early summer, I was giving a talk on gardening and allergies at Cal Poly University, in San Luis Obispo, a town of about 50 thousand people on California's central coast. I had gathered a large collection of plant samples to use in my talk and thought I should show some actual ragweed plants. For the next two hours I drove all over town, from one vacant lot to another, looking for ragweed and could not find a single plant! San Luis Obispo has plenty of pollen allergies, but not from ragweed. Like many other cities and towns, its allergies are caused by certain plants used in landscapes and gardens.

Just How Common Is Allergy Today?

Depending on what you read or whom you speak to, allergy affects as few as one in ten or as many as one third of all of us. The most commonly recognized signs and symptoms of allergy are nasal stuffiness and congestion; pale mucous membranes; sneezing; runny nose; red or watery eyes; dark circles under the eyes; plugged or stuffy ears; difficulty sleeping; loss of smell or taste; voice changes; postnasal drip; fatigue; scratchy or itchy throat; irritating, lingering cough; mouth breathing; itchy, dry skin; rash; or itchy noses, eyes, and ears. Do any of these sound familiar? Many people have allergies but simply never have been diagnosed.

Over 14 million people in the United States now have asthma. More than 35 million people in the United States suffer from chronic sinus problems. Some 50 million or more are affected by hay fever. One thing to keep in mind is that just because you don't have allergies now doesn't mean you never will. Many people never have an allergy until they are well past 50.

An Epidemic of Allergy

Allergies of all kinds have been on the increase in the United States and in urban environments worldwide. Deaths, particularly from asthma, have almost doubled every decade for the last 40 years. According to the National Institute of Allergy and Infectious Diseases, reports of asthma in the United States increased from 10.4 million to 14.6 million between the years 1990 and 1994. This is an alarming increase.

What is causing this terrible intensification? No one knows for sure. But consider this as a plausible explanation: Since the advent of the "Chemical Revolution" following World War II, exposure to man-made chemicals and potent chemical combinations has expanded wildly. After World War II there was a huge surplus of airplanes, and the United States Department of Agriculture (USDA) quickly made use of these extra planes to wage a huge chemical war against insects. Hundreds of thousands of square miles were blanket-sprayed with insecticides, exposing everyone in the path of these chemical applications to toxins. Even today, well-intentioned government agencies are still spraying "harmless" chemical insecticides over urban populations, as the recent medfly bombardment of the West Coast will attest. This heavy chemical exposure was previously unknown throughout all of mankind's history.

There has also been a great increase in the use of diesel engines in the last five decades, mostly in diesel trucks. Recent data suggest that constant exposure to diesel fumes leaves people much more susceptible to all types of allergies. Diesel waste gases and particulates themselves can trigger allergic attacks. In addition, the millions of tires on cars and trucks in our cities are constantly wearing down, and in the process they release a considerable amount of tiny airborne rubber particles into the air. These rubber particles are themselves potentially allergenic, and they increase the odds of exposed persons later becoming cross-reactive to pollens of other plants that are closely related to *Hevea,* the true rubber tree (see page 120).

To compound the problem, "Better Living through Chemistry" has been combined, in our urban environments, with a large increase in the use of seedless (litter-free), male-only plants in landscaping.

Nurseries have developed thousands of different seedless or "low-maintenance" varieties to supply these litter-free landscapes. Unfortunately, these seedless plants are usually all-male clones, which, while they don't produce seeds, do produce vast amounts of irritating airborne pollen. Our large urban landscapes are highly overpopulated with these heavy pollinating all-male trees, shrubs, and ground covers, and this combined with vast increases in the use of nonnative plant material—much of it highly allergenic and capable of producing massive amounts of airborne pollen—has in no small part contributed to the huge surge in allergy occurrence.

My theory is that this combination of urban pollution and greatly increased total pollen loads has caused the epidemic of allergy.

Horticulture's Dirty Little Secret: VOCs

Although it has been known for many years that certain trees actually cause air pollution and smog, this has been given very little attention. I suspect the same folks who want to hear nothing about allergy-free gardening also want little publicity about volatile organic compounds (VOCs).

VOCs are hydrocarbons which, when mixed with sunlight and nitrogen oxide, create ozone and carbon monoxide. Ozone and carbon monoxide are two of the main components of smog.

Most plants—trees in particular—contribute greatly to keeping our air clean by filtering out air pollutants. Trees remove gaseous air pollutants mostly by uptake through the many tiny openings (stomata) in their leaves. Trees and shrubs also remove the tiny airborne particulates that are another component of smog. Maples and plums are two of the very best smog removers. Trees also reduce the total amount of carbon dioxide and increase oxygen levels through photosynthesis.

Now here's the kicker: Some trees produce more VOCs than they remove. In fact, certain trees produce many times more VOCs than they consume. Interestingly, four of the worst VOC-producing trees—oak, carrotwood, eucalyptus, and sycamore—are also heavy allergenic pollen-producing trees. These trees, therefore, contribute to allergy in two ways.

The Future of Allergy-Free Gardening

I was excited when Dr. David Stadtner, the noted allergist, wrote back to me upon reading some of my first chapters and said that my work would help to alleviate much pain and suffering in the world, and that he thought my ideas were "revolutionary." It is indeed a horticultural revolution that I want to jump-start.

Many people have peculiar ideas about allergy. Large numbers of people, even today, still believe that allergies are all in our minds, that if individuals were just stronger mentally, if they had their act together, they wouldn't have any allergies. Amazingly, some of this flawed reasoning exists even in the medical field.

Within the area of commercial horticulture there has been stiff resistance to the ideas put forward in this book. Horticulture is big business. In California alone, over $10 billion was spent on gardening-related purchases in 1997. Vast sums of money are locked up in plant materials that are slammed in this text because they are highly allergenic and make people sick.

Landscapers' associations, I am happy to say, have shown great interest. Customers have been asking about allergy-free plants for some time now, and this has caught the landscapers' attention. The first article I published on this subject was in *California Landscaping*, the trade journal of the California Landscape Contractors Association. Nurserymen are also finally coming aboard. Recently I was asked to write a series of articles for *Pacific Coast Nurseryman Magazine*. I hope others will follow.

Education

Most gardeners ask for advice at their local nurseries. Retail nurserymen and -women need to become informed. The bulk of horticultural information is generated within our colleges and universities. When the connection between allergy and plants becomes a standard part of the curriculum of college horticulture programs, then, and only then, will this book have achieved success.

In our society today we profess (as well we should) to be highly committed to the rights of handicapped people. However, people with serious, sometimes life-threatening, allergies to plant odors and pollens get short shrift. People with allergies have been pushed around long enough. A real, significant reduction in the urban pollen load is long overdue.

I have great faith in those who really love to garden. My wife, Yvonne, and I used to own a retail nursery in Minnesota, and we noticed right away that almost all of our customers were wonderful people. Sure, there was the occasional grouch, but most who came to the nursery were fun, intelligent, interesting, down-to-earth folk. As one gardener to another, I ask all of you to get involved. Allergenic pollens cause much pain and misery, and it simply doesn't have to be this way.

Those of us concerned enough to put ideas into action can get it started, one plant at a time, by creating our own allergy-free gardens. We will be the trendsetters.

Community Involvement

Now is the time for us to fight back. To make major inroads toward reducing both the amount and the severity of allergy in our communities, people must take a stand. Localities must draw a firm line: "We will not plant any more fruitless mulberries, olives, pepper trees, or male-only pollinating shrubs and trees!"

In the allergy-free garden, we may have to learn to live with some seeds and spent flowers as a small price to pay for cleaner air.

I truly hope that the idea of *Allergy-Free Gardening* will spread from family gardens to city planners. In the long run, it can only be through cooperation and consideration for others that we will see vast urban landscapes that soften the concrete edges but cause little or no allergy.

The Basic Concepts of Allergy-Free Gardening

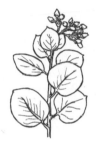

Nature has designed many dispersal systems for male pollen to get to female flower parts. Certain pollens are capable of causing much more allergy than others, and yet all pollen has the potential to cause some degree of allergy.

Allergy-Free Gardening has three aims: first, to reduce the number of plants used that produce highly allergenic pollen; second, to reduce the number of plants that release large amounts of less intense pollen; third, to reduce the number of plants used that cause allergy by their scent, or through contact with their foliage, stems, roots, or flowers.

Sex, Sex, and More Sex

How's that for cheap sensationalism? After editing this manuscript, my dad told me, "You need to write something about sex." Because my father is an old Swede, raised as a Lutheran, and known to be a bit of a prude at times, I was shocked. "Look," he told me, "you have been studying plant flowering systems for so long this whole business about sex and plants is perfectly normal to you. Most people, though, don't know that some plants are male and others are female. Most people don't realize plants have sex at all."

I suppose he's right. Plants do have sexes: some are male, some are female, and some are bisexual. In botany, the terms used for these flowering systems are almost always big twenty-dollar words, hard to remember and easy to confuse. The following list should be sufficient for you to understand the basic classifications used to sex flowering plants:

Perfect flowered. Many flowers, such as apple blossoms or roses, have both male and female parts all inside the same flowers. These flowers may also be called *bisexual, hermaphroditic,* or *complete.* The pollen in a perfect flowered plant doesn't have far to travel, and often, but not always, these plants cause little in the way of pollen allergies.

Monoecious flowered. *Monoecious* is Latin for "one house." In this system, there are separate male and female flowers; however, they are both on the same plant. Corn is a good example of a monoecious plant: the tassels are the male flowers and the ears of corn are clusters of female flowers. The pollen from the tassels drifts down to fertilize the female ears of corn. Oak and cypress are two examples of monoecious-flowered trees: they are pollinated by the wind, and each is capable of causing lots of allergy.

Dioecious flowered. In this system, plants have flowers that are all male or all female, and the plants themselves are either all male or all female. In most cases, the pollen from male plants is carried to the female plants by the wind. Dioecious plants include ash, willows, poplars, hollies, pepper trees, some maples, many kinds of palms, and many others. Pollen from dioecious males causes a great deal of allergy. Dioecious plants are often described as "separate-sexed."

Unisexual flowered. Used loosely, unisexual means that a species may have some flowers that are either only male or only female. Included here are terms such as *monoecious, dioecious, polygamodioecious, polygamomonoecious, gynodioecious,* and so forth. It is not within the scope of this book to closely examine these terms, because the idea of the book is to create something that makes the whole subject understandable. Nonetheless, any plant species that has unisexual flowers requires careful study by the allergy researcher.

Determining Allergy Potential

I used many criteria for determining the allergenicity of the plants in this book. In general, plants that spread their pollen mainly by the wind cause more than their share of allergy problems. Other plants rely on insects to pollinate them. Because these plants usually release less pollen into the air, these plants generally cause fewer allergies. However, allergists consider some of these plants to be *imperfectly insect-pollinated*. These plants are pollinated by insects, but still release plenty of pollen into the air and thus have a higher potential to cause allergy; an acacia tree is a good example of an imperfectly insect-pollinated plant.

Another factor to consider is the *relatives* of a plant. Plants are classified by botanists into large related groups called *families*. All too often, plants with notorious relatives are themselves allergy offenders. The

California pepper tree, for example, is a direct relative of poison ivy and poison oak. It's not surprising to discover that the pepper tree is also highly allergenic. Many families, such as the olive family *(Oleaceae)* and the cashew family *(Anacardiaceae)* have more than their share of allergenic members.

Size, shape, color, fragrance, or *lack of fragrance* must also be weighed when searching for problem plants. There are always exceptions, but in general, small flowers with little color are suspect. Off-white and greenish-colored flowers cause more allergies than all the others combined. On the other hand, blossoms shaped like little trumpets seldom cause much allergy because they are designed so that insects must actually crawl into them to contact the pollen.

The male parts *(stamens)* of the snapdragon flower, for example, are deep within the flower itself. An insect, usually a bumblebee, must push down the spring-loaded bottom lip of the flower and pry it open to get at the pollen. When the bumblebee backs out of the flower, the bloom snaps shut again without releasing pollen into the air. Combined with the snapdragon's attractive colors, subtle, alluring scent, and membership in a genus *(Antirrhinum)* generally free of known allergens, it isn't hard to see why the snapdragon rates as one of the best flowers for an allergy-free garden.

The actual *length of time* during the year that a plant releases pollen is another important consideration. Certain trees may expose us to allergenic pollen for as little as two or three days out of a year, while others (Arizona cypress is a prime example) bloom off and on throughout the year, and may release allergenic pollen for as long as six or seven months. Some eucalyptus trees are in bloom almost all year long, raining pollen almost continually on everything nearby.

The *specific gravity* of each species' pollen must be taken into account. Some pollen grains are heavy for their size, and heavy pollen will not fall far from the plant. Other pollens are extremely light and float easily in the wind; this lightweight pollen frequently causes problems.

The relative *dryness or stickiness* of a species' pollen must also be factored. Sticky pollen often sticks to something close to the source; dry pollen floats, to eventually land and stick on any available moist surface—often our mucous membranes.

The actual *shape* of each species' pollen grains is often a factor, because some grains are shaped like tiny cactus balls and can irritate membranes and skin simply by mechanical action. Other pollen grains, much more benign, are smooth-sided or have a waxy coating that keeps them from being easily absorbed.

Another often-overlooked question is, "On which year's wood does this tree or shrub produce flowers?" In some cases, as in boxwood, allergenic pollen can be produced only on old wood. In the case of boxwood, a hard yearly shearing ensures that we have only new growth each year and thus see little bloom (or pollen). In other cases, unfortunately, bloom is produced on new wood of the current season's growth and, in this case, it is next to impossible to prune away the allergy potential.

Fragrance in plants serves to attract pollinating insects, and often fragrant plants do not pose a pollen problem. On the other hand, the fragrance itself in many cases can cause allergic reactions to people who are sensitive to perfumes and odors.

Certain odors cause more problems than others do. As a rule of thumb, a light fragrance may be benign but a stronger fragrance may pose problems. Allergists refer to certain plants as having *negative odor challenges*, and anyone who is sensitive to too much perfume or cologne would be wise to avoid planting these.

I recently met a woman who had gone into anaphylactic shock after exposure to the fragrance of gardenia flowers. Many flower fragrances are created by airborne volatile oils, and some people are allergic to particular volatile oils. Few people, for example, are exposed to rose pollen, but no small number are allergic to the fragrance of strongly scented roses. Gardeners creating allergy-free landscapes must take the fragrance factor into consideration.

Night bloomers are plants that are most fragrant at night. Night blooming jasmine, angel trumpet, and four o'clocks are good examples. These night bloomers should not be placed near bedroom windows, or they may well contribute to allergy. Also a good many plants only release their pollen at night or very early in the morning. All plantings near or next to bedroom windows should get extra scrutiny. This is a prime location for the placement of plants with an allergy rating of 1 or 2.

Flower Position on Plant

The *position of the flower* on a plant can also make a difference when it comes to allergies. Many trees and quite a few shrubs are monoecious, having separate-sexed flowers on the same plant. Almost all of these monoecious flowered plants contribute to allergy, but some are far worse than others. In many monoecious plants, the unisexual flowers are on the same branches and the pollen doesn't have far to travel to reach a female flower. In other plants, the male flowers are on branches separate from the female flowers.

In certain monoecious systems, like corn, the male flowers are at the top of the plant and the female flowers are below them. In this case, the pollen simply falls down by gravity to reach the female flowers. In many other monoecious flowering systems, however (Italian cypress and castor bean are good examples), the male flowers are always found at the bottom of the plant and the females at the top. In this system, the pollen of the male flowers must float *up* to reach the female blooms. In the extensive list of criteria used to rate each species and cultivar in this text, monoecious systems, which feature the male flowers below the female, factor highly. These plants often have allergenic potential second only to certain male-only dioecious plants.

The Very Best Plants

In picking the very best materials for an allergy-free garden, priority is given to two groups of plants. First, those plants that produce large, very showy, lightly scented flowers, in which the male flower parts are either few in number or deeply recessed within the blossom, are almost certain to be perfectly pollinated by insects and rarely cause pollen problems.

The second type of plants that rate extremely well are those separate-sexed species in which the female plants are known and commercially named, or those in which the females of the species are easy to identify by sight. In separate-sexed dioecious plants, individual plants are either males or females. The males almost always are capable of causing problems, but the females have no pollen at all and usually make wonderful allergy-free landscape choices.

The Female Garden

Interestingly, many separate-sexed plants, such as ash, willow, mulberry, juniper, and maple, are always included in lists of plants that cause allergies, and people are almost always warned to avoid them. Nonetheless, the female-only plants are the only ones that don't ever produce pollen, and they can in fact be the very best.

Some have suggested that I have overreached with the title of this book, that there is no such thing as an allergy-free garden. However, it is quite possible to create an entirely all-female landscape, from the lawn to the shrubs to the trees. We can select female-only cultivars that do not cause contact allergies and do not present odor challenges. The right female garden would not release a single grain of pollen, ever! Such a garden would be truly allergy-free.

Pollinated female-only trees often set a lot of seed or fruit and can be messy. However, if only female trees are used, and the allergenic male pollinating trees are removed from the landscape, then the female trees will not set any seed. The result is a low-maintenance tree that does not cause allergies. A possible downside to a total female garden is that without pollinating male plants, there will be little or no fruit. Wildlife does depend on fruit from our landscapes, and there should usually be some low-allergy complete-flowered plants included that can set fruit. Crab-apple, cotoneaster, hawthorn, wild plum, and other low-allergy plants can fill this need.

Confusion and Plant Names

Always of concern are plants that have been well documented in medical literature over many years as causing allergy. There has been great confusion in this area, due largely to overuse and misuse of common names, as well as a lack of basic botanical understanding of complex plant flowering systems by many allergy writers. As one allergist said to me, "Most doctors don't know enough horticulture, and the horticulturists don't know beans about allergy."

A clear example of this confusion can be seen in the section of this text on cedar. There are actually only four species of true cedar, yet there are dozens of species of trees and shrubs that bear the common name "cedar." The true cedars pose a low allergy risk, but many of the misnamed "cedars" are among our very worst allergy offenders.

Another good example of confusion involves a tree called peppermint willow. Last year, I saw a long row of these trees being planted at a nearby college. I didn't recognize them and asked the landscapers what they were. They told me they were peppermint willows, and no, they didn't know the exact scientific name of the species, or if they were male or female cultivars. I searched through volumes on *Salix* (willow) and couldn't find this tree. Soon after, I saw more of these trees being planted, this time in several different locations closer to my own house. I looked harder and found the tree. Peppermint willows are not willows nor are they related to willow; they are *Eucalyptus nicholii*.

The confusion about the peppermint willow is interesting from both an allergy and a landscape perspective. First, had they been true deciduous willows, and female clones, they would have been excellent landscape choices for where they were planted. However, because they are actually evergreen *Eucalyptus*, the landscapers blew it on several counts.

Eucalyptus of all kinds cause allergy. This particular species will grow rapidly to 40 feet tall and wide. Because they are evergreen, they will not drop their leaves in fall. And because they were planted on the south side of buildings, these buildings will be in deep, cold shade all winter long; the sun shines low on the horizon during the winter, and all its intensity and warmth comes from the south. I am always amazed when I see landscapers planting large evergreen trees on the south side of any house or building, because this flies in the face of all gardening logic. Had these so-called willows truly been female willow trees, they would not have shed one grain of pollen and would have shaded the buildings during the hot summer; during the fall, they would have dropped their leaves and allowed the low winter sun to warm the classrooms.

Immediate and Delayed Allergic Reactions

Another reason for confusion about allergy and plants among lay persons is that allergy in almost any form can be what allergists call *immediate* or it can be *delayed*. If a fellow sticks his nose into a spray of bottlebrush flowers and almost instantly sneezes and feels bad, this is an *immediate* reaction and is easy to understand. However, if someone gets a big whiff of pepper tree pollen and feels fine until hours or even days later, when suddenly allergy develops, this is a *delayed* reaction and is much harder to gauge. Many plants produce these delayed reactions, and so mistaken assumptions are often made about what actually caused the allergy in the first place.

Diversity

Nature has given us a huge, diverse inventory of plants to use in our landscapes. All too often the same old plant materials are used over and over again in landscaping, resulting in an unfortunate blandness in many of our gardens. Relative to allergy, diversity is almost always a good thing. Too many of the same kinds of trees and shrubs in a landscape often contribute to individuals become hypersensitized to certain pollens. In the allergy rating system used in this text, overuse of the same plants rated 4 to 6 is asking for trouble. A few 4s, 5s, and even 6s in the landscape are seldom a problem.

Use a little extra imagination and plant more complex landscapes. These will be just as good (or better) looking and will cause fewer allergies. Plants rated 7, 8, or 9 should be used as little as possible. Most plants rated 8 to 10 really have no place in a healthy landscape. Plant materials rated 9 to 10 should be replaced, if at all possible, with cleaner substitutes. In many cases, people will discover that their own yards are loaded with high-allergy plants. Often these will be difficult or expensive to remove. I advise that you take them one at a time. Each heavy pollinator that goes leaves the air in your garden that much cleaner.

In a few cases of allergy rating, there is no clear-cut distinction on what a plant's exact rating number should be. In all cases where the computation of data is fuzzy about the exact number (for example, should it rate a 5 or 6?), the higher (or worse) rating has been used. With allergy, it is better to err on the side of safety.

Direct Exposure to Pollen

A male pepper tree in bloom in your own yard will expose you to more than ten times as much allergenic pollen as a similar pepper tree in a neighbor's yard down the street.

In 1972, a pollen scientist named Raynor demonstrated this concept of the importance of locality in allergy. He measured airborne pollen from a large field of timothy grass at different distances from the source. The closer to the field he measured, the greater the exposure to the pollen. Timothy pollen is exceptionally light and buoyant and well designed for travel by wind and air. In Raynor's study, he found that more than 99 percent of the timothy pollen was deposited less than six-tenths of a mile (about one kilometer) from the source. This study clearly demonstrates that the closer one is to the source, the greater the chance of exposure.

In my own studies, I have found time and again that the closer you are to a pollinating plant, the greater the chance of overexposure. Birch trees are well known to produce allergenic airborne pollen that can travel on the wind for many miles. Nonetheless, my observations of individual birch trees show that more than 99 percent of each tree's pollen falls out, lands, and sticks within 20 feet of the pollinating tree. The point here is, Avoid the pollen! Certain plants should never be planted near windows, doors, decks, or patios.

Weeds

There are many good books written about weeds and allergy, and only a few plants that are strictly weeds are included in this book. Pollen from many weeds can cause allergy, and it is very important that localities enforce rules about keeping vacant lots mowed down. All too often, these vacant lots, filled with allergenic weeds, are allowed to grow tall and flower, and are then mowed down only after they have released their pollen and produced another crop of weed seed for the next season. Keep vacant lots mowed often.

Although I am not a big advocate of herbicide use, occasionally we find it necessary to spray pernicious weeds like Bermuda grass or Johnson grass—both of them allergenic—with a nonselective herbicide. Take great care with chemicals, because exposure to many herbicides may cause allergy. Broadleaf weed killers, which often contain 2,4-D (a close cousin to Agent Orange), cause weeds to wilt quickly, and while they are in this stage, they become very attractive to livestock. Cattle are often poisoned by eating these recently sprayed weeds.

A note about pets: Our pets also can get allergies and dogs especially are often allergic to many of the same substances that may affect their owners. Cats, because they lick themselves so often, are highly susceptible to herbicide and insecticide poisoning.

Cultural Methods of Limiting Garden Allergy

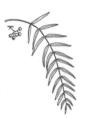

The most important thing a gardener can do to reduce the allergy potential of a garden is to plant those species and cultivars of plants that cause little or no allergy. Allergenic plants that already exist in the landscape may be removed, one at a time, and replaced with cleaner choices. In addition to the selection and planting of nonallergenic plants, however, other important things can be done to limit allergy in the home landscape.

Lawn Care

Lawns cause a large amount of allergy, but there are ways to limit pollen release in lawns. The actual allergic reaction to a lawn may be caused by several factors. A rotary power lawnmower stirs up a large amount of dust, pollen, and mold spores. The whirling blades also release into the air gaseous volatile oils that are exuded from the cut blades of grass. Also stirred up when lawns are mowed are tiny pieces of insect bodies. If you were to place a glass slide with a little petroleum jelly smeared on it next to a lawn being mowed, all these things (except the volatile airborne oils) would be stuck to the slide. All of these can cause allergy.

Hardware stores sell simple paper face-mask filters to cover the nose and mouth, and these are cheap and fairly effective at filtering out these allergenic materials.

In the case of those who are especially allergic to grass pollens, wearing a mask filter while mowing the lawn may not be enough to protect them from the allergens released. Also, these masks cannot protect the delicate and susceptible membranes of the eye. These gardeners would be wise to hire someone else to do the mowing, or to replace the lawn with a low-allergy ground cover.

Most lawn grasses release their pollen from about 3 A.M. to 8 A.M. With this in mind, it is never a good idea to mow lawns early in the morning. Many maintenance gardeners mow lawns, edge, weed whip, and rake leaves quickly, and are on to the next job. In the trade these guys are known as "mow, blow, and go" gardeners. They often start mowing lawns very early in the morning, then tidy up with a leaf blower—further stirring up just released pollen and dust. If you employ a maintenance gardener, ask him to do your yard later in the day. At the least, close the windows for a few hours until all that pollen has settled down.

Neighbors may unintentionally contribute to your allergy. When neighbors let their lawns grow tall and unkempt, airborne grass and weed pollen increase, making allergic individuals living nearby suffer. If you are highly allergic to grass, ask that neighbors keep their lawns mowed regularly.

Shrubs

Many landscape shrubs, used as foundation plantings or as hedges, produce small flowers that cause allergy. The more often these shrubs are sheared, the less the allergy potential. In some cases, as with boxwood, *Euonymus*, and many other common allergenic shrubs, one good hard shearing a year ensures that there will be little bloom. This helps a great deal. Even with shrubs like privet, which blooms on new wood, frequent shearing helps to cut down on the total pollen exposure.

Plant Identification

If you buy a house with a landscape and garden already in place, you may not know exactly what kinds of plants you have growing in your new yard. Ask an expert. Never be embarrassed to admit your ignorance; there are thousands of plant species, and no one can know them all.

A horticultural student may be employed for an hour or two to identify unknown plants, or take your samples to a local nursery, where a good staff can usually figure out what they are.

A visit to an arboretum is another fine way to learn to identify plants. Good arboretums have extensive plantings and usually do a decent job of clearly tagging most of the plant material.

Trees and Pruning Away Allergy

Because many trees grow large and tall, often towering above everything else in the garden, if they produce allergenic pollen they have a serious effect on the overall air quality of your garden. With many trees, especially deciduous (non-evergreen) trees, a yearly hard pruning, in which the ends of all branches are cut back, results in a tree that—for the next season—grows only vegetatively. It will produce only leaves, not allergy-producing flowers.

The worst allergy trees often produce flowers that are so small and colorless they are never even noticed, but these are the flowers that are least wanted. Hard, yearly pruning often gets rid of these tiny flowers and keeps a potentially highly allergenic tree from ever causing a problem.

Trees and Sex Changes: Grafting and Budding

In some cases, a young existing tree can be cut back and nonallergenic branches (called *scions*) grafted to it. For example, an allergy-causing Norway maple may be cut back and *top-grafted* with a type of maple known to be strictly female and productive of no pollen. Using this method, known as *top working*, a male poplar can be changed into a female. There are dozens of other species of trees where this is possible.

With some species of trees, *budding* is easier than grafting. Many good books on gardening explain how to graft or bud, but getting an old, experienced garden hand to actually show you how is always the best way to learn.

Keeping Trees and Shrubs Healthy

A good gardener develops a feel for her own garden. She knows almost instinctively when to water and fertilize. This feeling comes with experience. A safe, easy, and effective way to feed almost anything, especially anything in a container, is to put 8 ounces of water-soluble, all-purpose fertilizer in a clean 40-gallon plastic trash can, then fill the can with water, all the way to the top. With most water-soluble fertilizers, this gives you a liquid nutrient in the 200 to 400 parts per million (ppm) range, which is pretty near perfect liquid feed. (When using a 30-gallon trash can, use 6 ounces of fertilizer.) Every time you water your plants, you'll be simultaneously feeding them. This is how the pros fertilize plants in wholesale growing nurseries, and you always have some fertilizer handy.

Trees and shrubs often need extra attention. Sometimes the simple addition of a good layer of mulch will do wonders toward keeping plants healthy. Mulch is anything used to cover the soil: bark, leaves, old hay, cardboard, rocks. Thick mulch keeps the soil warmer in winter and cooler in summer, holds down the weeds, and helps to keep the soil moisture from evaporating.

In dry years, plants may well need a good weekly soaking; in wet years, they need a little extra fertilizer. The better care that is given them, the fewer insects and diseases they will have, and this will cut down on allergenic exposure to mold and insect dander.

Insects and Diseases

For one reason or another, despite being given plenty of attention, certain trees, shrubs, or other garden plants fail to thrive in some gardens. Plants that are not growing well quickly become targets for pests, diseases, or insects. I have seen a rabbit walk down a long row of small shrubs and stop to nibble only the plant already weakened from frost.

Mildew, rust, black spot, canker—there are hundreds of plant diseases. Aphids, scale, spider mites, thrips, and all manner of six- or eight-legged pests seek out and prey on those plants that are failing to thrive.

As insects suck the juices out of a plant, they secrete a sticky feces, called *honeydew*, and *mold* grows on this honeydew. Mold produces millions of airborne spores that cause allergy, and the insects themselves cause additional allergy. Allergies to insects are actually quite common.

A large sickly tree or hedge can pollute the entire garden airspace with potent allergens. In a well-designed, allergy-free garden, we try to work with nature, not against it. If our soil is alkaline, we don't plant acid-loving plants. They won't thrive. If we have a hot, dry climate and sandy soil, we don't plant those species native to the cool mountains, like azaleas and *Camellias*. A long walk around the neighborhood can be a good education about what grows best in that location.

This is not to say that we shouldn't try to grow difficult plants, that we should not experiment; certainly we should. Nonetheless, when a tree, shrub, vegetable, annual, or perennial fails to thrive and gets diseased and buggy, don't fall into the pattern of reaching for the spray gun. Knock the bugs off with a stiff stream of water from the hose, and if the bugs keep coming back to the same plant, dig it up and replace it with a better-suited one.

Insecticides and Herbicides

We all have our own opinions about the safety and use of pesticides. In the past, I used a great deal more of these chemicals than I do now. I grow a large number of roses, and I would rather dig one up and trash it, than have to spray it over and over. Likewise, we have many fruit trees, and in recent years we have learned to tolerate a few wormy apples rather than keep up this constant chemical battle.

We have begun to experiment, often with good success, with IPM, or integrated pest management. In IPM, the idea is to control insects, not to eradicate them. We have started to release beneficial insects like ladybugs, green lacewings, and many kinds of predatory and parasitic wasps. These are all useful alternatives to insecticides.

Don't fool yourself; pesticides, particularly the chemical ones, cause allergy. Not only do they cause allergy, but often a single overexposure to a pesticide can leave individuals hypersensitive to many substances that never bothered them before. It is no accident that so many Hispanic farmworkers suffer from countless allergies; they are frequently exposed to potent chemical pesticides. Use all pesticides sparingly, and never when the wind is blowing.

Homemade insecticides. A very effective insecticide can be made by mixing several teaspoons of liquid dish soap and 3 teaspoons of vegetable or mineral oil into 1 gallon of warm water.

For a somewhat more effective (and far more expensive) soap, substitute a commercially produced insecticidal soap. If warm-blooded pests like rabbits are a problem, add a few drops of hot pepper sauce to your homemade sprays.

If you've never tried simple sprays like these, do so. They often work well and they are nontoxic.

Tips for Reducing Allergen Exposure

If you are highly allergic to grasses, limit the bread you eat in spring and summer, and you'll probably feel better and have more energy. Many allergists have noticed increased allergy to grass pollens among patients who eat wheat products. Wheat, of course, is essentially a type of grass.

Keep the cats and dogs outside. It will be better for all concerned.

Allergy from dust and dust mites is often worst in winter, when houses are shut up tight and people stay inside too much. Open a window and let in fresh air. Put on a heavy coat, gloves, and cap and go for a long brisk walk, even in the winter.

Using clotheslines. During the summer, don't hang wet clothes outside to dry overnight or early in the morning; they will be covered with grass pollen. Hang clothes out when the sun is shining brightly. Also, if the day is especially windy, don't hang clothes outside or they will be covered with pollen. On a bath towel, this same pollen could be rubbed into someone's eyes.

Eczema and other skin rashes are often caused by contact allergy. Pollen itself, especially from oak and ash, may cause rash. Remember that all allergic reactions are not immediate.

Allergy to rubber is on the increase. This one could kill you. If you have allergies already, think twice before wearing rubber or latex gloves. Limit the use of all rubber products. Read the section under *Hevea brasiliensis* for more on rubber allergies.

Avoid latex sap. Any plants with white, milky sap are suspect. The "latex" is frequently poisonous and often can cause skin rash, swelling, or irritation. Teach children never to taste plant latex saps.

Don't smell the flowers. Many flowers, especially those rated 2–4 in this book, usually cause allergy only if you directly inhale their fragrance—and pollen. Don't stick flowers in other people's faces and don't let them do this to you. Remember, not all reactions are immediate.

Limit cut and dried flowers. Flowers rated 6 and above should never be used in the house as cut flowers. Be careful of dried flowers. Many times these varieties cause allergy while growing, and they can cause it while dried, too. Allergic response to the odor of dried silver dollar eucalyptus leaves is fairly common, as is allergy to the dried seed pods of *Lunaria annua*, money plant or honesty.

Exercise to keep allergy at bay. In cities where children stay inside watching endless hours of TV, allergies are common. Exercise and fresh air are important in keeping healthy, especially for children. Any exercise is better than none. (Exercise in itself, particularly vigorous exercise, can sometimes cause a type of allergy. See an allergist about exercise-induced allergies, but remember any exercise is good; it need not be sweaty and vigorous.)

Monitor pollen counts. The best time to go for a walk is in the middle of the day. Pollen counts tend to rise early and late in the day; they are often lowest at midday.

Stay inside on windy days. The worst time to go for a walk is on a hot, dry, windy day, because this is when there is the most pollen in the air.

Walk in the rain. Unless you are particularly allergic to mold spores, cool, rainy, or damp days are days with little airborne pollen and are good days to take an extra long walk.

Limit ferns as houseplants. If you have more allergy in winter, you are probably allergic to molds and spores and should not keep ferns in the house. If you are especially allergic to molds and spores, it might be wise to keep very few plants inside, especially in winter.

Watch the daisies. Plants that have daisy-like flowers often are related to ragweeds and can cause allergy. However, as you browse through this book, you will find many other flowers that look like daisies, but are not related to either true daisies or to ragweeds. These species are perfectly fine for the allergy-free garden. Two examples of unrelated look-alikes are ice plant and pincushion flower (*Scabiosa*). Both have daisy-like flowers but neither causes allergies.

Get allergy shots. Allergy shots to develop immunity usually work. Unfortunately with some HMOs it is difficult to get a referral to an allergist to undergo the series of shots. Insist on your rights. Sometimes the effects of these inoculations wear off after eight or ten years and they must be repeated.

In recent years, allergists have gotten much better at reducing allergy caused by cat dander. The new shots for cat-allergy work wonders for many people who, in the past, could not be in the same house with a cat.

Not all allergists are created equal. If you are not getting results with your allergist, find a new one. A good allergist can do wonders.

Choose Christmas trees wisely. Allergy to pine pollen is neither common nor usually severe, but some people are allergic to the smell of a pine tree in the house and are miserable every Christmas. A substitute for a pine Christmas tree might be a noble fir. Fir is a pine relative, but lacks some of the strong piney smell.

Another alternative is a large potted Norfolk Island pine (*Araucaria heterophylla*), used as a "living Christmas tree." This tree looks like a pine but is not related nor does it have the same strong smell. Keep this tree as a potted plant and do not plant it in the yard. When full grown, it causes allergies; as a potted plant, it never blooms and is fine.

Attract wild birds to the garden. A healthy population of wild birds in the garden helps to lower allergy potential because of the huge number of insects they eat. I have seen a small flock of common bushtits, tiny, dusky-brown birds, alight on a shrub afflicted with aphids, and in a matter of minutes eat up virtually every aphid in sight.

There are hundreds of species of insect-eating wild birds, and they are always welcome in the garden.

Surf the Internet. There is much fine information about allergy and plants on the Internet, but there is also much baloney. At least one-third of all the Internet allergy-plant information I have found is in error. (Garbage in, garbage out.)

In the last year, there have been a few good new plant-allergy sites. More information about this book and sources of all-female plants can be found at *www.allergyfree-gardening.com* and at *www.allergyfreegarden.com*.

Plant Listings

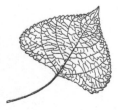

All plants are listed in alphabetical order by their scientific name, genus first, in italics. If the plant listed is of a particular species, the exact species name is given following the genus. If a whole group of plants is discussed, only the genus is given. A few genera have only one species: *Ginkgo biloba* is a good example. In many other genera, there are many different species. *Eucalyptus*, for example, has hundreds of different species. In this text, where there are long lists of different species of the same genus, the genus is abbreviated using only its first letter. Thus, in a list of MAPLES (*Acer*), the text reads: *Acer argutum, A. rubrum, A. saccharinum, A. tataricum,* etc.

After the scientific name, the common name or names by which the plant is known are listed in capital letters, also in alphabetical order.

Cultivated Varieties

In addition to genera and species, there are hundreds of thousands of cultivated varieties or cultivars known to horticulture. An example of this is the domestic apple, *Malus domestica*, of which there are over 7,000 cultivars. Where a cultivar is listed, the exact name of the cultivar will always be enclosed in single quotation marks. Thus, if we listed the apple tree *Malus domestica* 'McIntosh', *Malus* would be the genus; *domestica* would be the species; and 'McIntosh' would be the cultivar.

Hybrids

When hybrids are discussed, the female plant (the seed parent) is listed first. A hybrid cross between a RED MAPLE and a SILVER MAPLE is listed as *Acer rubrum* × *saccharinum* when the seed parent is RED MAPLE (*A. rubrum*) and the pollen parent is SILVER MAPLE (*A. saccharinum*).

Cross-Referencing of Names

Every attempt has been made to cross-reference common names with scientific names. For example, *Aptenia cordifolia* is a ground cover plant with little red flowers. However, it is quite possible that you only know the plant by its common name RED-APPLE ICEPLANT. If you look up RED-APPLE ICEPLANT in the text, it will direct you to *Aptenia cordifolia*.

Hardiness Zones

An attempt has been made to give a cold hardiness rating to each plant, and each plant is described as perennial, annual, shrub, vine, ground cover, or tree. Plant hardiness zones used in this book are based on the standard United States Department of Agriculture (USDA) 1–10 zoning system. Zone maps for the United States and Europe appear in the insert. In this system, the coldest areas (mountaintops, most of Alaska) are zone 1. Zone 10 is the warmest, most frost-free zone and exists mostly in southern areas, close to the oceans. The actual hardiness (to cold) of a species is affected by its size, age, type of soil, exposure to wind, drought, and many other factors. Often a plant can be grown successfully one zone colder than its normal range if all other conditions are favorable.

Gardeners sometimes confuse the terms "hardy" and "tender." In horticulture, a hardy plant is one that can withstand a great deal of frost and cold. A tender plant, on the other hand, cannot take either extreme cold or frost.

Poisonous Plants

In this text, I have included reference to poisonous plants, including plants such as the varnish tree, which are poisonous to the touch, and also many others that are poisonous only if eaten. Many plants that are poisonous if eaten do not necessarily cause allergies and the rating of a plant reflects only its allergy potential. Being poisonous does not by any means make a plant an allergy problem; still, it is good to know which ones could be dangerous.

See the Glossary for detailed explanations of the botanical and horticultural terms used in this text.

To my readers: If you discover a plant-related allergy that I may have overlooked, please contact me and share the information. I am always on the lookout for additional data and I value your input. I also welcome letters and e-mail, and I will try to answer them all in a timely fashion. All new useful information will find its way into the next edition of *Allegy-Free Gardening.*

My e-mail address: *tloallergyfree@earthlink.net*

II

Alphabetical Listing of Plants Rated for Allergy

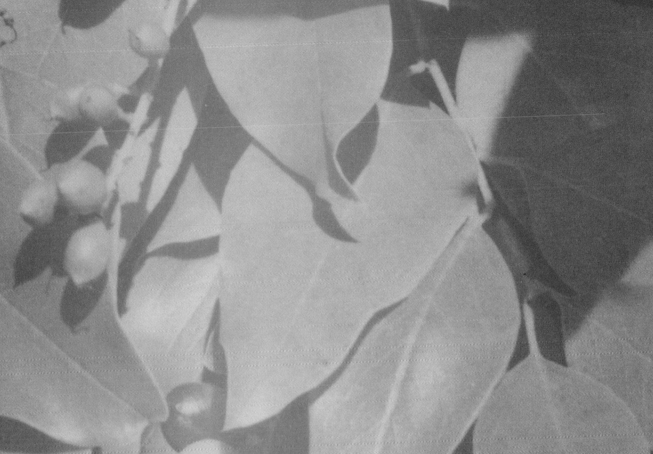

Prunus lyonii
CATALINA CHERRY

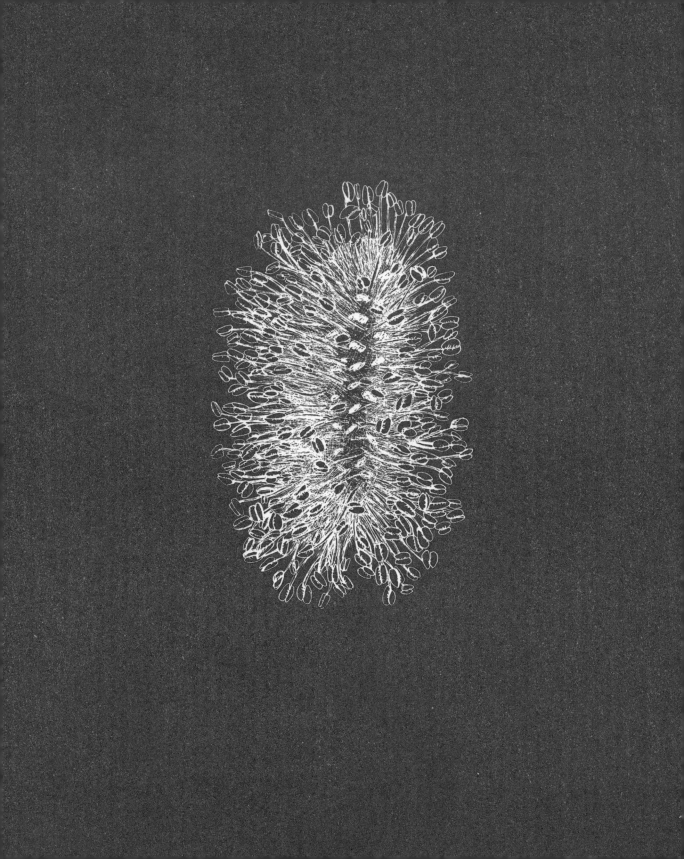

A

Allergy Index Scale: *1* is Best, *10* is Worst.

✳ for *1* and *2*　　✴ for *9* and *10*

📷 See insert for photograph

AARON'S BEARD.
See *Hypericum.*

Abelia. 5
Evergreen flowering shrubs hardy in plant zones 8 to 10. There are numerous species of *Abelia* and all have many small, white flowers, often tinged with pink. Easy to grow, all *Abelia* thrive in full sun to partial shade. The many flowers attract large numbers of honeybees and release little pollen. *Abelia* is a HONEYSUCKLE relative; individuals allergic to HONEYSUCKLE (see *Lonicera*) may experience cross-allergic reactions, although allergy to *Abelia* is much less common. In a few cases, skin rash caused by contact with the leaves has been noted.

Abeliophyllum distichum. 7
WHITE FORSYTHIA. A deciduous flowering shrub, hardy to zone 5. An OLIVE family member. Dormant branches are often cut and brought into the house to bloom. This is not advisable if you have allergies.

Abelmoschus esculentus. 3
OKRA. A common vegetable with handsome flowers that resemble *Hibiscus*, to which it is related. The plants need good soil, ample water, and warmth to bear well. The prickly leaves are known to cause contact skin rash.

Abies. ✳ 2
FIR, SILVER FIR, BALMIES, BALSAM FIR, SANTA LUCIA FIR, NIKKO FIR, ALGERIAN FIR, SPANISH FIR, GRAND FIR, CORK FIR, RED FIR, NOBLE FIR. Large, slow-growing evergreen, coniferous trees with classic "Christmas tree" shape. There are over 40 species; some are hardy to zone 1. Most FIRS do not grow well in hot, dry areas or in hot, smoggy cities. One species, *A. nordmanniana*, the NORDMANN FIR, from Asia Minor and Greece, grows well in most areas of California if supplied with plenty of water. All true FIRS produce pollen, but it has a waxy covering and rarely causes allergy.

Abies balsamea

Abronia. ✳ 1
SAND VERBENA. A perennial native of coastal areas, SAND VERBENA grows best in sandy soil and is tolerant of seaside conditions. Large clusters of white, pink, or red tubular, sticky flowers on low, spreading plants.

Abrus precatorius. Not rated.
ROSARY PEA. A vine with pea-like flowers producing attractive scarlet, black-spotted seeds, occasionally used as beads. These seeds are extremely poisonous; one seed can kill a child.

Abutilon. 3
CHINESE LANTERN, FLOWERING MAPLE. Tall, evergreen vinelike shrubs hardy only in the mildest climates. Easy to grow; many different varieties with a wide array of colors.

ABYSSINIAN BANANA.
See *Ensete.*

Acacia. 📷 shrubs 8, trees ✴10
AUSTRALIAN WILLOW, BLACKWOOD ACACIA, GOLDEN WATTLE, MIMOSA, MULGA, RIVER WATTLE, SILVER WATTLE, WHITETHORN. Common evergreen shrubs and trees from warm areas all over the world, especially Australia. Hardy in zones 9 and 10,

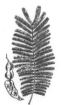

Acacia decurrens

they are very common in California and Florida. *Acacia* trees cover themselves with thousands of little yellow flowers in early spring. Easy to grow and fast growing, they cause plenty of allergies. *Acacia* leaves are poisonous.

ACACIA, SMOOTH ROSE.
See *Robinia*.

Acaena.   ❋ 2
SHEEP BUR. Small, low-growing perennials from New Zealand. Not hardy in cold winter areas, they are grown for their pale green leaves. After flowering, they produce burrs, which stick to clothes.

Acalypha. 📷   *males 8, females* ❋ 1
CHENILLE PLANT. A tender houseplant with large leaves and long, drooping clusters of chenille-like flowers. *Acalypha* is a separate-sexed species, however, and virtually all of the plants sold in the United States, Canada, and Europe are female clones, which cause no allergy.

Acanthophoenix.   6
BARBEL PALM. Subtropical palm trees.

Acanthus mollis.   ❋ 1
BEAR'S BREECH, SNAIL'S TRAIL. A big, shade-loving perennial with large leaves; hardy to zone 3 if mulched heavily in fall. BEAR'S BREECH often thrives where nothing else will grow. Tall spikes of white or purple flowers. Must be protected from snails and slugs.

ACEITUNO.
See *Simarouba*.

Acer.
MAPLE. A large group of deciduous trees and large shrubs. Various MAPLES are hardy in all zones. MAPLES do well in most areas, but few are well suited for desert landscapes, because all require plentiful water. Many cause allergy, but some species

are among our very finest choices for allergy-free landscapes. Some maple species are separate-sexed, other species are not.

Where the sex of the trees is not constant, it is not possible to rate the cultivars individually; these are marked 'not rated.' They are not recommended for planting in allergy-free gardens.

A. argutum.   8
POINTED-LEAF MAPLE.

A. buergeranum.   7
TRIDENT MAPLE.

A. campestre.   7
HEDGE MAPLE.

A. cappadocicum.   7
CAUCASIAN MAPLE.

A. carpinifolium.   *males 8, females* ❋ 1
HORNBEAM MAPLE.

A. circinatum.   5
VINE MAPLE.

A. cissifolium. 📷   *males 8, females* ❋ 1
IVY-LEAFED MAPLE.

A. crataegifolium.   7
HAWTHORN-LEAF MAPLE.

A. davidii.   6
DAVID'S MAPLE.

A. diabolicum.   *males 8, females 3*
HORNED MAPLE. Tiny stinging hairs on the seeds cause rash.

A. distylum.   6
LIMELEAF MAPLE.

A. × Freemanii.
FREEMANII MAPLES are natural hybrids of RED MAPLE and SILVER MAPLE.

A. × *F.* 'Armstrong'.   5
A tall, broad, hardy tree with some pollen.

A. × *F.* 'Autumn Blaze'.   7

A. × *F.* 'Autumn Fantasy'.   ❋ 1
No pollen.

A. × *F.* 'Celebration'.   8

A. × *F.* 'Celzam'.   8

A. × *F.* 'Indian Summer'.   ❋ 1
Fast-growing, big tree; great scarlet fall color
and no pollen.

A. × *F.* 'Jeffersred'.   7

A. × *F.* 'Marmo'.   8

A. × *F.* 'Morgan'.   ❋ 1

A. × *F.* 'Scarlet Sentinel'.   *Not rated.*

A. ginnala.   4
Small tree with fragrant flowers.

A. glabrum.   7
ROCK MAPLE, SIERRA MAPLE.

A. griseum. 📷   6
PAPERBARK MAPLE.

A. japonicum.   5
JAPANESE MAPLE. Many kinds.

A. macrophyllum.   8
BIGLEAF MAPLE. The numerous seeds of this species
have tiny stinging hairs that cause contact rash.
Plenty of pollen here, too.

Acer macrophyllum

A. mandshuricum.   7
MANCHURIAN MAPLE.

A. negundo.   *males* ❋ 10, *females* ❋ 1
ASH-LEAFED MAPLE, BOX ELDER. Fast growing, deciduous trees with leaves more like the ASH than
the MAPLE. Some BOX ELDERS cause severe allergy;
the female trees cause none at all.

A. n. 'Auratum'.   ❋ 1
No pollen.

A. n. 'Aureo marginatum'.   ❋10

A. n. 'Baron'.   ❋10
Male clone.

A. n. 'Rubescens'.   ❋ 1

A. n. 'Variegata'. 📷   ❋ 1
VARIEGATED BOX ELDER. A handsome tree with
unusual colored leaves and no pollen.

A. n. 'Violaceum'.   ❋10
A male clone.

A. oblongum.   7
EVERGREEN MAPLE.

A. opalus.   7
ITALIAN MAPLE.

A. palmatum.   5
JAPANESE MAPLE. There are several hundred named
cultivars of this small, handsome, deciduous tree.
All cause limited allergy.

A. paxii.   6
EVERGREEN MAPLE. Not hardy in cold areas.

A. pensylvanicum.   6
STRIPED MAPLE. Grows well only in the shade.

A. platanoides.   8
NORWAY MAPLE. A large, common urban tree.
There are many varieties sold; all can cause allergy.

A. pseudoplatanus.   8
SYCAMORE MAPLE. A very common, widely adapted, large, deciduous urban tree.

A. rubescens.   7
TENDER MAPLE. From Taiwan.

A. rubrum.
RED MAPLE, SCARLET MAPLE. A large group of handsome trees that grows fast and likes plenty of water. They vary in allergenic potential.

Acer rubrum

A. r. 'Autumn Flame'.   8

A. r. 'Autumn Glory'.   ❊ 1
Very good orange fall color and no pollen.

A. r. 'Autumn Spire'.   ✹ 9

A. r. 'Bowhall'. 📷   ❊ 1
Pyramidal form with good orange-red fall color and no pollen.

A. r. 'Columnare'; also 'Pyramidale'.   8

A. r. 'Davey Red'.   ❊ 1
Good fall color; can withstand more cold than most—hardy into zone 2.

A. r. 'Doric'.   ❊ 1
Brilliant deep red fall color and no pollen.

A. r. 'Embers'.   ❊ 1
Vigorous tree with a broad crown, great fall color, and no pollen.

A. r. 'Festival'.   ❊ 1

A. r. 'Firedance'.   8

A. r. 'Flame'. See 'Autumn Flame'.

A. r. 'Franksred'. See 'Red Sunset'.   ❊ 1

A. r. 'Karpick'.   8

A. r. 'Landsburg'. See 'Firedance'.

A. r. 'Northwood'.   8

A. r. 'October Brilliance'.   8

A. r. 'October Glory'. 📷   ❊ 1
Good lawn tree that does not cast a dense shade; dependable bright red-crimson fall color and no pollen. A fine tree.

A. r. 'Red Skin'.   ❊ 1
Very good fall color and no pollen.

A. r. 'Red Sunset'.   ❊ 1
Thick leaves which turn a reddish maroon color in fall and no pollen in spring.

A. r. 'Schlesinger'.   *Not rated.*

A. r. 'Shade King'.   *Not rated.*

A. r. 'Tiliford'.   ✹ 9

A. saccharinum. 📷   *males* ✹ *9, females* ❊ *1*
SILVER MAPLE. The SILVER MAPLES make up a large group of common, fast-growing deciduous trees, hardy in all zones. They will often grow where other maples will not. Their fast growth leads to weak wood and large broken branches are common. Most varieties should be avoided in the allergy-free land-scape, especially 'Silver Queen' and 'Skinner's Cutleaf Silver Maple', both of which are male.
    One SILVER MAPLE can be rec-ommended, however. *A. sacchar-inum* 'Northline' is a variety that produces no pollen, grows slower than most, has a wide-spreading habit, and is among the hardiest of all maples. 'Northline' turns a bright yellow color in the fall.

Acer saccharinum

A. saccharum.   7
SUGAR MAPLE.

A. tataricum. 📷   *5*
TATARIAN MAPLE.

A. t. ginnala.   *6*
AMUR MAPLE.

★There are other, less-often-used maples than those listed here. None recommended for the allergy-free garden.

ACEROLA.
See *Malpighia glabra.*

Achillea.   *7*
YARROW. Several species of hardy, easy-to-grow, yellow- or white-flowered perennials. They grow best in full sun and are often used for dried flowers.

Achimenes.   ✳ *1*
ORCHID PANSY. Small tender perennial with many varieties and wide range of colors.

Ackama.   *8*
Several species of small trees native to New Zealand; occasionally used in zone 10.

Acmena smithii.   *5*
LILLY-PILLY TREE. Small, evergreen tree with small pink flowers, edible berries. Hardy only in zone 10.

Acnistus australe.   *3*
Tall perennial for zones 7–10 that bears pendulous, trumpet-shaped lavender flowers.

Acoelorrhaphe wrightii.   ✳ *1*
PAROUOT PALM, PAUROTIS WRIGHTII. A shade-loving palm native to Florida and hardy in most southern states.

Acokanthera.   ✴ *9*
AFRICAN WINTERSWEET, BUSHMAN'S POISON. Two species of poisonous evergreen shrubs with fragrant white or pink flowers, occasionally used as a hedge or foundation plant in zone 10. Seeds and fruit are extremely poisonous if eaten, and the sap can cause severe skin rashes.

ACONITE.
See *Aconitum.*

Aconitum.   *4*
ACONITE, MONKSHOOD. Common, poisonous, hardy, easy-to-grow perennial for moist, shady areas. *Aconitum* is one of the most highly poisonous plants and even a few leaves or flowers, if eaten, could be fatal.

Acorus gramineus.   *6*
Grasslike perennial hardy in most zones. Used as ground cover in rock gardens.

Acrocarpus fraxinifolius.   *3*
PINK CEDAR. A briefly deciduous tree for zone 10. Not a true CEDAR but a member of the LEGUME family. Small red flowers appear in spring on this fast-growing tree. Not good in windy areas.

Acrocomia.   *5*
GRU-GRU PALM. Hardy only in coastal areas of zone 10, this palm has small, sweet, edible fruits.

Actinidia.   *males 5, females* ✳ *1*
KIWI. Several species. One, *A. arguta*, is hardy. The plants are sold as male or female. To get fruit you need both. The males can cause some allergy; the females have no pollen and cause no allergies.

Actinorhytis.   *8*
Tropical and subtropical palms.

ADAM'S NEEDLE.
See *Yucca.*

Adenium obesum.   *6*
Tender, odd-shaped shrub mostly grown in containers. Sap can cause rashes.

Adiantum.   *4*
MAIDENHAIR FERN. Ferns do not have pollen but produce spores that can cause allergies. The MAID-

ENHAIR is one of the better ferns, because it produces only small amounts of spores.

Adromischus. ✳ 1
PLOVER EGGS. Desert succulent grown for its thick leaves.

Aechmea. ✳ 2
AIR PINE. A bromeliad; tender except in warmest zones.

Aegopodium. 3
BISHOP'S WEED. A very hardy, perennial ground cover which grows well in the shade; a good substitute for IVY. May get weedy.

Aeonium. ✳ 1
Large group of tender succulents for zones 9 and 10, or houseplants elsewhere.

Aeschynanthus (Trichosporum). ✳ 2
BASKET PLANT, LIPSTICK PLANT. Houseplants grown for their unusual foliage.

Aesculus. 📷 7
BUCKEYE, HORSE CHESTNUT. Large, deciduous, flowering trees with poisonous seeds and pollen that is occasionally fatal to honeybees. There are many kinds of *Aesculus*, none good for the allergy-free landscape.

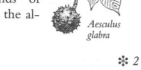

Aesculus glabra

Aethionema. ✳ 2
STONECRESS. Small, hardy, flowering perennial that grows best in sandy soil with a high pH.

AFRICAN BOXWOOD.
See *Myrsine*.

AFRICAN BREAD TREE.
See *Treculia*.

AFRICAN CORN LILY.
See *Ixia*.

AFRICAN DAISY.
See *Arctotis; Dimorphotheca; Osteospermum*.

AFRICAN EVERGREEN.
See *Syngonium podophyllum*.

AFRICAN LINDEN.
See *Sparmannia africana*.

AFRICAN RED ALDER.
See *Cunonia*.

AFRICAN SUMACH.
See *Rhus*.

AFRICAN VIOLET.
See *Saintpaulia ionantha*.

AFRICAN WINTERSWEET.
See *Acokanthera*.

Agapanthus. 📷 ✳ 2
LILY-OF-THE-NILE. Large, easy-to-grow perennials with white or blue flowers. Most *Agapanthus* are evergreen and none are hardy too far from the coast. LILY-OF-THE-NILE makes a good container plant outdoors.

Agapetes serpens. ✳ 1
An evergreen shrub for the cool areas of zones 9 and 10, with showy red hanging flowers in spring. Does best in moist, acid soil.

Agastache. 3
GIANT HYSSOP. A group of about 30 species of tall perennials, some native to United States. *A. cana* is grown in zones 9–10 for its dense clusters of rosy-pink flowers. Members of the MINT family, these plants are attractive to butterflies and bees.

Agathis robusta. 8
DAMMAR PINE, QUEENSLAND KAURI. Tall, narrow evergreen tree with bright green leaves; hardy only in zones 9–10. It needs fertile soil and ample water to thrive. Occasionally substituted for *Podocarpus*.

Agave.   4

CENTURY PLANT, RHINO'S HORN. Big, bold succulents hardy only in the warmest areas, or grown as houseplants for sunny rooms. Some *Agave* species grow far too large for the average landscape, and many have stiff leaves tipped with very sharp dangerous spines. Do not use the spine-tipped species near walkways or where children play. Plants may not flower for many years and then usually die after blooming. The attractive *A. attenuata*, or RHINO'S HORN, is spineless and makes a fine and unusual houseplant for a sunny room. The sap of certain *Agave,* especially *A. Americana* (CENTURY PLANT) can cause severe contact skin rash. Landscapers removing old CENTURY PLANTS often contract this blistering rash. All parts of some species of *Agave* are poisonous.

Ageratum.   5

Summer annual for all zones, bearing pink, white, or, most popular, blue flowers.

Aglaomorpha.   4

A tropical fern used in the greenhouse and as a houseplant. Ferns should not be used as hanging plants, because they may drop spores.

Aglaonema.   6

A rather common tropical evergreen perennial houseplant that can be allergenic when in bloom.

A. modestum.   ❋ 2

CHINESE EVERGREEN. A common, easy-to-grow houseplant that has been found by the National Aeronautics and Space Administration (NASA) to be especially good at cleaning up or "scrubbing" indoor air pollution.

Agonis flexuosa.   6

PEPPERMINT TREE, AUSTRALIAN WILLOW. Medium-sized evergreen type of MYRTLE tree, hardy in zones 9–10.

Agrimonia eupatoria.   ❋ 10

AGRIMONY. Native, tall hardy herbs sometimes grown in shady herb gardens for medicinal uses.

Several species, most with small yellow flowers and fuzzy or hairy leaves. This plant can cause severe skin rashes.

AGRIMONY.

See *Agrimonia eupatoria*.

Agropyron.   6

QUACKGRASS, WHEATGRASS. Hardy grasses that grow well in the Rocky Mountain area and are the cause of some allergy. One species, *A. repens*, commonly called QUACKGRASS, is a low-pollen producing species and as such it may have value in lawns of the future. In general the WHEATGRASSES do not usually produce highly allergenic pollen, making it a genus of grass that deserves further attention for its potential as a lawn grass.

Agrostemma githago.   4

CORN COCKLE. Annual herb grown for its purple flowers; the black seeds are poisonous.

Agrostis.   ❋ 9

BENT GRASS, REDTOP. Hardy lawn grasses, which must be kept mowed very low to avoid flowering.

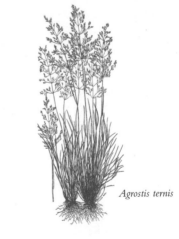

Agrostis ternis

Ailanthus.   ❋ 9

STINK TREE, TREE-OF-HEAVEN. A weedy tree with malodorous flowers that produce plenty of allergenic pollen. These trees are more appreciated in their native China, hence the name TREE-OF-

HEAVEN. Here they grow in waste places where other trees fail. This is said to be the tree in the book *A Tree Grows in Brooklyn*.

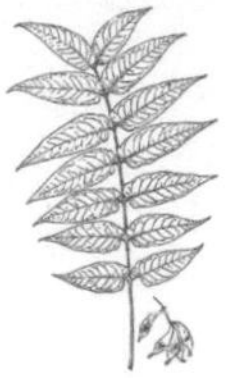

Ailanthus altissima

Aiphanes. *6*
Tropical and subtropical palms.

AIR PINE.
See *Aechmea*.

Ajuga. ✻ *1*
CARPET BUGLE. A hardy, blue-flowered ground cover perennial, *Ajuga* thrives in moist shade, and is a good substitute for IVY.

Akebia quinata. 7
FIVE-LEAF AKEBIA. Fast growing perennial vine native to Japan. *Akebia* is hardy only in zones 9 and 10; it bears attractive leaves and small, edible fruits.

AKEE TREE.
See *Blighia sapida*.

ALASKA YELLOW CEDAR.
See *Chamaecyparis*.

Albizia julibrissin. 📷 *8*
MIMOSA, SILK TREE. A hardy Japanese native common in California; it thrives in areas with high summer heat. Leaves are poisonous.

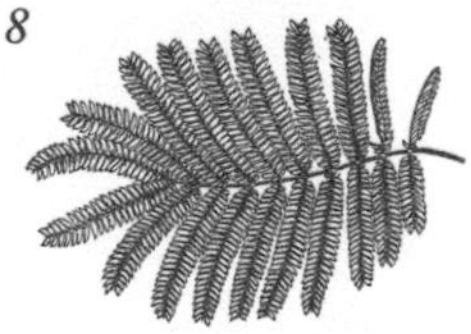

Albizia julibrissin

Alcea. 📷 ✻ *2, 3*
HOLLYHOCK. This old-fashioned tall perennial is hardy in all zones. The doubles are occasionally hard to find but worth the effort. The large, bristle-covered leaves occasionally cause contact skin rash for those with sensitive skin. HOLLYHOCK flowers produce a rather abundant low-allergenic pollen; these flowers should never be directly sniffed. The double-flowered varieties have a better allergy rating.

ALDER.
See *Alnus*.

Aleurites fordii. ✹*9*
TUNG OIL TREE. A small- to medium-sized evergreen tree for zones 9 and 10. Both pollen and sap are allergenic, and simple contact with the leaves could severely affect certain individuals, especially those with an allergy to rubber products. The seeds are poisonous and fatal to people and livestock.

ALEXANDER PALM.
See *Ptychosperma*.

ALEXANDRA PALM.
See *Archontophoenix*.

ALGAE.
A primitive, one-celled water plant. Marine algae is used to make a gelatinous substance called *carrageenan*, used in pharmaceuticals and foods like ice cream, cream, yogurt, salad dressing, frozen treats, and barbecue sauces. Carrageenan occasionally causes a powerful allergic reaction, mimicking rubber allergy.

ALGERIAN FIR.
See *Abies*.

ALGERIAN IVY.
See *Hedera canariensis*.

ALKALI GRASS.
See *Zigadenus*.

Allium. ✻ *2*
CHIVES, FLOWERING GARLIC, FLOWERING ONION, GARLIC. Hardy and easy-to-grow bulbs, *Alliums* do best in full sun in rich, moist soil. Some of the ornamental garlics and onions have a disagreeable odor when crushed.

Alloplectus (Hypocyrta) nummularia. ✻ *1*
GOLDFISH PLANT. Attractive small indoor potted plant which needs warmth and humidity to thrive.

ALLSPICE, CAROLINA.
See *Calycanthus floridus.*

ALMONDS.
See *Prunus communis.*

Alnus. 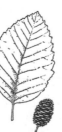 ✳9
ALDER. Large, hardy deciduous shade trees which grow very fast when given enough moisture. ALDER-caused allergies are very common and well known. ALDERS bloom very early in spring, occasionally as early as late December in zones 9 and 10. They shed a great deal of bright yellow, highly allergenic pollen.

Alnus rubra

Alocasia. ✲ 1
ELEPHANT'S EAR. A tender perennial grown for its large, bold leaves. It is used outdoors only in the warmest coastal zones.

Aloe. ✲ 1
Perennials and several species of small trees that are hardy outdoors in zones 9 and 10, and popular as houseplants elsewhere. Members of the LILY family, they are easy to grow.

Alopecurus. 8
FOXTAIL GRASS. Common forage grasses.

Aloysia triphylla. 3
LEMON VERBENA. Shrubby perennial in zones 9 and 10, prized for its fragrant leaves.

Alpinia. ✲ 2
GINGER. Easy-to-grow perennial in warm coastal areas.

Alstroemeria. 4
PERUVIAN LILY, SOUTH AMERICAN LILY. *Alstroemeria* is an easy-to-grow perennial for zones 4–10, producing showy flowers during much of the year. The flowers are very long-lasting when cut. The leaves occasionally cause an allergic skin rash, so use caution when handling them or working around them in the garden. The pollen is exposed but presents few problems unless directly inhaled.

Alternanthera ficoidea. 7
Shade plant grown as an annual in most zones, and used like *Coleus*, for its attractive leaves. Do not let it flower; keep the blooms clipped off because the flowers may be allergenic.

ALTHEA.
See *Hibiscus.*

ALUMINUM PLANT.
See *Pilea.*

Alyogyne huegelii. 3
BLUE HIBISCUS. A common tall perennial sub shrub in warm coastal areas. Blue, *hibiscus*-like flowers on a plant hardy to 20 degrees. The flowers attract hummingbirds.

Alyssum. 6
A low-growing perennial for all zones, with yellow, heavily fragrant flowers. The strong smell may bother some people. Contact with *Alyssum* flowers and leaves may irritate the skin.

ALYSSUM, SWEET
See *Lobularia maritima.*

Amaracus.
See *Origanum.*

AMARANTH.
See *Amaranthus.*

Amaranthus. 8
AMARANTH, LOVE-LIES-BLEEDING. Tall annuals grown in all zones for their long, drooping reddish flowers. They are closely related to common weeds known to cause much allergy.

Amarcrinum. ✲ 2
A tall, fragrant lily, easy to grow in mild winter areas.

AMARYLLIS.
See *Hippeastrum*.

Amaryllis belladonna
(Brunsvigia rosea). 📷   ✻ 2
NAKED LADY, BELLADONNA LILY. Hardy in zones 8 through 10 if protected in winter. NAKED LADY has big pink trumpet-shaped flowers that are borne when the plant has no leaves. Leaves grow after the flowers have bloomed. Clumps of NAKED LADY may last for many years. Some may find the unusual fragrance too strong when used in the house as a cut flower.

AMAZON VINE.
See *Stigmaphyllon*.

Ambrosia.   ✳ 10
RAGWEED. Some native and others accidental imports, RAGWEEDS thrive where man has neglected the land. They grow almost worldwide, but are most common in the midwestern United States. RAGWEEDS are also found in Eastern Europe and in parts of France. Most of the United Kingdom is free of *Ambrosia*.

On land untouched by human hand, RAGWEEDS are rarely found. These and many of the worst allergenic weeds flourish only where man has disturbed the soil and natural vegetation, and then left it in a disturbed state. Nature abhors bare ground and soon covers it with weeds. Ragweeds are common in burned-out soils, waste and dump areas, and wherever the ecosystem is out of balance.

One of the principles of sustainable agriculture is that the soil should always be covered, either by plants or mulch. Bare soil, exposed to the destructive effects of wind, rain, and sun, is soil being destroyed. If the cultural conditions are changed so that soil can sustain its fertility, friability, organic matter, earthworms, and all the other microorganisms that keep it healthy, then RAGWEEDS, CHEESEWEEDS, and TUMBLEWEEDS quickly disappear.

Ambrosia

To get rid of RAGWEED, chop it down before it can bloom and reseed. More important, work toward sustainability of the soil.

Farmers often spray RAGWEEDS with a herbicide containing 2,4-D (the same chemical as in dandelion killers). The sprayed RAGWEEDS quickly wilt and become highly attractive to livestock. Cattle in particular have frequently been poisoned with 2,4-D after grazing on recently sprayed weeds.

Amelanchier laevis.   3
SERVICE BERRY, SHADBUSH. A group of shrubs, small trees, and ground covers hardy to zone 3. SERVICE BERRY is among the first flowering trees to bloom in early spring and puts on a show of bright white blossoms, followed by small fruits which look and taste much like wild blueberries. Birds are very fond of these fruits—as is the author.

Amelanchier laevis

Ammophila.   ✳ 9
BEACHGRASS. Several species of imported grasses used to stabilize beaches. Once established, they often crowd out less aggressive native species and produce allergy.

AMOMYRTUS.
See *Luma apiculata*.

Ampelopsis brevipedunculata.   ✻ 2
BLUEBERRY CLIMBER. A deciduous vine for sun or shade, hardy in all zones; it grows strong and fast and needs good support. The fruits resemble BLUEBERRIES and are attractive to birds. *Ampelopsis* is a good substitute for ENGLISH IVY.

AMUR CHOKECHERRY.
See *Prunus maackii*.

AMUR CORK TREE.
See *Phellodendron*.

AMUR MAPLE.
See *Acer tataricum ginnala*.

Anacardiaceae.
CASHEW FAMILY. Large group of over 600 species of trees and shrubs, mostly evergreen but some deciduous, many with poisonous properties. This family of plants accounts for more cases of allergy than any other, and includes genra such as *Astronium, Cotinus, Harpephyllum, Laurophyllus, Lithrea, Mangifera, Pistache, Rhodosphaera, Rhus, Schinus, Semecarpus, Smodingium,* and *Spondias.* Individually rated.

Anacardium occidentale. ✳10
CASHEW. A large, spreading evergreen tree to 40 feet, grown as an ornamental in zone 10. It is native to tropical America and widely grown in tropics and subtropics; commercially in India. It is notable for its milky allergenic sap, yellowish pink flowers, and 3-inch-long edible red fruits called *cashew apples,* the seeds of which are cashew nuts.

Anacyclus depressus. 4
A perennial hardy in all zones with daisy-like flowers on a low-growing, spreading plant. It grows best on lighter soils.

Anagallis. 3
PIMPERNEL. Low-growing perennials or annuals for full sun in all zones. The small flowers are scarlet or blue. Plants are poisonous.

Anaphalis. ✳10
PEARLY EVERLASTING A perennial grown as cut flower and for long-lasting dried flowers. Avoid its use in the landscape and as a dried flower. *Anaphalis* is separate-sexed, but is not usually sold sexed.

Anchusa. ✳ 2
Hardy annuals or perennials similar to FORGET-ME-NOTS (*Myosotis*) but on much larger plants. It thrives in full sun and dry soil, where it produces its clusters of bright blue flowers in abundance.

Andrachne. 8
A native shrub occasionally used in landscaping in south-central areas of United States.

Andromeda. 4
BOG ROSEMARY. A hardy rock garden evergreen shrub with pale pink flowers for wet areas. See also *Zenobia.*

Andropogon. 7
BEARDGRASS, BIG BLUESTEM GRASS. A common grass that is the cause of some grass allergies.

Androsace. ✳ 2
ROCK JASMINE. A low-growing hardy perennial.

Andryala aghardii. 5
A small, low-growing yellow-flowered annual for rock gardens.

Anemone. 3
WINDFLOWER. Grown from seed, divisions, or tubers, *Anemones* are attractive garden flowers in all zones. In the garden these flowers present little allergy problem, but as cut flowers they are suspect. *Anemone* leaves and flowers are poisonous.

ANEMONE, BUSH.
See *Carpenteria californica.*

Anemopaegma chamberlaynii. ✳ 2
YELLOW TRUMPET VINE. Hardy only in zone 10; a good flowering vine for mild areas.

Anemopsis californica. ✳ 2
YERBA MANSA. A common western wildflower for wet places. The flowers look like small CONEFLOWERS with white petals (actually bracts). The leaves of YERBA MANSA are long and wide. As a wildflower it ranges from California to Texas and has long been used by inhabitants of the Southwest as an old folk remedy plant. The root is used to make a tea said to help relieve asthma.

Anethum. 3
DILL. A garden annual, easily grown from seed.

ANGEL TRUMPET.
See *Brugmansia; Datura.*

Angelica. 6
Biennial for all zones that thrives in rich, moist soils. Contact with the leaves of *Angelica* may cause skin rashes.

ANGEL'S HAIR.
See *Artemisia*.

ANGEL'S TEARS.
See *Narcissus triandrus; Soleirolia soleirolii*.

Angophora costata. 5
GUM MYRTLE. Evergreen tree for zones 9 and 10.

Anigozanthos. ✳ 2
KANGAROO PAW. Tender evergreen perennial for light soils with full sun and good drainage.

Anisacanthus. ✳ 2
DESERT HONEYSUCKLE. A perennial shrub for mild winter areas of zones 8–10. It bears bright orange flowers much of the year.

ANISE.
See *Foeniculum; Pimpinella*.

ANISE TREE.
See *Illicium anisatum*.

Annona cherimola. 📷 3
CHERIMOYA. A small, deciduous tree for warm coastal areas of zone 10. It has large attractive leaves and big, green, delicious fruits. CHERIMOYA is easily grown from the large black seeds. The leaves and stems of *Cherimoya* are quite poisonous.

Anredera (Boussingaultia). 7
MADEIRA VINE. Evergreen vines hardy to zone 8, or in colder zones if the tubers are dug and stored over winter. *Anredera* is notable for its heart-shaped leaves and clusters of fragrant white flowers.

Antennaria. males 5, females ✳ 1
PUSSY TOES, LADIES'-TOBACCO. A group of small deciduous perennial herbs, native to North and South America, and to North Europe and Asia. A few species are hardy in all zones. Dioecious, separate-sexed plants, especially *A. dioica*. The male plants are smaller than the females and in some species, male plants are unknown. Not usually sold sexed.

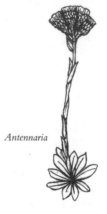

Antennaria

Anthemis. 7
DOG FENNEL, MARGUERITE DAISY. Hardy in all zones, this daisy-like perennial has been known to cause skin rash from contact with the leaves.

Anthoxanthum. ✳10
SWEET VERNAL GRASS, VERNAL GRASS. A European grass introduced and naturalized in the United States and the cause of widespread allergy, especially early in the spring.

Anthriscus. 3
CHERVIL. An annual herb for all zones, CHERVIL grows best in partial shade.

Anthurium. 📷 ✳ 2
Houseplants.

Antiaris. ✳10
Tropical trees or shrubs.

Antidesma. ✳9
CHINESE LAUREL. An evergreen tree for zone 10.

Antigonon. ✳ 2
CORAL VINE. Deciduous vine for zones 9 and 10, bearing long clusters of red flowers. It does well in desert areas, and should be mulched in colder areas.

Antirrhinum majus. ✲ 1
SNAPDRAGON. A hardy annual for all zones that thrives in cooler weather. Many sizes and colors are available.

Aphanamixis. ✺ 9
Seldom-seen, dioecious, zone 10 trees.

Aphananthe. ✺ 10
MUKU TREE. Several species of fast-growing ELM-related trees from Korea, eastern China, and Japan, occasionally used in landscaping in the United States. Hardy to zone 6, the MUKU TREE is one of the few ELM relatives that has separate male-only flowers, and because of this it releases large amounts of pollen into the air. ELM allergy is common and often severe.

Aphelandra. ✲ 2
Houseplant with big, striped leaves that does best in filtered light.

Apium graveolens. 5
CELERY. There are many documented examples of allergy to eating CELERY, as well as numerous examples of skin rashes caused by contact with leaves in sensitive individuals. CELERY is related to certain common allergenic weeds, such as QUEEN ANNE'S LACE, and cross-reaction allergies are common, especially during the fall peak of the RAGWEED bloom. Persons with RAGWEED allergies would be wise to avoid eating CELERY in the late summer and fall months.

Apocynum. 4
DOGBANE. A hardy perennial herb. The sap may cause rash in sensitive persons. Poisonous.

Aponogeton distachyus. ✲ 2
CAPE PONDWEED, WATER LILY, WATER HAWTHORN. Aquatic plants for lakes, ponds, and small pools.

APPLE.
See *Malus.*

APRICOT.
See *Prunus armeniaca.*

Aptenia cordifolia. 📷 ✲ 1
RED-APPLE ICEPLANT. Low-growing evergreen perennial for zones 9 and 10. It bears small red flowers, and is very easy to grow from cuttings inserted directly into the soil.

Aquilegia. ✲ 1
COLUMBINE. Hardy perennials for all zones, COLUMBINES are good garden and woodland flowers. Poisonous.

ARABIAN TEA.
See *Catha edulis.*

Arabis. ✲ 1
ROCKCRESS. A hardy perennial for all zones, often used as a rock garden plant. Easy-to-grow, attractive flowers are usually white or pink.

Arachis hypogaea. 3
PEANUT. Annual legume needing a warm summer, sandy soil, and a long growing season to produce well. All parts of the plant are edible, but allergy to eating peanuts is common and often severe. Allergy to pollen of peanuts, however, is quite rare.

Aralia. 5
A group of spiny deciduous shrubs or small trees with big, bold leaves. Hardy into zone 5.

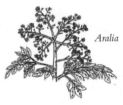
Aralia

ARALIA, FALSE.
See *Dizygotheca.*

ARAR TREE.
See *Tetraclinis.*

Araucaria. 8
BUNYA-BUNYA, MONKEY PUZZLE TREE. Large group of nonnative evergreen trees; some hardy into zone 5. *A. heterophylla*, the NORFOLK ISLAND PINE, is often grown as a houseplant tree. Kept in a container, most *Araucaria* will never bloom or cause allergies. Planted in the ground, however, they are not good choices for allergy-free landscapes.

Some species are separate-sexed and, in the future, female-only plants may be available. Because young *Araucaria* trees do not bloom, a small NORFOLK ISLAND PINE can be a good substitute for a real PINE Christmas tree for those with odor and perfume allergy to PINE.

Araujia. 3
WHITE BLADDER FLOWER. Easy-to-grow, woody vine for zones 8 to 10.

ARBOR SANCTA.
See *Melia*.

ARBORVITAE.
See *Platycladus; Thuja*.

Arbutus. 📷 3
MADRONE, STRAWBERRY TREE. Several species of native trees and shrubs hardy into zone 4. Attractive bark, small to medium size, and attractive fruits make these popular landscape choices. Drought tolerant.

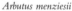

Arbutus menziesii

Archontophoenix. 📷 6
ALEXANDRA PALM, KING PALM. Hardy only in warmest areas of zones 9 and 10, these are handsome palms that unfortunately cause some allergy.

Arctocarpus communis. ✳ 2
BREADFRUIT. Grown mostly in the West Indies, Polynesia, and eastern India, the BREADFRUIT tree is a large evergreen with huge leaves and giant, bland fruits. The seeds are roasted and eaten like chestnuts. A low allergy risk.

Arctostaphylos. 3
MANZANITA, BEARBERRY. Evergreen shrubs and increasingly popular ground covers. Hardy into zone 5, MANZANITA is native to the dry areas of the West. Easy to grow in well

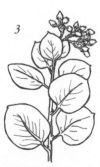

Arctostaphylos

drained soil, they do best in full sun. Many varieties have been developed for use as ground covers, and all of these are good choices where adaptable.

Arctotheca calendula. 7
CAPE WEED. Gray-leafed ground cover for zones 9 and 10, CAPE WEED spreads fast in full sun and is soon covered with yellow daisy-like flowers.

Arctotis. 6
AFRICAN DAISY. An annual and perennial that is easy to grow. It is available in many colors.

Ardisia. 3
SPICEBERRY. Evergreen shade-loving shrub or ground cover that requires ample moisture to grow well.

Areca. 6
BETEL NUT PALM. Tropical and subtropical palms.

Arecastrum romanzoffianum. 📷 6
QUEEN PALM. Occasionally sold as *Cocos plumosa*.

Arenaria. 3
SANDWORT. Hardy perennial ground cover occasionally used as lawn substitutes. Good in rock gardens.

Arenga. 5
Tropical and subtropical palm tree. Monocarpic, they only bloom once, then die after blooming. While blooming, they release abundant amounts of pollen.

Argemone. ✳ 2
PRICKLY POPPY. Annual or biennial for all zones. Very drought-tolerant, tall plant with prickly stems and big, showy white poppy flowers. Native to dry areas in the desert. *A. mexicana* has orange flowers. Poisonous.

Arikuryroba schizophylla. 6
Small subtropical palm trees, occasionally grown in Florida.

Aristolochia. 3
DUTCHMAN'S PIPE VINE. Hardy in most zones and easy to grow, *Aristolochia* thrives in either full sun

or deep shade. The odd-shaped flowers resemble a curved tobacco pipe. Very poisonous.

Armeria. 📷 ✳ 1
SEA PINK, THRIFT. A low-growing evergreen perennial native to coastal areas. Hardy in all zones. Very good plants for edging flower gardens. Easy to grow and often in bloom with many pink, red, or rose-colored flowers.

Armoracia rusticana. ✳ 2
HORSERADISH. Easy-to-grow, very hardy perennial grown for its pungent roots, which are used as a condiment.

Arnica. ✺ 10
Relatives of *Senecio* (which see). A group of about 30 species of hardy perennial herbs and flowers. All are poisonous if eaten and many species are capable of causing severe allergic skin reactions. The pollen of *Arnica* species is also highly allergenic, especially for anyone already allergic to the RAGWEEDS, to which *Arnica* is closely related.

Aronia arbutifolia. ✳ 2
RED CHOKEBERRY. Deciduous shrub native to the eastern United States and hardy to zone 4. Easy to grow and tolerant of wet soils, it has attractive autumn color and red berries that attract birds.

Arrhenatherum elatius. 4
TALL OATGRASS. A meadow grass, used mostly for pastures. TALL OATGRASS produces little pollen and is unimportant in causing allergy. This grass may find greater use as a lawn grass in the near future.

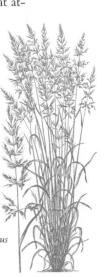

Arrhenatherum elatius

ARROW GRASS.
See *Triglochin*.

ARROW ROOT.
See *Zamia*.

ARROWHEAD VINE.
See *Syngonium podophyllum*.

ARROWWOOD.
See *Viburnum; Zamia*.

Artemisia. ✺ 9
ANGEL'S HAIR, DUSTY MILLER, SAGEBRUSH, SOUTHERNWOOD, TARRAGON, WORMWOOD. Many species of evergreen or deciduous shrubs or woody perennials, hardy in all zones. *Artemisias* are close relatives of ragweeds, and many people have strong allergic reactions to all of them, both from their odors and from their abundant pollen. Many more species of *Artemisia* are being used now, due to the popularity of native landscaping.

Artemisias are often called SAGE and as such are occasionally used in cooking. However, true culinary sage is actually a type of *Salvia* (which see) and is not related to *Artemisia*. Many species of *Artemisia* are poisonous if eaten, including their seeds, flowers, and leaves. Certain types of *Artemisia* are used in herbal medicinals; use *Artemisia* very carefully, if at all. If you are allergic to the RAGWEEDS, it would be wise to avoid any contact with the *Artemisias*.

One species, *A. absinthium*, a fragrant herb, was used to flavor a liqueur called *absinthe*. Popular in the late 1800s, many people, including the painter, Vincent van Gogh, were addicted to absinthe. Van Gogh's heavy absinthe consumption is said to have caused much of his famously erratic behavior. Absinthe was made illegal in France in 1912 and in the United States in 1915.

ARTICHOKE.
See *Cynara*.

ARTILLERY PLANT.
See *Pilea microphylla*.

Arum.   4

Large-leafed perennials, hardy to zone 6. Grown mostly as curiosity plants, some *Arum* bear very malodorous flowers. Recently a GIANT ARUM with a 6-foot-tall purple flower bloomed at the Huntington Gardens in Los Angeles. Huge crowds came to see this CORPSE FLOWER. The smell of the flower was compared to the inside of a filthy dumpster, or to that of a rotting carcass. The smell alone could cause allergy for some. Don't plant this one too close to the house. Poisonous.

Aruncus sylvester.   ✲9

Tall white-flowered annual with ferny foliage that grows best in moist, shady spots.

Arundinaria.

See BAMBOO.

Arundo donax.   8

GIANT REED. Hardy perennial for all zones. *Arundo* may become invasive.

Asarina antirrhinifolia.   ✲ 2

Tall annuals with colorful flowers that resemble SNAPDRAGONS.

Asarum.   ✲ 1

WILD GINGER. Hardy perennial that produces red flowers on low-growing plants. GINGERS require ample moisture and rich soil to thrive.

Asclepias.   3

BUTTERFLY WEED, GOOSE PLANT, MILKWEED. Hardy in full sun in all zones, the many species of this genus are toxic if eaten; cattle in particular are often poisoned from eating MILKWEED.

ASH.

See *Fraxinus.*

ASH-LEAFED MAPLE.

See *Acer negundo.*

ASH, MOUNTAIN.

See *Sorbus.*

Asimina triloba.   3

PAW PAW. Small, large-leafed, deciduous native fruit tree for moist areas of zones 5–8. The bland, custardlike fruit are borne on attractive trees.

Asparagus.   5

Ornamental and edible perennials. Ornamental asparagus is not nearly as hardy as the edible variety. ASPARAGUS FERN, not a true fern, is a popular houseplant. These are complete flowered and rated lower for allergy, at 3. The edible asparagus is separate-sexed, and most commercial varieties are males. People living near fields of asparagus are at risk from the pollen of the mature plants. People who handle a great deal of cut *Asparagus* can get skin rashes, and this is fairly common in *Asparagus* canning plants. Some people also report allergic reactions to eating *Asparagus.*

ASPEN.

See *Populus.*

Asperula azurea.   3

A hardy blue-flowered fragrant annual grown from seed.

Asperula odorata.

See *Galium odoratum.*

Asphodelus albus.   3

A white-flowered lily.

Aspidistra elatior.   ✲ 1

CAST IRON PLANT. An evergreen perennial, hardy to zone 7 and grown as a houseplant elsewhere. It will grow well in deep shade and needs little care.

Aspidium.

See *Rumohra.*

Asplenium.   4

BIRD'S-NEST FERN, houseplants. Outdoors in mild areas in shade with plenty of moisture. Spores from ferns can cause allergies, but usually the spores do not travel far from the parent plant. Unless used in overhead hanging baskets, most ferns do not present much of a problem in the allergy-free garden. (See also FERNS.)

ASSYRIAN PLUM.
See *Cordia.*

Aster.   doubles 6, singles 8
Hardy perennials for all zones, *Asters* are common garden flowers in a wide array of colors. Some make fairly large shrubs. *Asters* have a bad name in allergy studies and they do not make good cut flowers for the allergic household. Nonetheless, not all *Asters* produce the same amounts of pollen. A few plants in a large garden should not present much of a problem. Fully double-flowered varieties have far fewer exposed pollen parts.

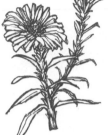
Aster

ASTER TREE.
See *Olearia.*

Asteriscus maritmus. 📷   6
Easy-to-grow, mound-forming perennials with yellow flowers. Full sun in zones 8–10.

Asterogyne.   5
Tropical and subtropical palms.

Astilbe.   6
Shade-loving perennials hardy in all zones, they are long-lived in cold-winter areas. *Astilbe* needs rich, moist soil to thrive.

Astrantia.   4
MASTERWORT. Shade-loving, large-flowered perennial or annual from seed.

Astrocaryum.   7
Palm. *A. mexicanum* grows in parts of zone 10.

Astronium.   ✳10
Numerous species of small allergenic trees native to South America, occasionally found planted in zones 9 and 10. In particular, *A. balansae,* a 30-foot evergreen tree with long compound leaves like sumac, is often used in landscaping.

Athrotaxis.   8
Evergreen coniferous tree from Tasmania used in zones 9–10. Related to *Cryptomeria,* these cause allergy.

Athyrium.   6
LADY FERN. Hardy fern for moist, shady areas. Grows to 4 feet.

ATLAS BROOM.
See *Cytisus.*

ATLAS CEDAR.
See *Cedrus atlantica.*

Atriplex.   ✳9
DESERT HOLLY, QUAILBUSH, SALTBUSH. Native desert perennials or large shrubs. Easy to grow and drought tolerant, these cause allergies.

Attalea.   7
Tropical and subtropical palms.

Aubrieta.   ✳ 2
Hardy, low-growing perennial for rock gardens or along rock walls.

Aucuba japonica. 📷   *Varies by cultivar.*
GOLD DUST PLANT. A small group of Asiatic evergreen shrubs hardy in zones 5 through 10, and used as a greenhouse plant in colder climates. Aucuba grows well in deep shade and has large, toothed, often variegated leaves. These are separate-sexed plants; males cause allergies, females do not. Look for named varieties or those already producing large red berries. The varieties 'Longifolia', 'Nana', 'Serratifolia', 'Fructu Albo', 'Pictura', 'Aureo-maculata', and 'Sulphur' are all females and have excellent allergy ratings. The

variety 'Crotonifolia' is a male and should be avoided. 'Variegata' can be either male or female. Don't buy 'Variegata' unless it is tagged as a female, or if it has red fruit.

Aulax. ❋ 2
Three species of South African evergreen shrubs with white or yellow flowers.

AURICULA.
See *Primula auricula.*

Aurinia saxatilis. 3
BASKET OF GOLD. Hardy perennial for all zones. May winter-kill in cold areas if not mulched. Bright yellow flowers are borne on low-growing plants ideal for the rock garden.

AUSTRALIAN BLUEBELL CREEPER.
See *Sollya heterophylla.*

AUSTRALIAN BOTTLE PLANT.
See *Jatropha.*

AUSTRALIAN BUSH CHERRY.
See *Syzygium.*

AUSTRALIAN FUCHSIA.
See *Correa.*

AUSTRALIAN PINE.
See *Casuarina.*

AUSTRALIAN WILLOW.
See *Acacia; Geijera parviflora.*

Austrocedrus. males ❋ 9, females ❋ 1
CHILEAN INCENSE CEDAR. Shrubs or small trees for zone 8, where summers are cool. Separate-sexed, dioecious plants, but not yet sold sexed. Females are excellent choices for the allergy-free garden.

AUTUMN CROCUS.
See *Colchicum autumnale.*

Avena. Not rated.
OATS. A common grain that may cause allergy but usually less so than corn, wheat, or barley. Wild varieties cause more allergy.

Averrhoa. ❋ 1
Two species of small Asian evergreen fruiting trees, occasionally found in zone 10 in Florida.

AVOCADO.
See *Persea americana.*

AZALEA.
See *Rhododendron.*

Azara. 4
Large, shade-loving evergreen flowering shrubs for zone 9 and 10. The flowers are small, yellow, and very fragrant; it may not be a good choice for those sensitive to odors.

Azoria vidalii. ❋ 2
Hardy perennial for shady, moist spots bears large, bell-shaped flowers on erect stalks. Needs protection in most cold-winter areas.

AZTEC LILY.
See *Lilium.*

B

Allergy Index Scale: *1* **is Best,** *10* **is Worst.**

❄ for *1* and *2* ✸ for *9* and *10*

📷 See insert for photograph

BABASSU.
See *Orbignya.*

Babiana. ❄ *2*
BABOON FLOWER. South African native for zones 4–10; grown from corms. It bears spring-blooming flowers of red, blue, lavender, and white.

BABOON FLOWER.
See *Babiana.*

BABY BLUE EYES.
See *Nemophila.*

BABY'S BREATH.
See *Gypsophila.*

BABY'S TEARS.
See *Soleirolia soleirolii.*

Baccharis pilularis. 📷 ✸ *10*
COYOTE BRUSH. Hardy in zones 6–10. Perennial shrubby ground cover or large loose bush. COYOTE BRUSH is very closely related to RAGWEED, and allergies are common and often severe. All varieties of *Baccharis* ground cover sold are all-male cultivars and are especially potent. COYOTE BRUSH became a very popular ground cover in California during the drought years of 1987–1995 because it is very drought tolerant; allergy to this plant is on the rise. All plants are poisonous.

BACHELOR'S BUTTON.
See *Centaurea.*

BACHELOR'S BUTTON, YELLOW.
See *Polygala.*

Bactris. *5*
SPINY-CLUB PALM. Small palms from tropical America.

Bacularia. 7
Tropical and subtropical palms.

BAHIA GRASS.
See *Paspalum.*

Balaka. *6*
Tropical palms.

BALD CYPRESS.
See *Taxodium distichum.*

BALLOON FLOWER.
See *Platycodon grandiflorus.*

BALM-OF-GILEAD.
See *Cedronella; Populus candicans.*

BALMIES.
See *Abies; Populus balsamifera.*

BALSAM.
See *Impatiens balsamina.*

BALSAM FIR.
See *Abies balsamea.*

BAMBOO. ❄ *2*
Giant grasses. Many people are allergic to grass pollen, and allergies to BAMBOO pollen are not unusual in the tropics; however, most BAMBOO does not flower when grown in the United States (except Hawaii). (I had a planting of GOLDEN BAMBOO,

a 3-foot-tall variety, that grew many years and never flowered.) There are many varieties of bamboo and most can be cut to the ground every year; they will regrow without flowering. Some of the more exotic and expensive species, such as BLACK BAMBOO, are usually kept confined to a large pot.

BAMBOO PALM.
See *Rhapis.*

Bamburanta.
See *Ctenanthe.*

BANANA.
See *Musa; Ensete.*

BANANA SHRUB.
See *Michelia.*

BANANA YUCCA.
See *Yucca.*

Banksia. 3
Large group of evergreen trees and shrubs mostly grown in Australia.

Baptisia australis. ✳ 2
WILD INDIGO. Tall perennial for full sun, hardy in all zones. Spikes of indigo blue flowers resemble SWEET PEAS.

BARBADOS CEDAR.
See *Cedrela.*

BARBADOS CHERRY.
See *Malpighia.*

BARBADOS NUT.
See *Jatropha.*

BARBASCO.
See *Jacquinia.*

BARBEL PALM.
See *Acanthophoenix.*

BARBERRY.
See *Berberis.*

BARLEY.
See *Hordeum.*

BARREL CACTUS.
See *Echinocactus; Ferocactus.*

BARREL PALM.
See *Colpothrinax wrightii.*

BASEBALL PLANT.
See *Euphorbia obesa.*

BASIL.
See *Ocimum.*

BASKET FLOWER.
See *Hymenocallis.*

BASKET OF GOLD.
See *Aurinia saxatilis.*

BASKET PLANT.
See *Aeschynanthus.*

BASSWOOD.
See *Tilia.*

Bauhinia. 4
ORCHID TREE. Medium-sized evergreen or deciduous flowering tree for zones 9 and 10. The flowers resemble ORCHIDS. Easy to grow from seed. Poisonous.

BAY.
See *Laurus; Umbellularia.*

BAY LAUREL.
See *Umbellularia californica.*

BAY, RED.
See *Persea borbonia.*

Bay star vine.
See *Schisandra.*

Bayberry.
See *Myrica.*

Beach aster.
See *Erigeron.*

Beach naupka.
See *Scaevola.*

Beach wormwood.
See *Artemisia.*

Beachgrass.
See *Ammophila.*

Bead plant.
See *Nertera granadensis.*

Bead tree.
See *Melia; Pithecellobium guadalupense.*

Beans.
See *Phaseolus.*

Bearberry.
See *Arctostaphylos; Rhamnus; Salix.*

Beard tongue.
See *Penstemon.*

Beardgrass.
See *Andropogon; Polypogon.*

Bear's breech.
See *Acanthus mollis.*

Bear's foot fern.
See *Humata tyermannii.*

Bear-tongue lily.
See *Clintonia.*

Beaucarnea recurvata. *males 6, females* ❋ *1*
Bottle palm, ponytail. Tall succulent with large, woody base. Hardy only in zone 10. Separate-sexed but not usually sold sexed.

Beaumontia grandiflora. ❋ *2*
Easter lily vine, herald's trumpet. Evergreen vine for zones 9 and 10 with large, fragrant, trumpet-shaped white flowers with bright green veins. Needs good soil and plenty of water. Flowers on old wood only, so do not prune too heavily. Protect from wind.

Beauty bush.
See *Kolkwitzia amabilis.*

Beautyberry.
See *Callicarpa bodinieri giraldii.*

Bee balm.
See *Monarda.*

Bee gum.
See *Nyssa sylvatica.*

Beech.
See *Fagus.*

Beef plant.
See *Iresine herbstii.*

Beefwood.
See *Casuarina stricta.*

Beetlewood.
See *Ostrya.*

Beets, sugar beets.
See *Beta vulgaris.*

Begonia. 📷 *fibrous 4, tuberous 3*
Annual and perennial shade-loving flowers. *Begonias* from seed are called fibrous begonias. Tuberous begonias are grown from fleshy tubers. *Begonias* are all monoecious, but the male flowers are situated above the female blooms. The petals are large, richly

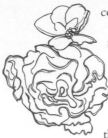

Begonia

colored, and attractive to insects. The small fibrous begonias shed more pollen than the larger tuberous kinds. In large-flowered *Begonias*, the male flowers are often single while the female are usually fully double. *Begonias* are not high allergy plants but they expose the gardener to more incidental pollen than would *Impatiens*. Good for hanging baskets in all but the hottest areas.

Belamcanda chinensis. ✹ 2
BLACKBERRY LILY, LEOPARD FLOWER. Rhizomatous perennial, hardy in all zones, bearing stalks of orange-red flowers. The seeds resemble BLACKBERRIES.

BELLADONNA LILY.
See *Amaryllis belladonna.*

BELLFLOWER.
See *Campanula.*

Bellis perennis. 📷 6
ENGLISH DAISY. Low-growing perennials hardy in all zones.

BELLS OF IRELAND.
See *Moluccella laevis.*

BELLY PALM.
See *Colpothrinax wrightii.*

Beloperone.
See *Justicia.*

BENJAMIN BUSH.
See *Lindera.*

BENT GRASS.
See *Agrostis.*

Bentinckia. 7
Tropical palms.

Berberis. 3
BARBERRY. Deciduous and evergreen spiny shrubs, some hardy in all zones. A useful plant, easy to grow in tough landscape situations. Poisonous.

Bergenia. 📷 ✹ 2
Evergreen shade perennial hardy in all zones. Its large, cabbage-like leaves and small pink, rose, or white flowers are susceptible to snails and slugs.

BERMUDA GRASS.
See *Cynodon dactylon.*

BERMUDA PALM.
See *Sabal.*

Bertholletia excelsa. ✹ 1
BRAZIL NUT, CREAM NUT, PARA NUT. A large, evergreen tree from tropical South America and the West Indies, grown for its seeds. Not grown in the United States, except in the mildest parts of zone 10. Trees have very large, 20-inch-long, leathery leaves and creamy white flowers. Fruits are round, 5 inches in diameter; the large seeds are the BRAZIL NUTS of commerce. The trees are entirely insect pollinated and are not known to cause allergy. They are fairly easy to grow from seed.

BE-STILL PLANT.
See *Thevetia.*

Beta vulgaris. ✹ 1
BEETS, SWISS CHARD. Garden vegetables. Beets should always be harvested long before they flower (if left to flower, they are no longer edible). The flowers may cause allergies but this is rare, because most are never allowed to bloom. BEETS have a very good allergy rating under regular culture.

Allergy to SUGAR BEET flowers is common and growing in incidence as the acreage of this crop is increased. People living close to SUGAR BEET fields are at most risk. Allergy rating for fields of sugar beets is high.

BETEL.
See *Piper.*

BETEL NUT PALM.
See *Areca.*

BETHLEHEM SAGE.
See *Pulmonaria.*

Betula. 📷 7
BIRCH. Although airborne BIRCH pollen causes allergy, the actual bloom time of most BIRCH trees is not long, usually finished within a few days. An occasional tree in the landscape (planted far from doors or windows) does not pose too much of a problem. However, people who are allergic to ALDER (see *Alnus*) may also become allergic to BIRCH. BIRCH trees rate better than ALDERS because BIRCH usually mature to be smaller trees, shed less pollen, and have a shorter pollen season. BIRCH trees bloom early in spring and occasionally flower again in late summer or fall. These shallow-rooted trees need plenty of water.

Betula papyrifera

BEVERLY HILLS ARBORVITAE.
See *Platycladus orientalis.*

Bidens ferulifolia. 6
YELLOW-FLOWERED DAISY. Mexican annual; easy to grow from seed.

BIG BLUESTEM GRASS.
See *Andropogon.*

BIG-CONE SPRUCE.
See *Pseudotsuga.*

BIG-LEAF HYDRANGEA.
See *Hydrangea macrophylla.*

BIG SAGEBRUSH.
See *Artemisia.*

BIG TREE.
See *Sequoiadendron giganteum.*

BIGLEAF MAPLE.
See *Acer macrophyllum.*

Bignonia.
The old name for many different species of flowering trumpet vines, some hardy and others tender. Most are fast growing and showy, but many TRUMPET VINES can cause contact skill allergies. For allergy ratings, see also *Anemopaegma; Distictis; Campsis; Clytostoma; Pandorea; Macfadyena; Pyrostegia.*

Billbergia. ❋ 2
VASE PLANT. A bromeliad.

BILBERRY.
See *Vaccinium.*

BIRCH.
See *Betula.*

BIRCH BARK CHERRY.
See *Prunus serrula.*

BIRD-CATCHER TREE.
See *Pisonia.*

BIRD-OF-PARADISE.
See *Strelitzia; Heliconia.*

BIRD-OF-PARADISE BUSH.
See *Caesalpinia.*

BIRD-ON-THE-WING.
See *Polygala.*

BIRD'S-EYE BUSH.
See *Ochna serrulata.*

BIRD'S EYES.
See *Gilia.*

BIRD'S-FOOT FERN.
See *Pellaea.*

BIRD'S-FOOT TREFOIL.
See *Lotus corniculatus*.

BIRD'S-NEST FERN.
See *Asplenium*.

BIRTHWORT.
See *Aristolochia*.

Bischofia javanica. ✳10
A large evergreen tree for zone 10. Separate-sexed, yet not sold sexed. The sap may cause rash and *Bischofia* may be especially bad for people with an allergy to latex.

BISCOCHITO.
See *Ruprechtia*.

BISHOP'S HAT.
See *Epimedium*.

BISHOP'S WEED.
See *Aegopodium*.

Bismarckia nobilis. 📷 *males* ✳ *9, females* ❋ *1*
A tropical palm tree occasionally grown in southern Florida and in California. These tall, very handsome fan palms are separate-sexed; the males cause allergy, the females do not.

BITTERROOT.
See *Lewisia rediviva*.

BITTERSWEET.
See *Celastrus*.

BITTERWOOD.
See *Simarouba*.

BLACK CALLA.
See *Arum*.

BLACK-EYED SUSAN.
See *Rudbeckia*.

BLACK-EYED SUSAN VINE.
See *Thunbergia*.

BLACK LOCUST.
See *Robinia*.

BLACK PALM.
See *Normanbya*.

BLACK PEPPER.
See *Piper*.

BLACK SALLY.
See *Eucalyptus*.

BLACK SNAKEROOT.
See *Cimicifuga*.

BLACK WALNUT.
See *Juglans*.

BLACKBEAD TREE.
See *Pithecellobium guadalupense*.

BLACKBERRY.
See *Rubus*.

BLACKBERRY LILY.
See *Belamcanda chinensis*.

BLACKBOY.
See *Xanthorrhoea*.

BLACKWOOD ACACIA.
See *Acacia*.

BLADDER FLOWER.
See *Araujia*.

BLADDERNUT.
See *Staphylea*.

BLANKET FLOWER.
See *Gaillardia*.

BLAZING STAR.
See *Chamaelirium luteum; Mentzelia.*

Blechnum (Lomaria).   4
Dwarf tree ferns.

BLEEDING HEART.
See *Dicentra.*

Bletilla striata.   � 1
CHINESE GROUND ORCHID. Lavender-orchid flowers on a hardy perennial plant (if mulched); does
best in shady, moist, rich soil.

Blighia sapida.   8
AKEE TREE. Four species of evergreen tropical trees,
some grown in parts of zone 10.

BLISTER CRESS.
See *Erysimum.*

BLOOD-LEAF.
See *Iresine herbstii.*

BLOOD LILY.
See *Hippeastrum.*

BLOOD-RED TRUMPET VINE.
See *Distictis.*

BLOODROOT.
See *Sanguinaria canadensis.*

BLUE BLOSSOM.
See *Ceanothus.*

BLUE BONESET.
See *Eupatorium.*

BLUE CROWN PASSION FLOWER.
See *Passiflora.*

BLUE CURLS.
See *Trichostema lanatum.*

BLUE DAWN FLOWER.
See *Ipomoea.*

BLUE DICKS.
See *Dichelostemma.*

BLUE DRACAENA.
See *Cordyline.*

BLUE-EYED GRASS.
See *Sisyrinchium.*

BLUE FESCUE.
See *Festuca glauca.*

BLUE GINGER.
See *Dichorisandra.*

BLUE GRAMA GRASS.
See *Bouteloua gracilis.*

BLUE GUM.
See *Eucalyptus.*

BLUE HIBISCUS.
See *Alyogyne huegelii.*

BLUE LACE FLOWER.
See *Trachymene coerulea.*

BLUE MARGUERITE.
See *Felicia amelloides.*

BLUE MIST.
See *Caryopteris.*

BLUE PALMETTO.
See *Rhapidophyllum hystrix.*

BLUE SPIRAEA.
See *Caryopteris.*

BLUE STAR CREEPER.
See *Laurentia fluviatilis.*

BLUE STEM, BIG BLUESTEM GRASS.
See *Andropogon*.

BLUE THIMBLE FLOWER.
See *Gilia capitata*.

BLUE VERVAIN.
See *Verbena*.

BLUE YUCCA.
See *Yucca*.

BLUEBEARD.
See *Caryopteris*.

BLUEBELL.
See *Endymion; Mertensia; Scilla*.

BLUEBELL, MOUNTAIN.
See *Mertensia*.

BLUEBELL, TEXAS.
See *Eustoma*.

BLUEBERRY.
See *Vaccinium*.

BLUEBERRY CLIMBER.
See *Ampelopsis brevipedunculata*.

BLUEGRASS.
See *Poa*.

BLUEWINGS.
See *Torenia*.

Boehmeria.   8
A large genus with numerous species of herbs, shrubs, and small trees, all of which can cause allergy. *B. nivea*, the CHINESE SILK PLANT, is occasionally grown in California.

BOG ROSEMARY.
See *Andromeda polifolia*.

BOKHARA FLEECEFLOWER.
See *Polygonum*.

BONESET.
See *Eupatorium*.

BORAGE.
See *Borago officinalis*.

Borago officinalis.   3
BORAGE. Annual herb for all zones. Sun or shade, easy to grow.

Borassus.   males ✺ 9, females ✳ 1
DOUB PALM, PALMYRA PALM, TALA PALM, TODDY PALM, WINE PALM. A group of tropical and subtropical separate-sexed fan palms, some used in zone 10, especially in Florida. Some are very large, growing to over 100 feet. Females of this group produce large seeds, which are used for a popular Asian drink called "toddy." The males of this family cause allergies; the females cause none. Not usually sold sexed.

Boronia.   3
Small evergreen shrub bearing small, fragrant leaves and pink flowers. *Boronia* needs light soil and even moisture to thrive.

BOSTON FERN.
See *Nephrolepis exaltata* 'Bostoniensis'.

BOSTON IVY.
See *Parthenocissus*.

BO-TREE.
See *Ficus religiosa*.

BOTTLE PALM.
See *Beaucarnea recurvata; Colpothrinax wrightii*.

BOTTLE PLANT.
See *Jatropha*.

BOTTLE TREE.
See *Brachychiton populneus; Firmiana simplex*.

BOTTLEBRUSH.
See *Callistemon; Melaleuca.*

Bougainvillea. 📷   ❋ 1
Popular flowering evergreen vines and shrubs for
zones 9 and 10; used in colder zones as container
plants. Most commonly seen with red or purple
flowers, but dozens of new colors are available. The
plants need warmth, and the roots are especially
sensitive to being moved, so transplant carefully.
The color in *Bougainvillea* comes mostly from colored leaves, called bracts, not from the actual flowers themselves, which are small and usually yellow.
A fine choice for an allergy-free landscape where
it will grow, or as a good, sunny window houseplant elsewhere. In Japan, *Bougainvillea* is trained
into stunning bonsai plants.

Boussingaultia.
See *Anredera.*

Bouteloua gracilis.   8
BLUE GRAMA GRASS. Lawn grass for cool areas; best
kept mowed at less than 1.75 inches.

Bouvardia.   ❋ 2
Evergreen shrub native to desert areas, bearing
red, pink, and rose-colored tubular flowers.

BOWDOCK.
See *Maclura pomifera.*

BOWER VINE.
See *Pandorea.*

BOWSTRING HEMP.
See *Sansevieria.*

BOWWOOD.
See *Maclura pomifera.*

BOX ELDER.
See *Acer negundo.*

BOX HOLLY.
See *Ruscus.*

BOX, JASMINE.
See *Phillyrea decora.*

BOX, SWEET.
See *Sarcococca.*

BOXWOOD.
See *Buxus; Myrsine; Paxistima.*

BOYSENBERRY.
See *Rubus.*

Brachychiton (Sterculia)

B. acerifolius.   3
FLAME TREE. Red flowering tree for zones 9 and 10.

B. populneus.   4
BOTTLE TREE. A large evergreen tree for zones 9
and 10, similar to CAMPHOR TREE, with 3-inch-long
woody seed pods.

B. discolor. 📷   ❋ 10
The HAT TREE or QUEENSLAND LACEBARK, is a a
very large tree with big leaves and clusters of large
trumpet-shaped flowers. The leaves and very large
seed pods of this tree have tiny stinging hairs that
cause severe skin irritation. It should be avoided.

Brachycome iberidifolia.   5
SWAN RIVER DAISY. A small annual bearing blue,
pink, or rose-colored flowers. Easy to grow.

Brachysema lanceolatum.   4
SWAN RIVER PEASHRUB. Drought-tolerant evergreen for full sun; it bears red flowers over an extended bloom period. *Brachysema* grows well in
hot, dry areas.

BRACKEN FERN.
See *Pteridium aquilinum.*

BRADFORD PEAR.
See *Pyrus.*

Brahea (Erythea)

B. armata. 📷   ❈ 2
MEXICAN BLUE PALM. A palm for warmer areas of zone 10; good blue leaf color.

B. edulis.   ❈ 2
GUADALUPE FAN PALM, ROCK PALM. Slow-growing palm for zones 9 or 10. Edible fruit.

B. elegans.   ❈ 2
FRANCESCHI PALM. Graceful palm for zone 10.

BRAKE.
See *Pteris.*

BRAMBLE.
See *Rubus.*

Brassaia actinophylla.   3
SCHEFFLERA, QUEENSLAND UMBRELLA TREE. Popular in Florida, Hawaii, and California.

Brassavola.   ❈ 2
Greenhouse orchids with fragrant, spiderlike white or green flowers.

BRASS BUTTONS.
See *Cotula squalida.*

Brassica.   *Group rated 3–6*
BROCCOLI, BRUSSELS SPROUTS, CABBAGE, CAULIFLOWER, MUSTARD, RAPE, RUTABAGA, TURNIPS, WILD MUSTARD. There are reports of allergy in Sweden to people living near RAPE fields, although this is not common.

BRAZIL NUT.
See *Bertholletia excelsa.*

BRAZILIAN FLAME BUSH.
See *Calliandra tweedii.*

BRAZILIAN GOLDEN VINE.
See *Stigmaphyllon.*

BRAZILIAN PEPPER TREE.
See *Schinus terebinthifolius.*

BRAZILIAN PLUME FLOWER.
See *Justicia.*

BRAZILIAN SKY FLOWER.
See *Duranta.*

BREAD TREE.
See *Treculia.*

BREADFRUIT.
See *Arctocarpus communis.*

BREATH–OF–HEAVEN.
See *Coleonema.*

BRIDAL ROBE.
See *Tripleurospermum.*

BRIDAL VEIL.
See *Tripogandra multiflora.*

BRIDAL VEIL BROOM.
See *Genista.*

BRIDAL WREATH.
See *Spiraea.*

Brimeura amethystina.   ❈ 2
Bulb hardy in all zones; it bears blue bell-like flowers.

BRISBANE BOX.
See *Tristania conferta.*

BRISTLEGRASS.
See *Setaria.*

Briza maxima.   5
RATTLESNAKE GRASS. Annual grass with nodding seeds. Sounds like rattlesnake rattles when shaken.

BROCCOLI.
See *Brassica.*

Brodiaea.   ✿ 1
Hardy corms for all zones. Easy to grow and may naturalize. (See also *Triteleia.*)

BROME GRASS.
See *Bromus.*

Bromelia (Guzmania; Neoregelia; Nidularium; Tillandsia; Vriesea).   ✿ 2
BROMELIAD. Perennials of the pineapple family, with strap-shaped leaves and showy single flower clusters growing in the center of the plant. Houseplants in most areas except warmer areas of zone 10. Drought-tolerant plants, easy to grow in pots.

Bromus.   ❋ 9
BROME GRASS. An important pasture and hay crop and the cause of many allergies. *B. secalinus*, however, sheds little pollen and causes little allergy. The use of this species should be encouraged.

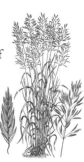
Bromus inermis

BRONZE DRACAENA.
See *Cordyline.*

BROOKLIME.
See *Veronica.*

BROOM.
See *Corema; Cytisus; Genista.*

BROOM PALM.
See *Coccothrinax.*

Broussonetia papyrifera. 📷
males ❋ 10, females ✿ 1
PAPER MULBERRY. A medium to large fast-growing, deciduous tree or large shrub, hardy to zone 4. It is characterized by its heart-shaped leaves and smooth gray bark. The cause of widespread and severe allergy, it should be removed from the landscape. If planted in your landscape, remove it. Some landscape trees labeled as FRUITLESS MULBERRY may actually be all-male clones of PAPER MULBERRY, although many erroneously believe them to be seedless varieties of RED or WHITE MULBERRY. (See also *Morus.*)

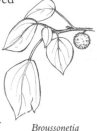
Broussonetia papyrifera

Browallia.   ✿ 2
Attractive blue flowers on small annual plant. Needs warmth and moisture.

Brugmansia. 📷   4
ANGEL TRUMPET, DATURA. An evergreen sub shrub that can be trained as small tree. For zone 10 or greenhouse; houseplant with good light. It bears large, night-fragrant, trumpet-shaped flowers of white, salmon, pink, or orange. Provide shelter from the wind, which can damage large, soft leaves. Very easy to grow from cuttings. Do not plant ANGEL TRUMPET under bedroom windows. All parts of these plants are mildly poisonous and contain a powerful, unpleasant hallucinogenic drug.

Brunfelsia pauciflora calycina. 📷   ✿ 2
YESTERDAY-TODAY-AND-TOMORROW. An evergreen shrub, slow-growing, for warm areas of zone 9 and all of zone 10. Related to nightshade, it does best in acid soil with plenty of iron and moisture. When in full bloom three colors of flowers—blue, purple, and white—are on the bush at same time. The small, round seed pods are poisonous if eaten.

Brunnera macrophylla.   ✿ 2
BRUNNERA. Hardy perennial for all zones. *Brunnera* grows well in the shade beneath deciduous trees.

Brunsvigia rosea.
See *Amaryllis belladonna.*

BRUSSELS SPROUTS.   ✻ *1*
See *Brassica.*

Buchloe dactyloides. males ✳ *10, females* ✻ *1*
BUFFALO GRASS. Drought-tolerant lawn grass native

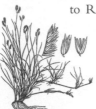

to Rocky Mountain areas. Keep this lawn mowed short to prevent allergies. New all-female cultivars, grown from sod or plugs, are low-growing and drought-tolerant, need little mowing, and produce no pollen. They are excellent choices for the allergy-free lawn.

Buchloe dactyloides

BUCKEYE.
See *Aesculus; Ungnadia.*

BUCKTHORN.
See *Hippophae; Rhamnus.*

BUCKWHEAT.
See *Eriogonum.*

BUCKWHEAT TREE.
See *Cliftonia monophylla.*

BUCKWHEAT, WILD.
See *Eriogonum.*

Buddleia. 📷   5
BUTTERFLY BUSH. Tall fast-growing perennial, shrub, or small tree, hardy in all zones. Some species are poisonous.

BUFFALO BERRY.
See *Shepherdia.*

BUFFALO GRASS.
See *Buchloe dactyloides.*

BUGBANE.
See *Cimicifuga.*

BUGLE LILY.
See *Watsonia.*

BUGLOSS.
See *Anchusa.*

Bulbinella floribunda.   5
Perennial tuberous flowers for zones 9 and 10. Easy to grow.

BULL BAY.
See *Magnolia grandiflora.*

BULRUSH, LOW.
See *Scirpus.*

BUNCHBERRY.
See *Cornus.*

BUNNY EARS.
See CACTUS.

BUNYA-BUNYA.
See *Araucaria.*

Bupleurum rotundifolium.   6
Grown as annual from seed for its large leaves and little yellow flowers.

Buphthalmum speciosum.   7
Quite tall yellow daisy, grown as an annual from seed.

BURDEKIN PLUM.
See *Pleiogynium.*

BURMESE PLUMBAGO.
See *Ceratostigma.*

BURNING BUSH.
See *Euonymus; Kochia.*

BURRO TAIL.
See *Sedum.*

Bursera.   **6**

ELEPHANT TREE, GUMBO-LIMBO TREE. Subtropical trees occasionally grown in zone 10.

Burseraceae.   **6**

TORCHWOOD. Many species of tropical and subtropical trees and shrubs.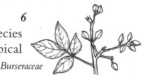

Burseraceae

BUSH ANEMONE.
See *Carpenteria californica.*

BUSH CHERRY.
See *Syzygium paniculatum.*

BUSH MORNING GLORY.
See *Convolvulus.*

BUSH PALM.
See *Sabal.*

BUSH POPPY.
See *Dendromecon rigida.*

BUSHMAN'S POISON.
See *Acokanthera.*

BUSY LIZZY.
See *Impatiens.*

BUTCHER'S BROOM.
See *Ruscus.*

BUTCHER'S VINE, CLIMBING.
See *Semele androgyna.*

Butia capitata (Coccus australis). 📷   **6**

JELLY PALM, PINDO PALM. A tall (to 20 feet), hardy palm with a thick trunk, this palm grows slowly and is hardier than most. It produces edible sweet yellow fruit.

BUTTER DAISY.
See *Verbesina.*

BUTTERCUPS.
See *Eranthis hyemalis; Ranunculus; Thalictrum.*

BUTTERFLY BUSH.
See *Buddleia.*

BUTTERFLY FLOWER.
See *Schizanthus.*

BUTTERFLY ORCHID.
See *Orchids.*

BUTTERFLY PALM.
See *Chrysalidocarpus.*

BUTTERFLY PEA.
See *Clitoria.*

BUTTERFLY VINE.
See *Stigmaphyllon.*

BUTTERFLY WEED.
See *Asclepias.*

BUTTERNUT.
See *Juglans.*

BUTTONBALL TREE.
See *Platanus.*

BUTTONWOOD.
See *Platanus.*

Buxus. 📷   **7**

BOX, BOXWOOD. Numerous species of evergreen shrubs and small trees, often used for low hedges. The very small, rounded leaves and dense growth habit make BOXWOOD a good hedge plant. BOXWOOD flowers are small, greenish, and inconspicuous; however, they do cause allergies. BOXWOOD flowers on old wood, so if hedges are kept closely sheared, the plants will not flower. All parts of the plant are highly poisonous if eaten.

C

Allergy Index Scale: *1* is **Best**, *10* is **Worst.**

❇ for *1* and *2*　　❋ for *9* and *10*

📷 See insert for photograph

CABBAGE.　　　　　　　　　　　　　　　❇ *1*
See *Brassica.*

CABBAGE, FLOWERING.　　　　　　　　❇ *1*
See *Brassica.*

CABBAGE PALMETTO.
See *Sabal.*

CABBAGE TREE.
See *Cordyline; Cussonia spicata.*

CACAO TREE.
See *Theobroma cacao.*

CACTUS FAMILY. 📷　　　　　　　　　❇ *1*
A large group of spiny, succulent plants, some very cold hardy and others frost tender. Almost all cactus need fast-draining, light soil, warmth, full sun, and little water in the summer. Because they are pollinated at night by moths, cactus flowers, though often rare, are usually showy and highly attractive. Some members of the *Euphorbia* genus look like CAC-

Cactus

TUS, but are not similar either botanically or in allergen potential. True cactus, although often covered with sharp spines, some often tiny, is a very fine choice for allergy-free landscaping.

Caesalpinia.　　　　　　　　　　　　　　*3*
BIRD-OF-PARADISE BUSH, POINCIANA. Deciduous or evergreen small tree or shrub. Leguminous plants that grow well in hot low-desert areas. All parts of these plants, especially the seeds, are poisonous if eaten.

CAJEPUT TREE.
See *Melaleuca.*

Caladium bicolor.　　　　　　　　　　　*4*
Big, fancy-leaved tuberous perennial for mild winter areas. Houseplants elsewhere. The flowers may cause allergies, yet flowers are seldom seen on these plants, which are grown only for their leaves.

CALAMINT.
See *Satureja.*

CALAMONDIN.
See *Citrus.*

Calamus.　　　　　males ❋ *9,* females ❇ *1*
Large group of tropical palms. Separate-sexed trees.

Calathea.　　　　　　　　　　　　　　　❇ *1*
ZEBRA PLANT. Houseplants. Many species, most with large, unusual leaves.

Calceolaria.　　　　　　　　　　　　　　❇ *2*
Perennials; some hardy in all zones. Small, pouch-like yellow-orange flowers.

Calendula officinalis. 📷　　　　　　　　*6*
CALENDULA, POT MARIGOLD. Annual grown in all zones. Edible yellow or orange flowers. Easy to grow. Do not use as cut flowers.

CALICO BUSH.
See *Kalmia latifolia.*

CALICO FLOWER.
See *Aristolochia*.

CALIFORNIA BAY.
See *Umbellularia californica*.

CALIFORNIA CHRISTMAS TREE.
See *Cedrus deodara*.

CALIFORNIA FAN PALM.
See *Washingtonia filifera*.

CALIFORNIA FUCHSIA.
See *Zauschneria*.

CALIFORNIA GERANIUM.
See *Senecio*.

CALIFORNIA HOLLY.
See *Heteromeles arbutifolia*.

CALIFORNIA HOLLY GRAPE.
See *Mahonia*.

CALIFORNIA LAUREL.
See *Umbellularia californica*.

CALIFORNIA NUTMEG.
See *Torreya*.

CALIFORNIA POPPY.
See *Eschscholzia californica*.

CALIFORNIA WAX MYRTLE.
See *Myrica*.

CALLA LILY.
See *Zantedeschia*.

Calliandra. *6*
A large genus of evergreen, flowering shrubs. *C. tweedii*, the TRINIDAD FLAME BUSH is a graceful, evergreen shrub with bright red powderpuff flowers. Hardy in zones 9 and 10. An attractive shrub, but keep this one away from the house.

Callicarpa bodinieri giraldii. *3*
BEAUTYBERRY. Hardy, deciduous shrub for zones 5–8. Small lilac-colored flowers followed by purple fruit, which persist into winter.

Callicoma. *8*
An Australian evergreen shrub or small tree, hardy in zones 9–10. Leaves toothed, glossy above, and hairy below.

Calliopsis. .
See *Coreopsis*.

Callirhoe involucrata. ❊ *2*
A poppy-like trailing mallow, grown from seed. Good in hot sunny areas. Purple-red flowers.

Callisia. *5*
Houseplants related to WANDERING JEW. May cause allergies in dogs, especially red, watery eyes.

Callistemon. ✹*9*
BOTTLEBRUSH. Evergreen trees or shrubs. Many species. Hardy into warmer areas of zone 8. Most have bright red clusters of flowers that look like baby-bottle brushes. Some confusion in the trade with the genus *Melaleuca*, to which they are related. Native to Australia, BOTTLEBRUSH pollen is heavy and does not travel far; however, up close it can be a very potent allergen. People with allergies should never attempt to smell one of these flower clusters or the result may be fast and severe.

If BOTTLEBRUSH is kept in the back of the landscape or planted far from doors, windows, patios, or swimming pools, it is much less of a problem.

Callistephus chinensis. *6*
CHINA ASTERS. Annual in all zones. Do not use these for cut flowers.

Callitris. ✹*9*
CYPRESS PINE. Group of species from Australia, occasionally grown in zones 9 and 10. Not a true pine.

Calluna. *double-flowered 4, single-flowered 5*
HEATHER, SCOTCH HEATHER. A species of flowering shrub native to Europe and Asia Minor, grown in zones 5–10 in the United States. To thrive, heathers need acid soil (peat or sand is best) and a good supply of water. They are low-growing plants with tiny leaves and masses of small pink, white, or purple flowers. Heather grows best in full sun or partial shade in hot summer areas. There are several cultivars with double flowers. 'County Wicklow' has double pink flowers, 'Else Frye' has double white flowers, 'Tib' has double rosy-purple flowers.

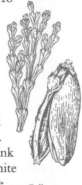

Calluna

Calocedrus decurrens (Libocedrus). 8
INCENSE CEDAR. Large evergreen tree, not a true CEDAR. This tree is often used when small as a pyramidal arborvitae but it quickly outgrows the ordinary yard and is far too large for most gardens. Smell is pungent and will affect some with perfume or PINE-type sensitivities. Pollen is a problem.

Calochortus tolmiei. ❋ 2
CAT'S EARS, MARIPOSA LILY, PUSSY EARS. Lily-like native corms, hardy in all zones.

Calodendrum capense. 📷 4
CAPE CHESTNUT. Profuse blooming lilac-colored flowers in late spring. Grown in California and Florida. A slow-growing beautiful tree to 40 feet. *Citrus* relative, despite its disparate appearance.

Calonyction aculeatum.
See *Ipomoea alba*.

Calothamnus. 8
NET BUSH. Evergreen Australian shrub similar to BOTTLEBRUSH.

Caltha palustris. ❋ 1
MARSH MARIGOLD. Perennial; hardy in all zones. Grows well next to streams, ponds, moist areas.

Calycanthus floridus. 📷 3
CAROLINA ALLSPICE. Deciduous shrub hardy into zone 4. Purple fragrant flowers. *C. occidentalis*, the SPICE BUSH, is hardy to zone 5. A West Coast native, it can be trained into small tree.

Calypso bulbosa. ❋ 1
Pink-flowered orchid which grows best in the shade of trees. This hardy little plant needs humus-rich soil with good moisture.

Calyptrogyne. 5
Small group of Mexican palms.

CAMAS.
See *Camassia; Zigadenus*.

Camassia. 3
CAMAS. Perennial bulb, hardy in all zones. Grows best in heavy soil with abundant moisture. Blue or white lily-like flowers.

Camellia. 📷
double-flowered ❋ 1, single-flowered 3
Of the many species, the most common and popular is *C. japonica*, an evergreen shrub or small tree. Camellia flowers are white, red, pink, or mixed and resemble TUBEROUS BEGONIAS. Hardy into zone 6, *Camellias* are grown in cool greenhouses worldwide. Cult-ure is exacting; they need acid soil, rich in humus; perfect drainage, but also constant moisture; lots of iron. Keep a deep mulch of leaf litter around the base.

Camellia

Camellia flowers may be singles, semi-doubles, or full doubles. In some fully double varieties, the flowers have no stamens (the male parts) and so have no potential to release pollen. *Camellias* belong to the TEA family and, although sometimes difficult to grow, they're worth the effort. The full doubles, known as formal doubles, are excellent choices for the allergy-free landscape; the single-flowered varieties only slightly less so.

CAMOMILE.
See *Chamaemelum nobile.*

Campanula. ❄ *1*
BELLFLOWER, CANTERBURY BELL. Annuals and perennials for all zones. Many species, generally with blue or lavender flowers. Grow best in filtered shade inland and full sun near the coast. Keep well watered in summer.

CAMPHOR TREE.
See *Brachychiton acerifolius; Cinnamomum camphora.*

CAMPION.
See *Lychnis; Silene.*

Campsis. 📷 *5*
COW ITCH VINE, TRUMPET CREEPER, TRUMPET VINE. Hardy vine into zone 3, where it may die back to ground and regrow in spring. Several species, most have large orange flowers. Vigorous climbers cling to brick, wood, and stucco surfaces. Contact with the leaves can cause skin rash, inflammation, and blistering in some individuals. Use care when pruning.

Camptotheca acuminata. 7
Deciduous tree, native to China. Sometimes grown in California.

Canarium ovatum. *males 7, females* ❄ *1*
PILI NUT. A big (to 65 feet) evergreen tree grown mostly in the Philippines at low elevations, for the hard-shelled, fat-filled nuts. PILI NUT trees are separate-sexed; the males produce airborne pollen. The female trees (which bear nuts) cause no allergies.

CANARY BIRD BUSH.
See *Crotalaria.*

CANARY BIRD FLOWER.
See *Tropaeolum.*

CANARY GRASS, CANARY REED GRASS.
See *Phalaris.*

CANDLE BUSH.
See *Cassia alata.*

CANDLE PLANT.
See *Senecio.*

CANDLEBERRY.
See *Myrica.*

Candollea cuneiformis.
See *Hibbertia.*

CANDYTUFT.
See *Iberis.*

CANDYWEED.
See *Polygala.*

CANE PALM.
See *Chrysalidocarpus.*

Canella. *4*
WILD CINNAMON. Evergreen tree occasionally grown in warmer areas of Florida and California.

Canna. 📷 *3*
Hardy in all zones, but the tuberous roots should be lifted and stored in the coldest climates. Tall, broad-leafed plants with terminal flower clusters of many colors. Easy to grow, but does best with full sun and good moisture.

Cannabis sativa. *males 6, females* ❄ *1*
MARIJUANA. An annual plant, occasionally grown (illegally) in gardens. Separate-sexed; male plants shed airborne pollen profusely and cause limited allergy.

CANTERBURY BELL.
See *Campanula.*

Cantua buxifolia. *3*
FLOWER-OF-THE-INCAS, MAGIC FLOWER. Tender perennial shrub that does best in light shade. Drought tolerant. Long, pendulous, tubular flowers; plants should be staked for support. Grown in cool greenhouses outside of zone 10.

CAPE CHESTNUT.
See *Calodendrum capense.*

CAPE COWSLIP.
See *Lachenalia.*

CAPE DAISY.
See *Venidium.*

CAPE FORGET-ME-NOT.
See *Anchusa.*

CAPE FUCHSIA.
See *Phygelius capensis.*

CAPE HONEYSUCKLE.
See *Tecomaria capensis.*

CAPE MARIGOLD.
See *Dimorphotheca; Osteospermum.*

CAPE MYRTLE.
See *Myrsine.*

CAPE PITTOSPORUM.
See *Pittosporum.*

CAPE PLUMBAGO.
See *Plumbago auriculata.*

CAPE PONDWEED.
See *Aponogeton distachyus.*

CAPE PRIMROSE.
See *Streptocarpus.*

CAPE WEED.
See *Arctotheca calendula.*

Capsicum.   ❋ 1
Vegetable garden plants; BELL PEPPERS and hot CHILI
PEPPERS. Members of the POTATO family. Flowers,
usually white but sometimes purple, do not release
pollen into the air. PEPPERS are nutritious and the
plants can be ornamental if grown well. All PEPPERS
do best with full sun, rich, well-drained soil, plenty

of fertilizer, and water. BELL PEPPER fruits will often
sunburn if the leaf canopy is not thick enough. To
grow enough and large enough leaves, use a fertilizer with plenty of nitrogen.

Caragana arborescens.   4
SIBERIAN PEASHRUB. Large, deciduous, yellow-
flowered shrub hardy into coldest zones.

CARAWAY.
See *Carum carvi.*

CARDINAL CLIMBER.
See *Ipomoea.*

CARDINAL FLOWER.
See *Lobelia.*

CARDOON.
See *Cynara.*

Carex. 📷   ❋ 9
SEDGE. Large group of grasslike plants, all of which
cause allergies. Some are separate sexed.

Carica papaya.   *males 8, females* ❋ 1
PAPAYA. Tropical evergreen fruit tree. Separate-
sexed trees with airborne pollen. Females are excellent, pollen-free trees.

Carissa. 📷   ❋ 2
NATAL PLUM. Evergreen shrub for zones 9 and 10.
White flowers, red, edible but tasteless, fruit. Sap
may cause skin rash. A very good, low-pollen
shrub.

Carlina.   5
ANNUAL DAISY. Large flowers, one to a plant. Used
as dried flowers.

CARMEL CREEPER.
See *Ceanothus.*

CARNATION.
See *Dianthus.*

CARNAUBA WAX PALM.
See *Copernicia*.

Carnegiea gigantea. ✳ 1
SAGUARO CACTUS. Giant cactus, native to Southwest. White flowers bloom at night.

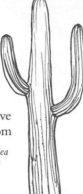
Carnegiea gigantea

CAROB.
See *Ceratonia siliqua floridus*.

CAROLINA ALLSPICE.
See *Calycanthus floridus*.

CAROLINA BUCKTHORN.
See *Rhamnus*.

CAROLINA JESSAMINE.
See *Gelsemium sempervirens*.

CAROLINA LAUREL CHERRY.
See *Prunus caroliniana*.

Carpentaria. 6
A palm from Australia, to 40 feet.

Carpenteria californica. ✳ 1
BUSH ANEMONE. Evergreen shrub native to the West Coast and hardy into zone 6. Does best in dry areas. Handsome shrub with fragrant white flowers.

CARPET BUGLE.
See *Ajuga*.

CARPET PLANT.
See *Episcia*.

Carpinus. 📷 8
HORNBEAM. Common, deciduous hardy trees with leaves similar to an ELM. All cause allergies.

Carpobrotus. ✳ 2
HOTTENTOT FIG, ICE PLANT, SEA FIG. Coarse, fast-growing perennial common along coastal areas. Flowers yellow- or rose-colored.

CARRAGEENAN.
See *Algae*.

CARRION FLOWER.
See *Smilax; Stapelia*.

CARROT.
See *Daucus*.

CARROTWOOD TREE.
See *Cupaniopsis anacardioides*.

Carthamus tinctorius. 5
FALSE SAFFRON, SAFFLOWER. Annual grown for safflower oil and also used as garden annual for its blue flowers. Full sun. Drought tolerant.

Carum carvi. ✳ 2
CARAWAY. Hardy herb for all zones. Used to flavor pickles and rye bread.

Carya. 📷 8– ✳10
HICKORY, PECAN. *C. illinoensis*, the PECAN, is hardy into zone 7 but produces its best crops of nuts in zone 9. It causes severe allergy. *C. ovata*, the SHAGBARK HICKORY, causes the most severe allergies of any HICKORY species. HICKORY is related to WALNUT, and cross-allergic responses between the two are common.

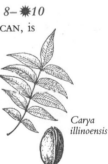
Carya illinoensis

Caryopteris. 4
BLUEBEARD, BLUE MIST, BLUE SPIRAEA. Hardy deciduous shrub with blue flowers. Full sun. Drought tolerant.

Caryota. 6
FISHTAIL PALMS, WINE PALM. Handsome palm tree for zone 10.

Cascara sagrada.
See *Rhamnus*.

CASHEW.
See *Anacardium occidentale*.

Casimiroa edulis. ❋ 2

SAPOTE. Evergreen fruit tree that grows anywhere LEMONS thrive. Large, round, edible fruit ripens in late summer. Large seeds. Trees grow fast and are easy to start from seed, although quality of the fruit is variable. The best fruit is from budded trees. Leaves and sap are poisonous.

Cassia. 6

CANDLE BUSH, SENNA. Many species of evergreen or deciduous shrubs and trees. Most *Cassias* have abundant bright yellow flowers. Mimosa-like plants. Oil of *Cassia* has been known to cause skin rash. Seeds are poisonous.

Castanea. 6

CHESTNUT. Large, hardy deciduous nut-bearing trees. Because of a widespread fungal disease, the AMERICAN CHESTNUT is almost extinct, but there are CHINESE and SPANISH CHESTNUTS that are immune to the blight. The pollen, although abundant, is mixed with nectar, sticky, mostly insect-pollinated, and does not travel far. It is only a problem when contacted directly.

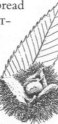

Castanea dentata

Castanopsis. 6

CHINQUAPIN. Many species of evergreen trees and shrubs. Hardy in zones 8–10.

Castanospermum australe. 3

MORTON BAY CHESTNUT. Large evergreen tree for zone 10. Bright red and yellow flowers. Seeds are edible.

CAST IRON PLANT.
See *Aspidistra elatior.*

CASTOR BEAN.
See *Ricinus communis.*

CASTOR-OIL PLANT.
See *Ricinus communis.*

Casuarina. ❋10

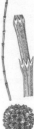

BEEFWOOD, SHE-OAK, HORSETAIL TREE. Australian evergreen tree much planted in zones 9 and 10. Cause of increasing allergy. Trees may naturalize in some areas and force out native species. Sometimes also called AUSTRALIAN PINE.

Casuarina equisetifolia

CAT GUT.
See *Tephrosia.*

CATALINA CHERRY.
See *Prunus lyonii.*

CATALINA IRONWOOD.
See *Lyonothamnus floribundus.*

CATALINA PERFUME.
See *Ribes viburnifolium.*

Catalpa. 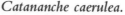 8

Large deciduous trees hardy in all zones. Many large white flowers followed by long bean-like seed pods. *Catalpas* are well known in allergy studies.

Catalpa speciosa

Catananche caerulea. 6

CUPID'S DART. Hardy perennial for all zones. Cornflower-blue flowers are often used as dried flowers, but these may cause allergy.

CATBERRY.
See *Nemopanthus.*

CATCHFLY.
See *Lychnis; Silene.*

Catha edulis. ❋ 1

ARABIAN TEA, CHAT, KHAT. Big evergreen shrubs for zones 9 and 10. Shiny green leaves with red stems and reddish bark. Small white flowers. Drought tolerant; tolerant of poor soil and wind. In Ethiopia and some other countries the fresh leaves are chewed for their stimulant properties, and the cured leaves are used for tea.

Catharanthus roseus. ⬚   ❊ *1*
ANNUAL VINCA, MADAGASCAR PERIWINKLE. Frost-tender perennial, usually grown as a heat-loving annual. These plants have been greatly improved in the last 20 years, largely due to the efforts of plant breeder Ronald Parker, a professor of horticulture at the University of Connecticut. Low-growing, spreading garden plants for hot, sunny areas. Many hybrid colors, including white with red eyes and red with white eyes. Beautiful, easy to grow, fairly drought tolerant. (Also see *Vinca rosea.*)

CATMINT.
See *Nepeta faassenii.*

CATNIP.
See *Nepeta cataria.*

CAT'S CLAW.
See *Macfadyena unguis-cati.*

CAT'S EARS.
See *Calochortus tolmiei.*

CATTAIL.
See *Typha.*

Cattleya.   ❊ *2*
An epiphytic orchid. Greenhouse plant, grown in bark mixture. *Cattleyas* are among the showiest of the orchids. Need warm nights, filtered light, and high humidity.

CAUCASIAN MAPLE.
See *Acer cappadocicum.*

CAULIFLOWER.   ❊ *1*
See *Brassica.*

Ceanothus.   *ground covers 5, shrubs 6, trees 7*
WILD LILAC. Mostly evergreen shrubs, ground covers, and small trees for zones 6–10. Native to Pacific coastal mountains. Many clusters of blue and occasionally white flowers. Drought tolerant. Need good drainage.

CEDAR.
See *Cedrus.*

CEDAR, ALASKA YELLOW.
See *Chamaecyparis.*

CEDAR, ARIZONA.
See *Cupressus arizonica.*

CEDAR, BATTLE AX.
See *Thujopsis dolabrata.*

CEDAR, CIGAR BOX.
See *Cedrela odorata.*

CEDAR, CLANWILLIAM.
See *Widdringtonia.*

CEDAR, COLORADO RED.
See *Juniperus scopulorum.*

CEDAR, DEERHORN.
See *Thujopsis dolabrata.*

CEDAR, ELM.
See *Ulmus crassifolia.*

CEDAR, GIANT.
See *Thuja.*

CEDAR, GROUND.
See *Lycopodium.*

CEDAR, HIBA.
See *Thujopsis dolabrata.*

CEDAR, INCENSE.
See *Calocedrus decurrens.*

CEDAR, JAPANESE.
See *Cryptomeria japonica.*

CEDAR, JAPANESE RED.
See *Cryptomeria japonica.*

CEDAR, MEXICAN.
See *Cupressus.*

CEDAR, MLANJE.
See *Widdringtonia.*

CEDAR OF GOA.
See *Cupressus.*

CEDAR OF LEBANON.
See *Cedrus libani.*

CEDAR, PINK.
See *Acrocarpus fraxinifolius.*

CEDAR, PLUME.
See *Cryptomeria japonica.*

CEDAR, PORT ORFORD.
See *Chamaecyparis.*

CEDAR, PORTUGUESE.
See *Cupressus.*

CEDAR, RED.
See *Juniperus virginiana.*

CEDAR, SALT.
See *Tamarix.*

CEDAR, SOUTHERN RED.
See *Juniperus silicicola.*

CEDAR, SPANISH.
See *Cedrela odorata.*

CEDAR, STINKING.
See *Torreya.*

CEDAR, TAIWAN.
See *Taxodium.*

CEDAR, TECATE.
See *Cupressus forbesii.*

CEDAR, WESTERN RED.
See *Thuja plicata.*

CEDAR, WEST INDIAN.
See *Cedrela odorata.*

CEDAR, WHITE.
See *Chamaecyparis; Juniperus; Thuja.*

CEDAR, WILLOWMORE.
See *Widdringtonia.*

Cedrela. 📷 ✱ 2
BARBADOS CEDAR, CIGAR BOX CEDAR, SPANISH CEDAR, TOONA TREE, WEST INDIAN CEDAR. An interesting group of about 20 species of subtropical timber trees, of the MAHOGANY family, deciduous and evergreen, some planted in California and Florida. Certain species of *Cedrela*, especially *C. odorata*, are called CEDARS although they are not related. *C. odorata* is hardy to zone 6 and the wood is used for making cigar boxes because it has a pungent smell that repels insects. Another, *C. toona*, commonly called the TOONA TREE, is an evergreen tree for zone 10 that has lightly fragrant loose clusters of white flowers.

Cedronella. 3
BALM-OF-GILEAD. Perennial sub-shrub from the Canary Islands, occasionally grown in California.

Cedrus. 📷
CEDAR, TRUE CEDARS. Four species of evergreen trees native to Africa and Asia. All four are pine relatives, and like the pines, although they shed abundant pollen, they are not responsible for much allergy. There is an occasional allergic response to the lumber, which is aromatic and used in making cedar chests and similar forms of furniture.

C. atlantica. ✱ 2
ATLAS CEDAR. Hardy to zone 7. Grows to 100 feet.

C. brevifolia. ✱ 2
CYPRESS CEDAR. Hardy to zone 7. It is similar to CEDAR OF LEBANON but with shorter leaves.

C. deodara. 📷
Males 5, females ✽ 1, monoecious trees 3
CALIFORNIA CHRISTMAS TREE OR DEODAR CEDAR. Hardy to zone 7. A tall, evergreen tree common in California cities, but native to the Himalayas. The trees have grayish needles and drooping, curved tops. Many were once sold as living Christmas trees in the Los Angeles area. Many named varieties sold. Some DEODAR CEDARS are separate-sexed, but none are sold sexed. At least one of them, *C. deodara* 'Repandens', also sold as *C. d.* 'Pendula', is a weeping, all-male form rated at 5. In the near future it may be possible to buy sexed cedars. It will be easy then to pick females, which would be near-perfect allergy-free trees.

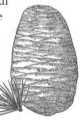

Cedrus deodara

C. libani. ✽ 2
CEDAR OF LEBANON. A tall, evergreen tree hardy in zones 6–10. Many varieties are sold. In Biblical times, there were vast forests of these lofty trees growing on the slopes of Lebanon. The prophet Ezekiel said they were so beautiful that they were the envy of all the trees in the garden of Eden. King Solomon used the wood of *C. libani* for the beams and panels in the temple in Jerusalem and in his grand royal palace.

Cedrus libani

Celastrus. males 7, females ✽ 1
BITTERSWEET. Hardy, deciduous vines for all zones. Does best in cold winter areas. Red seeds stay on plants for much of winter and are not especially prized by birds. These are separate-sexed plants, and only the females produce the berries. Seeds and leaves are highly poisonous if eaten. Female plants are pollen-less and excellent choices for the allergy-free landscape.

CELERY.
See *Apium graveolens*.

Celosia. 6
COCKSCOMB. Heat-loving annual for all zones. Red or yellow flowers in plume-like clusters, some tall and others short like combs of a rooster. Full sun. For best results set out transplants that are not yet in bloom. Do not use the tall varieties as cut flowers.

Celtis. 8
HACKBERRY, SUGARBERRY. Deciduous trees related to ELM. Hardy in all zones. More work needs to be done to determine which species produce the most airborne pollen, because some are much better (or worse) than others. All *Celtis*, however can contribute to allergy. In the United States allergy to *Celtis* is common. In other countries, Argentina for example, *Celtis* is considered a major allergy tree.

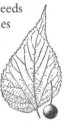

Celtis occidentalis

Centaurea. 4
BACHELOR'S BUTTON, DUSTY MILLER. Hardy annuals and perennials for all zones. There are over 500 species of *Centaurea*, but only a few are popular garden plants. Although relatives to the *Helianthus* family of DAISIES and SUNFLOWERS, the structure of *Centaurea* flowers does not pose much of an allergy risk. Avoid use as a cut flower in the house.

CENTIPEDE GRASS.
See *Eremochloa*.

CENTIPEDE PLANT.
See *Homalocladium platycladum*.

Centranthus ruber. ✽ 2
JUPITER'S BEARD, RED VALERIAN. An easy to grow perennial for zones 8–10. A European native, *Centranthus* has naturalized in many California locations. Drought tolerant and long-lived. Reddish flowers most common, but there are also white, which are more attractive than the red. The rather malodorous flowers shed little pollen.

CENTURY PLANT.
See *Agave americana*.

Cephalocereus senilis. ✻ *1*
OLD MAN CACTUS. Mexican native for zone 10. Tall (eventually to 40 feet), with long, gray hairs. Old plants have rose-colored flowers in April or May.

Cephalophyllum* 'Red Spike' *(Cylindrophyllum). ✻ *2*
Perennial ice plant with bright red flowers. Zones 9 and 10.

Cephalotaxus. 📷 *males 8, females* ✻ *1*
CHINESE PLUM YEW, PLUM YEW. Asiatic evergreen trees or shrubs hardy to zones 4 and 5. Plum-like edible fruit. Most species are separate-sexed plants, and only the females bear fruit. Common landscape shrubs in the southeastern United States, PLUM YEWS grow best in moist shady spots. Some named cultivars to avoid are all males: *C.* 'Harringtonia', *C.* 'pedunculata', *C.* Harringtonia 'Fastigiata', *C. koraiana*, and two others mistakenly sold as *Podocarpus, P. coraianus*, and *P. koraiana*. Because they are pollen-free, female plants are excellent in the allergy-free landscape.

Cerastium tomentosum. *3*
SNOW-IN-SUMMER. Low-growing perennial hardy in all zones. Short-lived ground cover with masses of white flowers.

Ceratiola ericoides. *males* ✹ *9, females* ✻ *1*
ROSEMARY. Not to be confused with *Rosmarinus officinalis*, the true culinary rosemary, *Ceratiola* is a low, evergreen, spreading, separate-sexed shrub native to the southern coastal plain, occasionally used in landscaping. Pollen-free female plants are good choices for the allergy-free garden.

Ceratonia siliqua. *males 8, females* ✻ *1*
CAROB TREE, ST.-JOHN'S BREAD. CAROB may be an all-male tree, an all-female tree, or both, which explains why some bear so many long seed pods while others (the males) have none. CAROB sheds abundant pollen, and the trees are messy. In some neighborhoods in zone 9 and 10 these trees are very common street trees, and in these locations allergy to CAROB is not rare.

Ceratopetalum. *8*
Five species of trees or shrubs from New Zealand occasionally grown in California.

Ceratostigma. *3*
One of several plants sold as *Plumbago*. Several species of evergreen shrubs or perennials for zones 5–10, these have bright blue flowers which are darker than the sky-blue of the CAPE PLUMBAGO, *Plumbago auriculata*.

Ceratozamia mexicana. *3*
A cycad grown in zone 10. Slow-growing, short, palm-like plant.

Cercidiphyllum japonicum.
males 8, females ✻ *1*
KATSURA TREE. Slow-growing, deciduous tree hardy to zone 3; native to Japan.

Cercidium. *5*
PALO VERDE. Deciduous tree native to desert areas of Southwest. These trees will grow in areas where no other tree will grow. Small yellow flowers, green bark, thorns.

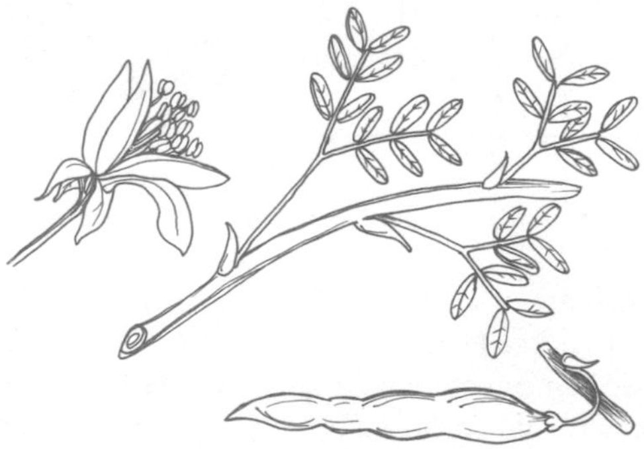

Cercidium

Cercis. *5*

REDBUD. Some species hardy into zone 5. Deciduous flowering tree with reddish flowers. The bark is occasionally used to relieve diarrhea, usually as a tea.

Cercocarpus. *4*

MOUNTAIN MAHOGANY. Evergreen or deciduous tall shrub or small tree native to West Coast. Hardy in all zones and quite drought tolerant. Good plants for cold, dry areas. Member of the ROSE family. Leaves are poisonous.

Cereus. ❄ *1*

NIGHT-BLOOMING CACTUS. With long, white, beautiful fragrant flowers. Zones 9 and 10. See also *Selenicereus.*

Cerinthe. ❄ *2*

Erect perennial hardy to zone 7; strong blue flower colors.

Ceropegia woodii. ❄ *1*

ROSARY VINE. Outdoors in warmest parts of zone 10 and houseplant elsewhere. Small evergreen vine with tiny leaves. Needs shade and abundant water.

Ceroxylon. *males 8, females* ❄ *1*

WAX PALM. A group of about 15 species that includes some of the world's tallest palms, some to over 185 feet. Native to Columbia and Peru, they are all separate-sexed. Not sold in the United States, the males are potent allergy trees; the females cause none.

Cestrum nocturnum. *4, for fragrance*

Tall evergreeen for zone 10, or easy-to-grow greenhouse plant in colder climates. Tends to get leggy in shade. Small white flowers have powerful fragrance that could bother those with sensitivities to perfumes and odors. Seeds are poisonous.

CEYLON GOOSEBERRY.
See *Dovyalis hebecarpa.*

Chaenomeles. ❄ *2*

FLOWERING QUINCE, QUINCE. Deciduous shrub hardy in all zones. QUINCE is one of the first shrubs to bloom in early spring, with showy bright pink, white, or red blossoms. Most have thorns but a few varieties are thornless. (FRUITING QUINCE is *Cydonia.*)

Chaenorrhinum. ❄ *1*

FALSE SNAPDRAGON. Annual or tender perennial from seed. Fine blue flowers.

CHAIN FERN, GIANT.
See *Woodwardia fimbriata.*

CHAIN PLANT.
See *Tradescantia.*

Chamaecyparis (Retinispora). *8*

ALASKA YELLOW CEDAR, FALSE CYPRESS, LAWSON CYPRESS, PORT ORFORD CEDAR, WHITE CEDAR. A large group of many species of hardy, evergreen trees and shrubs. Often commonly called CEDARS, these are actually closely related to CYPRESS instead. Several are from Japan, and some are native to the northwest coastal areas. All *Chamaecyparis* may cause allergy. Good substitutes are PINES, TRUE CEDARS, and selected female JUNIPER cultivars.

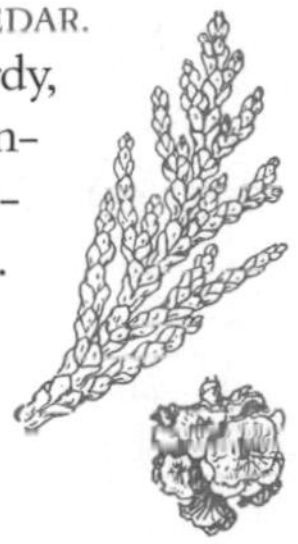

Chamaecyparis lawsoniana

Chamaedorea. *males 8, females* ❄ *1*

A large group of about 100 species of Mexican and tropical palms, all separate-sexed. Males cause allergy; females do not. One species is a common houseplant, *C. elegans*, the PARLOR PALM or GOOD-LUCK PALM. Your luck will be better if your PARLOR PALM is female. Occasionally sold under the invalid name of *Neanthe bella.*

Chamaelirium luteum. *7*

BLAZING STAR. A tuberous perennial lily, native to the south-central United States and occasionally planted in shady spots in the garden. Separate-sexed.

Chamaemelum nobile. 7

CHAMOMILE. Hardy low-growing evergreen perennial. Used for tea and occasionally grown as a substitute for lawns. Skin rash occasionally reported from using CHAMOMILE flowers as a hair wash or tonic, as are allergic reactions to drinking the tea. See also *Matricaria recutita*.

Chamaerops humilis. 📷
males ✹ *9, females* ❋ *1*

MEDITERRANEAN FAN PALM. The only palm tree native to Europe, this is among the hardiest all palms. Short, with a very thick trunk, this tree grows as far north as Seattle, Washington. Propagated from clumps that develop at the base. As a rule almost all fan palms are insect-pollinated and do not pose allergy problems. The MEDITERRANEAN FAN PALM is, however, an exception: it is a separate-sexed, wind-pollinated tree that, when mature, may cause allergy. Female trees bear no pollen and are good choices in the allergy-free landscape.

Chamelaucium uncinatum. 4

GERALDTON WAXFLOWER. Evergreen shrub native to Australia and grown in zones 9 and 10. Needle-like leaves and small pink flowers often used in flower arrangements. Needs fast-draining soil in full sun.

CHAMOMILE.
See *Chamaemelum nobile*.

Chamveyronia. 7

Tropical and subtropical palms.

CHASTE TREE.
See *Vitex*.

CHAT.
See *Catha edulis*.

CHECKERBERRY.
See *Gaultheria*.

Cheiranthus cheiri. 3

WALLFLOWER. Perennial, hardy into zone 6. Easy to grow in full sun. Prune to shape.

Chenopodium. group ✹ 9–10

GOOSEFOOT FAMILY. Many weeds, but some *Chenopodiums* are grown as herbs, vegetables, or ornamentals. Some common names are MERCURY, MEXICAN TEA, QUINOA, SPANISH TEA, WILD SPINACH, and WORMSEED. The crushed leaves of many *Chenopodiums* give off volatile organic compounds (VOCs), which can cause dizziness if inhaled. Contact with the leaves often results in allergic skin reactions. All species of *Chenopodium* cause pollen-related allergies, and many are poisonous.

CHENILLE PLANT.
See *Acalypha*.

CHERIMOYA.
See *Annona cherimola*.

CHERRY.
See *Prunus*.

CHERRY PALM.
See *Pseudophoenix*.

CHERRY, WEST INDIAN.
See *Malpighia glabra*.

CHERVIL.
See *Anthriscus*.

CHESTNUT.
See *Castanea*.

CHILEAN BELLFLOWER.
See *Lapageria rosea*.

CHILEAN GUAVA.
See *Ugni molinae*.

CHILEAN INCENSE CEDAR.
See *Austrocedrus*.

CHILEAN JASMINE.
See *Mandevilla laxa*.

CHILEAN WINE PALM.
See *Jubaea.*

Chilopsis linearis. 📷   5
DESERT WILLOW. Small, flowering, deciduous tree
native to western deserts. Easy to grow from seed
or hardwood cuttings,
this tree grows best in
hot, dry desert climates.
Many small CATALPA-
like flowers, which are used
in Mexico to make a cough
medicine. The flowers are also
occasionally used as a heart
stimulant medicine.

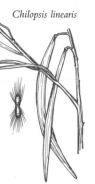

Chilopsis linearis

CHIMING BELLS.
See *Mertensia.*

Chimonanthus praecox.   3
WINTERSWEET, MERATIA. Deciduous shrub from
China, hardy into zone 6; needs winter cold to
thrive. Fragrant yellow flowers bloom very early in
the spring. Needs plenty of water.

CHINA ASTER.
See *Callistephus chinensis.*

CHINA BERRY.
See *Melia.*

CHINA FIR.
See *Cunninghamia.*

CHINA TREE.
See *Saponaria.*

CHINCHERINCHEE.
See *Ornithogalum.*

CHINESE BOTTLE TREE.
See *Firmiana simplex.*

CHINESE DATE.
See *Ziziphus.*

CHINESE ELM.
See *Ulmus parvifolia.*

CHINESE EVERGREEN.
See *Aglaonema modestum.*

CHINESE FIR.
See *Cunninghamia.*

CHINESE FORGET-ME-NOT.
See *Cynoglossum.*

CHINESE FOUNTAIN PALM.
See *Livistona.*

CHINESE GROUND ORCHID.
See *Bletilla striata.*

CHINESE HOUSES.
See *Collinsia heterophylla.*

CHINESE JUJUBE.
See *Ziziphus.*

CHINESE LANTERN.
See *Abutilon, Physalis.*

CHINESE LAUREL.
See *Antidesma.*

CHINESE MAIDENHAIR TREE.
See *Ginkgo biloba.*

CHINESE PARASOL TREE.
See *Firmiana simplex.*

CHINESE PISTACHE TREE.
See *Pistache.*

CHINESE PLUM YEW.
See *Cephalotaxus.*

CHINESE RICE PAPER PLANT.
See *Tetrapanax papyiferus.*

CHINESE RUKKIS TREE.
See *Eucommia ulmoides.*

CHINESE SCHOLAR TREE.
See *Sophora japonica.*

CHINESE SOAPBERRY.
See *Sapindus.*

CHINESE SWAMP CYPRESS.
See *Glyptostrobus lineatus.*

CHINESE TALLOW TREE.
See *Sapium sebiferum.*

CHINESE THREAD TREE.
See *Eucommia ulmoides.*

CHINESE VARNISH TREE.
See *Rhus.*

CHINESE WATER PINE.
See *Glyptostrobus lineatus.*

CHINQUAPIN.
See *Castanopsis.*

Chionanthus. 📷 *males ✹ 10, females ❋ 1*

FRINGE TREE. Two deciduous tree species, one native and one Chinese. Both are hardy in zones 5 to 10. FRINGE TREES are separate-sexed trees and both sexes flower profusely, similar to white lilacs. Members of the OLIVE family, these trees can cause severe allergy. The male trees have larger flowers and only the female trees produce clusters of the small olive-like fruits; females are pollen-free and good selections for the allergy-free landscape.

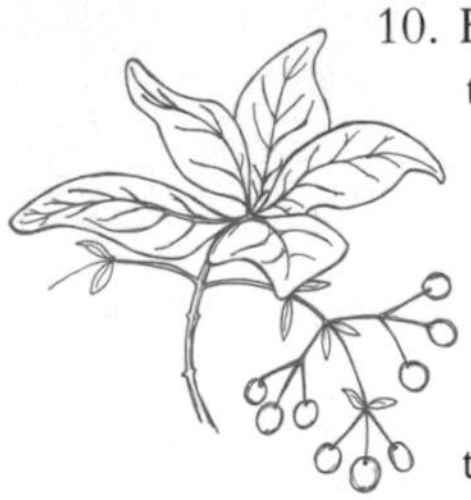

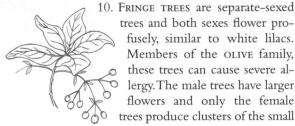

Chionanthus

Chionodoxa. *❋ 2*

GLORY-OF-THE-SNOW. Hardy bulb in all zones. Bright blue flowers on small plants bloom very early in spring and occasionally naturalize.

Chiranthodendron pentadactylon. *5*

MONKEY-HAND TREE. Fast-growing, large evergreen tree for zone 10. Small, red, TULIP-like flowers resemble small hands. Large green leaves.

Chitalpa. *6*

A hybrid cross between *Catalpa* and *Chilopsis.* Zones 9 and 10.

CHIVES.
See *Allium.*

Chloris. *8*

RHODES GRASS, FINGER GRASS. An imported grass that causes allergy, especially in the western United States. This species is spreading quickly and is taking over much native habitat along parts of the Pacific Coast.

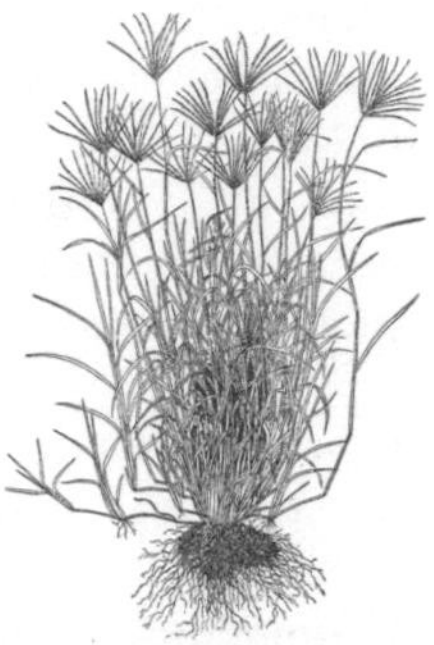

Chloris

Chlorophora. *✹10*

Several species of evergreen tropical trees, occasionally used in warmest areas of zone 10.

Chlorophytum comosum. *❋ 2*

SPIDER PLANT. Easy-to-grow houseplant. Sensitive to chlorine in water, which causes tip burn on the long strap-shaped leaves. Can be used as a ground cover in shady areas of zone 10. SPIDER PLANT was found by the National Aeronautic and Space Administration (NASA) to be the best houseplant for "scrubbing" indoor air pollution.

Choisya ternata. *3*

MEXICAN ORANGE. Evergreen shrub for zones 9 and 10. Fragrant white flowers.

CHOKEBERRY, RED.
See *Aronia arbutifolia.*

CHOKECHERRY.
See *Prunus virginiana.*

Chorisia. 7
FLOSS SILK TREE, KAPOK. Evergreen or briefly deciduous trees with stout, heavily thorned trunks. Hardy in zones 8–10. Showy large white or pink flowers. Sheds lots of silky down called *kapok*, which was used to stuff pillows and as insulation for vests, especially during World War II. KAPOK is known to cause allergies, including hay fever, asthma, and contact skin rash.

CHRISTMAS BERRY.
See *Heteromeles arbutifolia*.

CHRISTMAS CACTUS.
See *Schlumbergera*.

CHRISTMAS PALM.
See *Veitchia*.

CHRISTMAS ROSE.
See *Helleborus*.

CHRISTMAS TREES.
For comments, see page 22. See also *Abies; Cedrus; Pinus*.

Chrysalidocarpus. males ✳ 9, females ❀ 1
Twenty species of palms from the tropics. *C. lutescens*, the BUTTERFLY PALM, CANE PALM, or YELLOW PALM, is frequently used in Florida landscaping. Trees are separate-sexed and only the males cause allergy.

Chrysanthemum. 📷
double-flowered 4, single-flowered 7
COSTMARY, DUSTY MILLER, FEVERFEW, FLORIST'S CHRYSANTHEMUM, GARDEN CHRYSANTHEMUMS, MARGUERITES, OXEYE DAISY, PAINTED DAISY, SHASTA DAISY. A large group of over 200 species of annuals and perennials, including some of our most common garden flowers. Allergy to *Chrysanthemum* is common. Allergy to the insecticide *pyrethrum*, made from a type of *Chrysanthemum*, is also common. A few people are sensitive to the leaves of *Chrysanthemums* and may get skin rashes from handling the plants. Some people may also be allergic to their fragrance.

Chrysanthemums are *short-day plants* and bloom best in autumn, when day length is less than 12 hours. Pollen may cause allergy, especially in those already sensitive to RAGWEED. The double-flowered varieties shed less pollen than single-flowered types.

Chrysolarix.
See *Pseudolarix*.

Chrysophyllum cainito. ❀ 2
STAR APPLE. A tall evergreen tree of the American tropics, grown for its star-shaped sweet green or purple fruits.

CHUPAROSA.
See *Justicia*.

Cibotium. 7
Several species of TREE FERNS, some of which may reach over 12 feet. Popular landscape plants in Florida and California. These large ferns shed spores, which drop directly under the tree. Do not place them next to patios or directly over where people sit. Also do not position them next to windows, because the spores are minute enough to easily pass through most screens.

Cichorium intybus. 5
CHICORY. A hardy blue-flowered perennial, native of Europe, with thick, tuberous roots that are used to flavor coffee. Very easy to grow and often naturalizes.

CIDER GUM.
See *Eucalyptus*.

CIGAR BOX CEDAR.
See *Cedrela*.

CIGAR PLANT.
See *Cuphea*.

CILANTRO.
See *Coriandrum sativum*.

Cimicifuga. *3*
BUGBANE, COHOSH, SNAKEROOT. Hardy perennials for all zones. Used in shady gardens with moist soil; some species are native to eastern United States.

Cineraria. 📷 *6*
Short-lived perennials. Many hybrids with vivid colors, developed for shady moist areas. Popular potted flowering plants. See also *Senecio*.

Cinnamomum camphora. 📷 *8*
CAMPHOR TREE. Large evergreen tree of zones 9 and 10, the source of *camphor*. Leaves have a pleasing smell when crushed. CAMPHOR TREES are very popular street trees in much of California and Florida. During spring, these trees bear thousands of persistent, tiny yellowish flowers, which shed copious amounts of pollen that rarely drifts far from the tree.

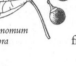
Cinnamomum camphora

CINNAMON FERN.
See *Osmunda*.

CINNAMON, WILD.
See *Canella*.

CINQUEFOIL.
See *Potentilla*.

Cirsium. ✳*9*
Various THISTLES; many cause allergies.

Cissus. *4*
Evergreen vine for zones 8–10. Vigorous growth and handsome leaves. Easy to grow. Some, especially *C. rhombifolia*, the GRAPE IVY, are used as houseplants. Some *Cissus* are separate-sexed.

Cistus. *3*
ROCKROSE. Evergreen shrub, hardy in zones 8–10. Good in full sun. Drought tolerant. Large showy white or purple flowers on easy-to-grow three to six foot bushes.

Citharexylum fruticosum. *5*
FIDDLEWOOD, FLORIDA FUDDLEWOOD. Small tree for zone 10, with small lightly fragrant flowers.

Citrus. *4–5*
CITRONS, GRAPEFRUITS, KUMQUATS, LEMONS, LIMES, ORANGES, TANGERINES. Long-lived, handsome evergreen trees for zones 9 and 10 in favored locations with good frost drainage. *Citrus* needs good soil drainage and summer irrigation to thrive. Most also need high summer heat to produce sweet fruit, especially GRAPEFRUIT. Mature trees bear fragrant, white blossoms during most of the year and most allergy to *Citrus* is in response to the heavy fragrance. Allergy to the pollen is less common. People living in or next to *Citrus* groves are more likely to develop sensitivity. The flowers of most tangerines and kumquats are smaller and much less fragrant, making them better choices for individuals with fragrance sensitivities.

Allergy to *Citrus* is neither particularly common nor severe. On rare occasions, however, some people develop *photodermatitis* from contact with *Citrus* plants or fruit. Photodermatitis is a rash caused by exposure to sunlight after contact with an allergen.

Cladrastis lutea. 📷 *5*
YELLOWWOOD. Deciduous native trees hardy in all zones. Long clusters of very fragrant white flowers late in spring. Young trees are slow to mature and may not bloom for many years.

Clarkia. ✳ *2*
GODETIA. Native annual for all zones. Full sun. Good cut flowers in red, white, pink, rose, and purple, both single- and double-flowered varieties. Fast-growing from direct seeding.

Claytonia. ✳ *1*
MAYFLOWER, SPRING BEAUTY. Small perennial with early spring bloom for moist, shady areas.

Clematis. *3*
Several hundred species of evergreen or deciduous hardy flowering vines. *Clematis* are among the most beautiful vines for winding up the trunks of trees,

climbing on a trellis, or growing up and through climbing roses. *Clematis* does best when the roots are kept cool (mulch) and the tops have warmth and sunlight. They should have fast-draining soil and do well in large pots. Acid soil should be limed before planting. There are some well-documented cases of skin rashes caused by contact with *Clematis* foliage. Slow-growing at first and hard to establish, *Clematis* is worth the effort. Poisonous if eaten.

Cleome spinosa. 4
SPIDER FLOWER. Tall, easy-to-grow summer annual.

Clerodendrum. 3
GLORYBOWER. Over 400 species of evergreen trees, shrubs, and vines, some hardy to zone 6. Unusual red, white, or red-and-white flowers, some resembling BLEEDING HEARTS (*Dicentra*).

Clethra alnifolia. 📷 4
Deciduous shrub native to eastern United States. Culture is similar to that of *Rhododendron*: shade, mulch, acid soil, good moisture, fast drainage. Small white flowers are richly fragrant. May pose problems for the odor-sensitive.

Clethra arborea. 4
LILY-OF-THE-VALLEY TREE. Evergreen tree for zones 9 and 10. White flowers closely resemble LILY-OF-THE-VALLEY, and the fragrance is also similar. Not a tree for the odor-sensitive individual.

Cleyera japonica. 📷 4
Handsome evergreen shrub, for zones 8–10, with small, white, fragrant flowers followed by clusters of dark red berries, which persist through winter. Culture similar to *Camellia*, to which it is related.

Clianthus puniceus. ❋ 2
PARROT BEAK. A shrubby evergreen vine or shrub from New Zealand, grown in zones 9–10. Small leaflets edge long leaves. Flowers are red, pink, or white, shaped like a parrot's beak. Full or part shade.

CLIFF-BRAKE.
See *Pellaea*.

CLIFF ROSE.
See *Cowania mexicana*.

Cliftonia monophylla. ❋ 2
BUCKWHEAT TREE. Small native evergreen tree for zones 7–10. Flowers are small, pink or white, and attractive to bees.

CLIMBING BUTCHER'S VINE.
See *Semele androgyna*.

CLIMBING FERN.
See *Lygodium japonicum*.

CLIMBING LILY.
See *Gloriosa rothschildiana*.

Clintonia. ❋ 2
BEAR-TONGUE LILY, COW-TONGUE LILY. Small tuberous, native lilies hardy to zone 4. Grow best in shady, moist situations.

Clitoria. ❋ 2
BUTTERFLY PEA. A large genus of perennial flowering vines, some of which can be grown in most zones. The double-flowering variety is hardy only in zones 8–10. Showy pea-like flowers.

Clivia. ❋ 2
KAFFIR LILY. Popular greenhouse plant, also used in well-protected, deep-shade landscapes in zones 9 and 10. Easy to grow under the right conditions. Flowers are bright orange, rarely yellow, on *Iris*-like plants with broad, strap-shaped leaves. Container plants flower best when root bound.

CLOVE.
See *Syzygium aromaticum*.

CLOVE PINK.
See *Dianthus*.

CLOVER.
See *Melilotus; Trifolium*.

CLUB MOSS.
See *Lycopodium*.

Clytostoma callistegioides.　　　　　❋ 2
VIOLET TRUMPET VINE. For zones 7–10, this vine dies back to ground outside of zone 10. Grown from cuttings of old wood.

Cnidoscolus. 📷　　　　　　　　　※10
SPURGE NETTLE. Large group of perennial herbs, shrubs, or small trees native to North and South America. All can cause skin rash and inhalant allergy.

COCA PLANT.
See *Erythroxylum coca*.

Coccoloba.　　　　　　　　　　　8
PIGEON PLUM, SEA GRAPE, SNAILSEED. Large group of tropical and subtropical evergreen trees, vines, and shrubs, some with edible fruit. A few are grown in southern Florida.

Coccos australis.
See *Butia capitata*.

Coccothrinax.　　　　　　　　　❋ 1
BROOM PALM, SILVER PALM. Slow-growing palms for sunny areas in zone 10. Good allergy choices.

Cocculus laurifolius.　　*males* ※ 9, *females* ❋ 1
CORAL BEADS, MOONSEED, SNAILSEED. Evergreen small tree, shrub, or vine-like plant, hardy in zones 7–10. Bears many small white flowers in early summer on plant covered with three-inch-long, deeply veined leaves. Separate-sexed plants; only females produce the red or black fruits. The female plants produce no pollen, but males produce a great deal of potentially allergenic pollen. Unfortunately, *Cocculus* is rarely sold sexed and so usually gets a poor rating.

　　The bark of *Cocculus* contains a powerful alkaloid poison, *coclaurina*, which has the same properties as the poison *curare*. It would make good sense to be especially careful not to get fresh sap in your eyes or in a cut or scratch on your hands. Take care when pruning.

COCKLE.
See *Silene*.

COCKSCOMB.
See *Celosia*.

COCKSPUR CORAL TREE.
See *Erythrina crista-galli*.

Cocos.
Individually rated.

C. australis.　　　　　　　　　6
PINDO PALM. Small palm tree with good, edible orange fruit. A better choice for a fruiting palm, however, would be the GUADALUPE PALM.

C. nucifera.　　　　　　　　　7
COCONUT PALM. Many palms are sold as *Cocos* species, but only *C. nucifera* is a true COCONUT PALM. These are the tall, coconut-bearing palms of the tropics. Monoecious, they do cause some allergy in areas where common.

C. plumosa.
See *Arecastrum romanzoffianum*.

COCOS PALM.
See *Syagrus*.

Codiaeum.　　　　　　　　　　4
CROTON. Several species of evergreen trees or shrubs from the tropics, grown in United States as houseplants. Large variegated colorful leaves. Need good heat and light to thrive in house. As houseplants these are rarely seen in bloom, yet the flowers may cause allergy. Remove blooms as soon as they appear. On large-leafed houseplants such as CROTON, the foliage should be wiped down with a moist cloth every week to cut down on allergenic house dust. Poisonous.

Coelogyne. ✽ *2*
Greenhouse orchid with showy white flowers, for partial shade. Grow these pseudobulbs in containers of orchid bark and feed them regularly.

Coffea arabica. ✽ *2*
COFFEE. Grown commercially for COFFEE BEANS. Can be grown outside in frost-free areas of zone 10, where it needs partial shade to thrive. An attractive small tree for greenhouse or houseplant use.

COFFEE FERN.
See *Pellaea.*

COFFEE TREE, WILD.
See *Colubrina arborescens.*

COFFEEBERRY.
See *Rhamnus californica.*

COHOSH.
See *Cimicifuga.*

COHUNE PALM.
See *Orbignya.*

Coix lacryma-jobi. 7
JOB'S TEARS. Perennial grasslike plant grown as annual in cold climates. Grows to 6 feet, with shiny white seed pods with bead-like seeds often used for bracelets and rosaries. Sun or part shade.

Colchicum autumnale. 3
AUTUMN CROCUS, MEADOW SAFFRON. Perennial corm, often used as a blooming houseplant; the plant will flower from a corm simply watered and set in a dish. As a garden plant *Colchicum* does not pose much potential for allergy. Because the corms contain the powerful drug *colchicine,* which is used in genetic experiments, it is wise for pregnant women not to handle them, and for them to be kept away from small children.

Coleonema (Diosma). 4
BREATH-OF-HEAVEN. Evergreen shrub for zones 9 and 10, with tiny leaves and many small fragrant white or pink flowers. Needs full sun and good drainage. Greenhouse plant in cooler regions. Popular landscape shrub in California.

Coleus hybridus. ✽ *1*
Perennials used as annuals in all zones. Good foliage plant for shady spots. Large colored leaves in a wide variety of colors available. Houseplant for sunny rooms. Easy to root from cuttings. A member of the MINT family.

Collinsia heterophylla. ✽ *1*
CHINESE HOUSES. California native annual, grown from seed. White or rose-colored snapdragon-like flowers.

Colocasia esculenta. ✽ *2*
ELEPHANT'S EARS, TARO. Zone 10 perennials with big tuberous roots and huge green leaves. Give them shade, plenty of moisture, and protection from the wind because the big leaves tear easily. Plants seldom flower. Poisonous.

Colpothrinax wrightii. ✽ *1*
BARREL PALM, BELLY PALM, BOTTLE PALM, CUBAN BELLY PALM. Central American and Cuban palms with trunks swollen in middle at maturity.

COLTSFOOT.
See *Galax; Tussilago.*

Colubrina arborescens. 8
WILD COFFEE TREE. Shrub or small evergreen tree for zone 10 and tropics.

COLUMBINE.
See *Aquilegia.*

Columnea. ✽ *2*
NORSE FIRE PLANT. Many species. Trailing houseplants with orange, red, or yellow flowers. Related to AFRICAN VIOLETS and have similar culture requirements.

Comarostaphylis diversifolia. 5
SUMMER HOLLY. Small evergreen tree native to California. Needs fast drainage and partial shade to thrive. Dark green leaves, small white flowers; red berries persist into winter.

COMFREY.
See *Symphytum*.

COMPASS PLANT.
See *Silphium*.

COMPTIE.
See *Zamia*.

Comptonia peregrina. 7
SWEET FERN. Hardy perennial native to eastern United States. Not a true fern. See also *Myrica*.

CONEFLOWER, PURPLE.
See *Echinacea purpurea*.

CONFEDERATE JASMINE.
See *Trachelospermum*.

Consolida ambigua. 3
LARKSPUR. Hardy annual for all zones. Many double-flowering varieties in white, blue, or purple. Grows to two feet, depending on variety.

Convallaria majalis. 4
LILY-OF-THE-VALLEY. Hardy perennial grown from pips. Grown as ground cover underneath taller, shade-loving plants. Very fragrant white flowers may cause allergy in fragrance-sensitive individuals. Plants are highly poisonous if eaten, especially the roots.

Convolvulus. �֎ 2
Several species of shrublike MORNING GLORY. Grows well in dry, sunny locations of zones 7–10.

COONTIE.
See *Zamia*.

Copernicia. �֎ 1
CARNAUBA WAX PALM, PETTICOAT PALM. A group of tall, handsome subtropical palms, some used in zones 9–10, especially in Florida.

COPPER LEAF.
See *Acalypha*.

Coprosma. males ✺ 9, females ✺ 1
A large group of evergreen shrubs and small trees native to Australia, New Zealand, and the Pacific Islands. *C. repens*, the MIRROR PLANT, is often used in landscaping in zones 7–10. Male and female flowers are borne on separate plants. The female plants, which can be identified by their small red or yellow berries, cause no allergy. Females are fine (they have small red or yellow berries), and the males are not. Generally not yet sold sexed, so whole group is usually suspect.

COQUITO PALM.
See *Jubaea*.

CORAL BEADS.
See *Cocculus laurifolius*.

CORAL BELLS.
See *Heuchera*.

CORAL PLANT.
See *Jatropha*.

CORAL TREE.
See *Erythrina*.

CORAL VINE.
See *Antigonon*.

CORALBERRY.
See *Symphoricarpos*.

CORDGRASS.
See *Spartina*.

Cordia. *5*
Large group of mostly tropical evergreen or decid-uous trees or shrubs occasionally used as green-house plants, houseplants, or landscape material in zone 10. *C. myxa*, the ASSYRIAN PLUM, is a small de-ciduous tree found in California.

Cordyline. *3*
CABBAGE TREE, DRACAENA, DRAGON TREE, GRASS PALM. Twenty species of large evergreen shrubs or small trees. Those grown outdoors in zones 9 and 10 are tall, and resemble *Yucca*, to which they are related. Small, fragrant white flowers.

Corema. ✳9
BROOM, CROWBERRY, POVERTY GRASS. Hardy ever-green separate-sexed shrubs used as ground cover.

Coreopsis (Calliopsis). 📷 *6*
PERENNIAL DAISY, TICKSEED. Yellow flowers on easy-to-grow, sun-loving plants. Double- and single-flowered varieties are available; doubles shed far less pollen.

Coriandrum. *5*
CILANTRO, CORIANDER. Aromatic herbs grown and used for seasoning. Small white flowers.

Coriaria japonica. ✳9
TANNER'S TREE. Group of shrubs and small trees, some hardy into zone 4. They bear many small greenish flowers and produce poisonous fruit.

CORK FIR.
See *Abies*.

CORK OAK.
See *Quercus suber*.

CORK TREE.
See *Phellodendron*.

CORKWOOD.
See *Leitneria*.

CORN.
See *Zea mays*.

CORN COCKLE.
See *Agrostemma githago*.

CORN LILY.
See *Ixia; Veratrum*.

CORN PLANT.
See *Dracaena*.

CORNELIAN CHERRY.
See *Cornus*.

Cornus. 📷 *5*
CORNELIAN CHERRY, CRACKER-BERRY, DOGWOOD, FLOWERING DOGWOOD, OSIER, RED OSIER. Large group of hardy decidu-ous shrubs and trees, many na-tive to the United States. On rare occasions implicated in al-lergy. Avoid direct contact with flowers.

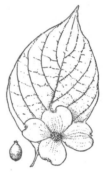
Cornus florida

Corokia cotoneaster. *3*
Small evergreen shrub native to New Zealand, hardy to zone 6. Oddly shaped branches with tiny leaves and small yellow flowers followed by orange berries. Needs little water and fast drainage.

Coronilla varia. *3*
CROWN VETCH. Hardy perennial legume used as hay crop or for ground cover in large, sunny areas. Pea-like flowers are usually purple. Dried flowers, as found in hay, can cause allergy, but fresh flowers rarely do so.

Corozo. *8*
OIL PALM. Tropical palm tree.

Correa. ✳ *2*
AUSTRALIAN FUCHSIA. Low-growing evergreen shrubs hardy to zone 8. Plants bear pink or red fuchsia-like flowers. Often used as ground covers,

they need fast drainage and should not be over-watered.

Cortaderia selloana. males 8, females ✽ 1
PAMPAS GRASS. Tall, clump-forming perennial grass with tall erect white or pink flower spikes. Hardy into zone 6, these occasionally naturalize in zones 8–10. PAMPAS GRASS is unusual in that, although it is a separate-sexed species, most individual plants are female and are able to set viable seed without pollination by a male plant. Female *Cortaderia* plants are excellent additions to the landscape.

Corylopsis. 📷 7
WINTER HAZEL. Deciduous shrubs and small trees, hardy to zone 4. Very early flowering, the yellow flowers appear on bare branches early in the spring. Branches of *Corylopsis* are often brought into the house to bloom in late winter, where they may cause allergy.

Corylus. 📷 8
FILBERT, HAZELNUT. Deciduous, hardy nut trees or shrubs, these are known to cause allergy, especially among individuals living close to FILBERT orchards.

Corynocarpus laevigata. 4
NEW ZEALAND LAUREL. Evergreen shrub or small tree, for zones 9–10. Dark green, glossy leaves and small, orange, 1-inch-long, ovoid fruits, which are very poisonous.

Cosmos. 📷 5
Tall flowering annuals of many colors. Easy and fast growing from seed.

COSTA RICAN HOLLY.
See *Olmediella betschlerana.*

Cotinus. 8
SMOKE BUSH, SMOKE TREE. Two species of unusual but attractive deciduous shrubs or small trees, hardy in all zones. Relatives of POISON IVY, the

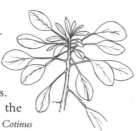
Cotinus

pollen of *Cotinus* is highly allergenic but, because the smoky-colored flowers are borne on old wood, the pollen can be avoided by hard yearly pruning. Contact with the sap of this plant is known to cause skin rashes.

Cotoneaster. ground cover 3, shrubs 5
A large group of evergreen and deciduous shrubs, trees, and ground covers, with small, grayish leaves, small white flowers, and clusters of orange-red berries that are attractive to birds. The low-growing ground-cover *Cotoneaster* cultivars shed less pollen than do the taller, shrubby plants. Berries and leaves are poisonous.

Cotoneaster

COTTON.
See *Gossypium hirsutum.*

COTTONWOOD.
See *Populus.*

Cotula squalida. 4
NEW ZEALAND BRASS BUTTONS. Low-growing evergreen perennial for zones 6–10. Yellow, buttonlike flowers and soft, gray-green feathery leaves. Ground cover in full sun or part shade with plenty of water.

Cotyledon. ✽ 2
Succulents for zones 9 and 10; houseplant elsewhere. Full sun or partial shade, easy to grow.

Cowania mexicana. ✽ 2
CLIFF ROSE. Hardy to zone 3. Native to western deserts and drought tolerant, this shrubby perennial can grow to 6 feet. Attractive little white or yellow flowers.

COW ITCH TREE.
See *Lagunaria patersonii.*

COW ITCH VINE.
See *Campsis.*

COW-TONGUE LILY.
See *Clintonia.*

COWBERRY.
See *Viburnum; Vaccinium.*

COWSLIP.
See *Primula.*

COWSLIP, CAPE.
See *Lachenalia.*

COYOTE BRUSH, COYOTE BUSH.
See *Baccharis pilularis.*

CRAB CACTUS.
See *Schlumbergera.*

CRABAPPLE.
See *Malus.*

CRABGRASS.
See *Digitaria sanguinalis.*

CRACKERBERRY.
See *Cornus.*

Crambe cordifolia.   5
Large shrubby perennial grown from seed as an
annual. Many small white flowers.

CRANBERRY.
See *Vaccinium; Viburnum.*

CRANESBILL.
See *Erodium; Geranium.*

CRAPE MYRTLE.
See *Lagerstroemia indica.*

Craspedia globosa.   5
Tall, round, yellow-flowering plants grown from
seed as annuals and used for dried flowers.

Crassula. 📷   ❋ 2
JADE PLANT. Succulent perennial, hardy in zones 9
and 10 and common as sun-loving houseplants.
Very easy to grow and drought tolerant.

Crataegus.   4
HAWTHORN. Many species of thorny, deciduous,
flowering trees, some hardy into zone 3. White,
pink, or red flowers are followed by small red
berries, which are attractive to birds. Double-flowered varieties shed less pollen than single-flowered. Allergy to HAWTHORN pollen is not common,
and when it occurs, is rarely severe. HAWTHORN
needs a period of winter chill to thrive; in warm
zone 10 in particular, they will grow, but not well,
and often are infested with aphids. Best grown in
zones 3 to 7.

CRAZYWEED.
See *Oxytropis.*

CREAM BUSH.
See *Holodiscus.*

CREAM NUT.
See *Bertholletia excelsa.*

CREEPING CHARLIE.
See *Pilea.*

CREEPING SAGE.
See *Salvia.*

CREEPING ZINNIA.
See *Sanvitalia procumbens.*

CREOSOTE BUSH.
See *Larrea tridentata.*

CRIMEAN LINDEN.
See *Tilia.*

Crinodendron (Tricuspidaria).   ❋ 2
FLOWERING OAK, LILY-OF-THE-VALLEY TREE. Evergreen trees native to Chile, and grown in zones 9
and 10. Grows well in shade with moist, acid soil.

Lots of attractive bell-shaped white flowers in summer, followed by many seed pods.

Crinum. 3
SPIDER LILY. Large lily-like flowers on bulb-grown plant. Perennial in zones 9 and 10, in partial shade or full sun. Fragrant flowers are borne atop long stems.

Crocosmia (Montbretia). 3
Hardy corm grows into zone 6, if mulched in winter. Will naturalize in mild areas. Orange, red, or yellow blooms make long-lasting cut flowers.

Crocus. ✳ 2
Low-growing, early-blooming spring flowers grown from corms. Many colors. Will naturalize where conditions are perfect. One species, *C. sativus*, is grown for the pollen, which is collected and sold as the spice, SAFFRON. (See also *Colchicum autumnale*.) Poisonous.

Crossandra infundibuliformis. ✳ 2
A houseplant with dark green leaves and showy orange or scarlet flowers. Needs a warm room and filtered sunlight.

Crotalaria. 4
CANARY BIRD BUSH, RATTLEBOX. Large group of evergreen perennials and shrubs for zone 10. Large, fast-growing plants must be pruned back often. Numerous small yellow-green flowers and gray-green leaves. Very poisonous.

CROTON.
See *Codiaeum*.

Croton japonicum.
See *Mallotus japonica*.

Croton megalobotrys. ❋9
Large, tropical evergreen tree. *C. monanthogynus*, known as PRAIRIE TEA, is an annual native of the southern United States and Mexico.

CROWBERRY.
See *Corema; Vaccinium*.

CROWFOOT.
See *Ranunculus*.

CROWN-BEARD.
See *Verbesina*.

CROWN-OF-THORNS.
See *Euphorbia milii*.

CROWN VETCH.
See *Coronilla varia*.

Cryosophila. ✳ 1
Several species of small palm trees grown in zones 9 and 10, occasionally sold as the genus *Acanthorrhiza*.

Cryptanthus. ✳ 1
EARTH-STARS. Fancy-leafed perennials in tropical zones and houseplants elsewhere, EARTH-STARS are members of the PINEAPPLE family.

Cryptocarya rubra. ✳ 2
Evergreen tree native to Chile, and hardy in zones 9 and 10. Copper-red new leaves and glossy green older leaves on an attractive tree, slow-growing to 60 feet.

Cryptomeria japonica. 📷 ❋10
JAPANESE CEDAR. Hardy to zone 5, this is not a true CEDAR but more closely related to CYPRESS. A tall evergreen Asian tree, it is native to Japan, where it is now considered the primary source of allergenic airborne pollen and, in Tokyo, the most common cause of both asthma and hay fever. Most of the recent severe *Cryptomeria* allergy in Japan is from a mass planting of these trees initiated by the Japanese Department of Agriculture.

Several kinds of *Cryptomeria* are sold in the United States, including a dwarf variety and one called 'Plume Cedar'.

Cryptotaenia. 4
Tall foliage plant, grown as annual in all zones. Small yellow flowers.

Ctenanthe. 3
BAMBURANTA. Grown in light shade in the warmest parts of zone 10, or as a houseplant elsewhere. Prized for its unusual, leathery leaves.

CUBAN BELLY PALM.
See *Colpothrinax wrightii.*

CUBAN ROYAL PALM.
See *Roystonea regia.*

CUCUMBER TREE.
See *Magnolia.*

Cudrania. 📷 *males* ✳ *9, females* ✳ *1*
Five species of deciduous spiny trees, vines, or shrubs from China and Australia, related to MULBERRY. Some are hardy to zone 5. *C. tricuspidata* is a small thorny tree occasionally used as a hedge plant. Separate-sexed, but not sold sexed. The pollenless females plants are a good choice for the allergy-free garden.

Cunninghamia. ✳9
CHINESE FIR. Three species of large, Asian, evergreen coniferous trees, hardy in zones 8–10, none of which is an actual FIR. They are closely related to *Cryptomeria japonica* (which see) and, like *Cryptomeria,* can cause allergy.

Cunonia capensis. *males* ✳ *9, females* ✳ *1*
AFRICAN RED ALDER. A large group of trees and shrubs mostly native to South America, some of which are seen in California. Almost all of the *Cunonias* pose allergy potential. Separate-sexed plants, not yet sold sexed. Females do not produce pollen and are good choices for the allergy-free landscape.

CUP FLOWER.
See *Nierembergia.*

CUP-OF-GOLD VINE.
See *Solandra maxima.*

Cupaniopsis anacardioides. 7
CARROTWOOD. Australian native evergreen tree much used as street tree in Florida and California. Wood just under the bark is carrot color. CARROTWOOD trees look similar in many ways to CAROB trees and like CAROB, they also cause allergy.

Cuphea. ✳ 2
CIGAR PLANT. Large group of Mexican native herbs and shrubs useful in the warmer zones. Small, tubular red flowers like little cigars. Sun or part shade. Easy to grow from cuttings.

CUPID'S DART.
See *Catananche caerulea.*

Cupressocyparis leylandii. 8
Evergreen hybrid tree, fast growing and often used for tall screens. In many areas this tree is dying off due to canker infection.

Cupressus. ✳10
CYPRESS. A large group of evergreen trees with short, needle-like leaves, often grayish green colored, similar to JUNIPERS, with which they are sometimes confused. Seeds form in round, golf-ball-sized brown pods. CYPRESS are used in landscaping in warm, Mediterranean regions, but are not hardy enough for use in either Northern Europe or the colder parts of the United States. They are drought tolerant and very common on the West Coast. All shed profuse amounts of allergenic pollen, and may do so throughout as much as six or seven months of the year in warm climates. Reactions to CYPRESS pollen are often severe.

C. forbesii.
TECATE CYPRESS. Large evergreen bush native to Southern California.

C. glabra, C. arizonica. 📷
ARIZONA CYPRESS. A large, gray-leafed shrub, to 40 feet tall and wide. Does well in the desert.

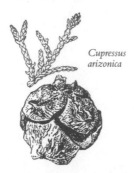

Cupressus
arizonica

C. macrocarpa.
MONTEREY CYPRESS. Tall, native tree growing along the central coast of California. Livestock have been poisoned by eating MONTEREY CYPRESS.

C. sempervirens.
ITALIAN CYPRESS. Tall, common, narrow landscape shrub, much overused in landscaping.

Cupressus
sempervirens

CURRANT.
See *Ribes.*

CUSHION PINK.
See *Silene.*

Cussonia spicata.   3
CABBAGE TREE. Small evergreen tree for zone 10, grown mostly for its large fancy leaves. Small yellow flowers on 6-inch-long spikes.

Cyanotis.   3
PUSSY EARS, TEDDY BEARS. Evergreen houseplants. Need good light indoors.

Cycas.   males 5, females ✳ 1
SAGO PALMS. Dwarf palms for zones 9 and 10. Often grown as container plants in greenhouses in colder climates. *Cycas* are separate-sexed trees and both sexes bear cones. Female trees can be distinguished by their much larger cones. Males cause limited allergy; females none. Plants are expensive, so when buying mature trees, insist on females, which cause no allergy.

Cyclamen.   ✳ 1
Tuberous perennials, some hardy into zone 4. Good flowering potted plants for the house but move them outside in the shade after they bloom. Red, pink, white, and salmon colored flowers. *C. hederifolium* is the hardiest. Outside all need shade, moisture, yearly fertilizer.

Cyclophorus.
See *Pyrrosia.*

Cylindrophyllum.
See *Cephalophyllum.*

Cymbalaria.   ✳ 1
Small, creeping perennials for zones 5–10. Little leaves and small purple flowers on this ground cover for shady, moist areas.

Cymbidium.   ✳ 1
Greenhouse orchids, grown in containers of bark, with regular water, feeding, and filtered shade. Good cut flowers.

Cynara.   3
ARTICHOKE, CARDOON. Perennial vegetables of the THISTLE family. ARTICHOKES are hardy in zones 9 and 10. CARDOON is grown for its edible leaf stalks; hardy zones 8–10.

Cynodon dactylon. 📷   ✴10
BERMUDA GRASS. A tough lawn grass for southern states that flowers even when quite short. The

flowers produce plenty of pollen of the worst sort. To reduce flowering and pollen production, keep BERMUDA GRASS lawns well fertilized, watered, and mowed often and low.

Hybrid BERMUDA GRASSES are better choices because they grow more slowly and flower less often. BERMUDA GRASS can also be a very difficult weed to eradicate when it spreads into perennial beds, because it spreads by underground rhizomes. Eradicate BERMUDA GRASS by applying a nonselective, systemic herbicide. BERMUDA GRASS that has spread to vacant lots has great potential to produce pollen; insist that owners of empty lots keep them mowed frequently.

Mow BERMUDA GRASS lawns late in the afternoon, because the pollen is most active early in the morning. In general, lawn grasses that do not flower unless they are tall are the best choices.

Cynoglossum.   ✳ 2
CHINESE FORGET-ME-NOT. Annual or short-lived blue-flowered perennial. Grows best in full sun, with abundant water.

Cyperus.   7
NUT GRASS, PAPYRUS, PERENNIAL SEDGE. Bog and pond plants often regarded as weeds.

CYPRESS.
See *Cupressus.*

CYPRESS CEDAR.
See *Cedrus brevifolia.*

CYPRESS, FALSE.
See *Chamaecyparis.*

CYPRESS PINE.
See *Callitris.*

CYPRESS, SWAMP.
See *Cyrilla racemiflora; Glyptostrobus lineatus.*

Cypripedium.   4
LADY SLIPPER ORCHIDS, LADY SLIPPERS. Native orchid bearing pink, white, or yellow flowers.

Moisture- and shade-loving hardy perennials, they look good planted with ferns and other shade lovers. Contact with the leaves and flowers of PINK LADY SLIPPER occasionally causes severe skin rash.

Cyrilla racemiflora.   ✳ 2
HE HUCKLEBERRY, IRONWOOD, MYRTLE, SWAMP CYPRESS, TITI. Neither a true CYPRESS nor an allergy plant, *Cyrilla* is hardy in zones 8–10. Small flowers are attractive to bees.

Cyrtanthus mackenii.   ✳ 1
FIRE LILY. Bulb, hardy in zones 9–10. Small, iris-like plants with white, red, or yellow flowers for moist shady areas.

Cyrtomium.   4
HOLLY FERN. Tall leathery-leafed fern for zones 8–10, grows to 3 feet in shady, moist locations.

Cytisus.   5
ATLAS BROOM, BROOM, SCOTCH BROOM. Lots of bright yellow flowers on these lacy-leaved sub shrubs. Protect from snails near the coast. All parts of these plants, seeds, leaves, flowers, are poisonous if eaten. Allergy to BROOM is uncommon, except in areas where there is a great deal of it growing. Occasionally naturalizes in mild winter areas.

D

Allergy Index Scale: *1* is Best, *10* is Worst.

✻ for *1* and *2*   ✽ for *9* and *10*

📷 See insert for photograph

Daboecia.   ✻ *2*
HEATHER, HEATH. Small evergreen flowering shrub of the HEATHER family, hardy in zones 6–10. Needs acid soil, good drainage, and ample water. Thrives in partial shade inland; full sun near the coast. Small, drooping pink, white, red, or rose-colored egg-shaped flowers.

Dactylis.   ✽ *10*
ORCHARD GRASS. A common forage grass in the southern and eastern United States, ORCHARD GRASS is one of the worst allergy grasses. If used, it should be pastured or cut early in the season as a hay crop to avoid flowering.

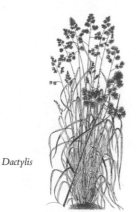

Dactylis

DAFFODIL.
See *Narcissus.*

DAGGER PLANT.
See *Yucca.*

DAHLBERG DAISY.
See *Dyssodia tenuiloba.*

DAHLIA. 📷   *6*
Perennial flowers from seed and tubers. Hardy to zone 7; DAHLIAS must be lifted and overwintered indoors in colder areas. They thrive in full sun. DAHLIAS come in a wide variety of sizes and colors, and are popular as cut flowers. DAHLIAS are related to RAGWEED and cross-allergic reactions occur. Full doubles do not shed much pollen, although single-flowered varieties produce pollen copiously. Some formal DAHLIAS produce no pollen and are good allergy-free plants.

Dais cotinifolia.   *3*
POMPOM TREE. South African native shrub or small tree, grown in full sun, in zones 9–10. Resembles CRAPE MYRTLE, with clusters of puffy pink flowers.

DAISY.
See *Anthemis; Bellis perennis; Bidens feruliflora; Carlina; Coreopsis; Euryops; Heliopsis; Tripleurospermum; Venidium; Verbesina.*

DAISY TREE.
See *Montanoa.*

DAISYBUSH.
See *Olearia.*

Dalea spinosa.   ✻ *2*
SMOKE TREE. A thorny native of the western deserts, zones 8–10, *Dalea* bears fragrant violet flowers. Summer deciduous, it drops its leaves in summer when the soil gets dry, then grows new leaves in autumn. Can be propagated from seed.

DALLIS GRASS.
See *Paspalum.*

DAME'S ROCKET.
See *Hesperis matronalis.*

DAMMAR PINE.
See *Agathis robusta.*

DANDELION.
See *Taraxacum officinale.*

DANEWORT.
See *Sambucus.*

Daphne odorata. 5
WINTER DAPHNE. Sweet-smelling, white-flowered small evergreen shrubs for shady areas with fast drainage, acid soil, and constant moisture. The sap and juice from the berries may cause dermatitis, and the fragrance may bother odor-sensitive individuals. Small fruits are highly poisonous if eaten.

Daphniphyllum. 8
Group of evergreen shrubs and trees native to Japan, Korea, and Australia, occasionally used in United States. Hardy into zone 7, all cause allergy. Dioecious, but not sold sexed.

DARNEL.
See *Lolium.*

Dasylirion. *males 8, females* ✳ 1
SPOON FLOWER. Desert natives related to *Agave*, these are separate-sexed and the males can cause allergy.

DATE PALMS.
See *Phoenix dactylifera.*

Datisca cannabina. ✳9
A tall perennial herb that closely resembles *Cannabis sativa*, or MARIJUANA.

Datura. ✳ 2
ANGEL TRUMPET, DEVIL WEED, JIMSON WEED, LO-COWEED, THORN APPLE. Perennial natives of dry areas. Big, white, trumpet-shaped flowers shed little pollen. Plants contain narcotic that produces dramatic, unpleasant reactions. (See also *Brugmansia.*)

Daucus. ✳10
CARROT, QUEEN ANNE'S LACE, WILD CARROT. A tall weed of waste areas, occasionally allowed to grow in the back of perennial borders; a common allergen.

Davidia involucrata. 📷 6
DOVE TREE. A medium-sized, beautiful deciduous shade tree from China, hardy in zones 5–10.

DAVID'S MAPLE.
See *Acer davidii.*

DAWN REDWOOD.
See *Metasequoia.*

DAYLILY.
See *Hemerocallis.*

DEAD NETTLE.
See *Lamium maculatum.*

DEADLY NIGHTSHADE.
See *Solanum.*

DEATH CAMAS.
See *Zigadenus.*

DEERHORN CEDAR.
See *Thujopsis dolabrata.*

DEERWOOD.
See *Ostrya.*

Delosperma. 3
SUCCULENT ICEPLANT. Trailing, white-flowered perennial for zones 9–10.

Delphinium. 3
Tall flowering perennials, some hardy to zone 2. Many species and colors, especially blues, purples, and whites; some western native species have red flower spikes. They thrive in full sun, rich, acidic soil, and ample moisture. *Delphinium* leaves and seeds are very poisonous. The annual

Delphinium menziesii

89

Delphinium is called LARKSPUR, and it is also poisonous, occasionally fatal, especially if eaten by cattle, sheep, or horses.

Dendrobium. ❋ 2
A group of tropical orchids that are popular as greenhouse plants. They are grown under cool, dry, and lean conditions until flower buds form; then watered and fed. One plant may produce hundreds of flowers.

Dendromecon rigida. 3
BUSH POPPY. West Coast native shrub with large yellow flowers. Does best in full sun; drought tolerant.

DEODAR CEDAR.
See *Cedrus deodara.*

Derris. 5
FLAME TREE, JEWEL VINE. A group of evergreen leguminous trees and vines; one source of the insecticide ROTENONE.

DESERT BROOM.
See *Baccharis.*

DESERT CANDLE.
See *Eremurus.*

DESERT HOLLY.
See *Atriplex.*

DESERT HONEYSUCKLE.
See *Anisacanthus.*

DESERT IRONWOOD.
See *Olneya tesota.*

DESERT OLIVE.
See *Forestiera.*

DESERT PALM.
See *Washingtonia.*

DESERT WILLOW.
See *Chilopsis linearis.*

Desmanthus. 6
A group of about 20 species of trees, shrubs, and herbs native to the Western Hemisphere and Madagascar, all of them suspect in allergy studies. One species, *D. illinoensis*, PRICKLEWEED or PRAIRIE MIMOSA, is a perennial with dense clusters of white flowers, native from Ohio to Florida and also in New Mexico. Occasionally used as a flowering perennial, it may naturalize.

Desmoncus. 8
A large group of tropical and subtropical palm trees, occasionally planted in Florida.

Deutzia. 3
Hardy deciduous flowering bushes with many small white, pink, or purple flowers.

DEVIL WEED.
See *Datura.*

DEVIL'S BACKBONE.
See *Pedilanthus tithymaloides.*

DEVIL'S IVY.
See *Epipremnum aureum.*

DEVIL'S WOOD.
See *Sambucus.*

Dianthus. 📷 3
CARNATIONS, PINKS, SWEET WILLIAMS. Many hardy species of annual and perennial herbs and flowers, popular as garden and cut flowers. Low pollen producers, but highly fragrant *Dianthus* may affect people with odor sensitivities. Grown from seed or cuttings, *Dianthus* thrive in full sun with regular watering, especially during cool weather. Pinch off old flowers or cut plants back after bloom.

Diascia. ❋ 2
TWINSPUR. Annuals and perennials.

Dicentra. 📷 4

BLEEDING HEARTS, DUTCHMAN'S BREECHES, GOLDEN EAR-DROPS, SQUIRREL CORN, STEER'S HEAD, TURKEY CORN. Hardy perennials for shady, moist spots. About 20 species in the genus, most are grown from corms or tubers. The unusual flowers, occasionally shaped like small red or pink hearts, produce little exposed pollen. *Dicentras* would be almost perfect allergy-free plants except that handling the leaves, flowers, or roots can cause skin rash in some people. All parts of *Dicentra* are poisonous if eaten.

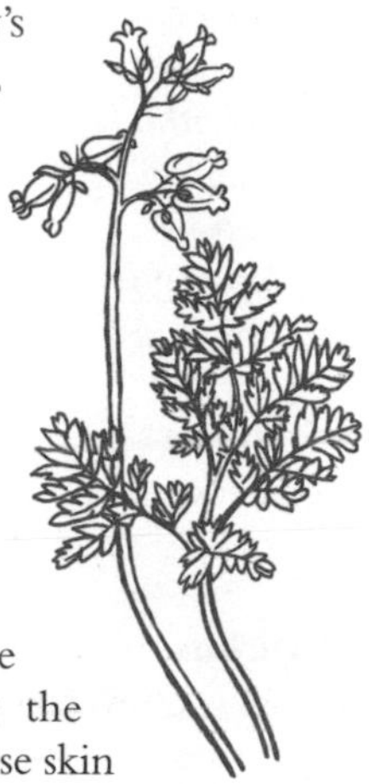

Dicentra

Dichelostemma. 3

BLUE DICKS, FIRECRACKER LILY, SNAKE LILY, WILD HYACINTH. Several species of perennials native to the West Coast.

Dichondra. ❊ 2

Nine species of small, creeping, or prostrate perennials. *D. micrantha* is occasionally used as a good, allergy-free lawn substitute (for small areas) in warm winter areas, mostly Florida and California. It grows best in full sun, but will tolerate some shade. *Dichondra* can be planted from seed, plugs, or flats; it spreads by surface root-runners. If heavily fertilized and watered, *Dichondra* can grow to 6 inches and require mowing. Soil is prepared as for planting a lawn, and seeded with 2 to 3 pounds of seed for every 1,000 square feet.

Dichorisandra. 4

BLUE GINGER. Perennial houseplants, related to WANDERING JEW. Small blue flowers.

Dicksonia. 5

TASMANIAN TREE FERN. Hardiest of the TREE FERNS, to about 20 degrees. May attain a height of 15 feet.

Dictamnus albus. 6

FRAXINELLA, GAS PLANT. Hardy perennial for all zones. Volatile oils in the plant will ignite in the air if a match is held close to a flower on a warm, still night. With this in mind, odor-sensitive individuals might want to avoid this plant.

Dictyosperma. 6

PRINCESS PALM, YELLOW PALM. Two species of palms, occasionally grown in zone 10.

Didiscus.

See *Trachymene.*

Dieffenbachia. 5

DUMB CANE. Large evergreen houseplant with big, often variegated leaves. Needs good light and should not be overwatered. DUMB CANES get their name because the sap, if ingested, irritates the tongue, mouth, and throat, making speech difficult. The effect can last up to 20 hours. The sap or juice can also cause skin rash. When grown as houseplants, these plants seldom bloom but if they do the flowers have good capacity for allergy. In a greenhouse they are more likely to flower and present allergy problems.

Dietes (Moraea). 📷 ❊ 2

FORTNIGHT LILY. Easy-to-grow, long-lived, clumping perennials with long strap-shaped leaves and flat, bright white flowers. Popular and common in zones 9–10.

Digitalis. ❊ 2

FOXGLOVE. Tall, hardy, flowering perennials or biennials which produce spikes of bell-shaped flowers in pastel colors. Source of the drug *digitalis*. All parts of this plant are highly poisonous. Easy to grow in full sun or partial shade. An annual variety is available. When used as cut flowers, they may shed pollen; FOXGLOVES are best kept in the garden.

Digitaria sanguinalis. 7

CRABGRASS. This weed grass blooms when still low and, although it does cause allergy, the plants do not produce much pollen.

Dill.
See *Anethum.*

Dillenia. 3
Large group of mostly Asian evergreen shrubs and trees, some grown in zone 10.

Dimorphotheca. 5
AFRICAN DAISY, CAPE MARIGOLD. Sun-loving, low-growing, spreading annuals for all zones.

Dioon. *males 5, females* ✤ 1
A cycad; less hardy than *Cycas revoluta.*

Dioscorea. ✤ 2
SWEET POTATO.

Diosma.
See *Coleonema.*

Diospyros. 📷 3
PERSIMMON. Many species of evergreen and deciduous trees in the EBONY family. Two species of deciduous fruit trees are used in the United States. Beautiful landscape trees, *Diospyros* is Latin for *two fires*, referring to the bright fiery color of the ripe fruits and also to the unusually good scarlet-orange fall color of the leaves. *D. virginiana*, the AMERICAN PERSIMMON, is a tall fruiting tree, native to the southeastern United States and hardy in zones 3–10. In zones 6 or 7, with good soil and regular water, this PERSIMMON may reach 100 feet, although 50 feet is average.

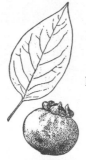
Diospyros virginiana

D. kaki, the JAPANESE PERSIMMON, is a shorter, rounder tree. The cultivar 'Fuyu' has orange fruits, flattened rather than round, which can be eaten any time after they turn orange. The fruits of the AMERICAN PERSIMMON must be dead ripe before eating; otherwise they are inedibly astringent. 'Fuyu' grows slowly but matures to a handsome, spreading small tree with netted bark and excellent fall color. Ornamental in all seasons.

Diplacus.
See *Mimulus.*

Dipladenia.
See *Mandevilla.*

Diplopappus.
See *Felicia.*

Disanthus. ✤ 2
Deciduous shrub from Japan, grown for its good fall color in zones 8–10.

Distichlis. *males* ✻ 9, *females* ✤ 1
SALTGRASS. Several species of low-growing, spreading grasses used to control erosion, especially in alkaline soils. SALTGRASS is separate-sexed and can be grown asexually from rhizomes; hence an all-female cultivar may be developed.

Distictis. 5
TRUMPET VINES. Evergreen vines for zones 8–10. Several related species, all producing large flowers on fast-growing vines. All may cause contact skin allergies, so use caution when pruning.

Dizygotheca. 4
FALSE ARALIA. Houseplant or zone 10 outdoors in shade.

Dock, dock sorrel.
See *Rumex.*

Dodecatheon. ✤ 1
SHOOTING STAR. Hardy perennials for all zones. Resembles *Cyclamen.*

Dodonaea viscosa. 8
HOP BUSH, HOPSEED. Arizona native evergreen shrub for zones 8–10.

Dog fennel.
See *Anthemis.*

Dog tooth violet.
See *Erythronium.*

DOGBANE.
See *Apocynum*.

DOGWOOD.
See *Cornus*.

Dolichos. 5
HYACINTH BEAN. Fast-growing flowering pea vines, easy to grow from seed. Perennial in mild areas.

Dombeya. 3
PINK BALL DOMBEYA. Tender winter-blooming evergreen shrubs, with large leaves and round clusters of pink or red flowers. *Dombeya* needs sun, warmth, and ample water to thrive.

DONKEY TAIL.
See *Sedum*.

Doronicum. 8
LEOPARD'S BANE. Hardy perennials with yellow daisy flowers borne on erect stems.

Dorotheanthus bellidiformis. 3
LIVINGSTONE DAISY. Profusely flowering, low and spreading annual ICEPLANT for all zones.

Doryanthes palmeri. ❋ 2
SPEAR LILY. Giant succulent resembling *Agave*. Flower spike may reach 10 feet.

DOUB PALM.
See *Borassus*.

DOUBLE COCONUT PALM.
See *Lodoicea*.

DOUGLAS FIR.
See *Pseudotsuga*.

DOUM PALM.
See *Hyphaene*.

DOVE TREE.
See *Davidia involucrata*.

Dovyalis hebecarpa. *Variable, according to sex*
CEYLON GOOSEBERRY, KEI APPLE, UMKOKOLO. Small group of subtropical spiny evergreen fruit trees, occasionally grown in zone 10. Trees are usually separate-sexed; male trees may cause allergy, females do not, and a few bisexual trees are less likely to produce severe allergy. The trees produce enormous yields of fruit the size of large marbles, with apricot-colored flesh and very sweet, intensely red juice, which is used for jelly and beverages.

Doxantha.
See *Macfadyena*.

Dracaena. 📷 ❋ 2
CORDYLINE, CORN PLANT, DRAGON TREE. Outside in zone 10; houseplants elsewhere. Palm-like trees and strap-shaped leafed, erect houseplants. *Dracaenas* (Latin for "little dragon") are superb for cleaning up indoor air pollutants such as carbon monoxide, benzene, and formaldehyde.

DRAGON TREE.
See *Cordyline; Dracaena*.

DRAGONHEAD, FALSE.
See *Physostegia virginiana*.

Drimys winteri. 7
PEPPER TREE, WINTER'S BARK. Small evergreen trees for zones 8–10. WINTER'S BARK has fragrant leaves and clusters of JASMINE-scented small white flowers. It thrives in sunny coastal areas, or in partial shade elsewhere.

Drosanthemum. 3
ICEPLANT. Perennial for zones 9–10. Drought-tolerant, it grows best in coastal regions.

Dryas. ❋ 2
Hardy, white- or yellow-flowered perennial used in sunny rock gardens or as a ground cover.

Drymophloeus. 8
A group of small palms, some grown in Florida.

Dryopteris.   5
WOOD FERNS. Hardy in most regions.

Duchesnea indica.   ✤ 1
INDIAN MOCK STRAWBERRY. Ground cover for small areas, *Duchesnea* bears yellow flowers and fruits that resemble STRAWBERRIES but are bland and tasteless. Attractive to birds.

Dudleya.   ✤ 1
LIVE FOREVER. Small perennial succulent for full sun and dry conditions in zones 9–10.

DUMB CANE.
See *Dieffenbachia*.

Duranta.   4
PIGEON BERRY, SKY FLOWER. Spiny, blue-flowered evergreen shrubs for zones 9–10. Small tubular violet flowers are followed by long, trailing clusters of small, yellow, poisonous fruit.

DUSTY MILLER.
See *Artemisia; Centaurea; Chrysanthemum; Senecio.*

DUTCHMAN'S BREECHES.
See *Dicentra*.

DUTCHMAN'S PIPE VINE.
See *Aristolochia*.

DWARF PALM.
See *Sabal*.

Dyssodia tenuiloba (Thymophylla).   6
DAHLBERG DAISY, GOLDEN FLEECE. Annual native of the Southwest, with yellow flowers and small needle-like leaves. It thrives in sandy soil and full sun.

E

Allergy Index Scale: *1* is Best, *10* is Worst.

✱ for *1* and *2*　　✻ for *9* and *10*

📷　See insert for photograph

EARTH-STAR.
See *Cryptanthus.*

EASTER LILY CACTUS.
See *Echinopsis.*

EASTER LILY VINE.
See *Beaumontia grandiflora.*

Echeveria.　　　　　　　　✱ *1*
HENS-AND-CHICKS. Easy-to-grow, drought-tolerant succulent for zones 8–10. Good in pots.

Echinacea purpurea. 📷　*5*
PURPLE CONEFLOWER. Hardy perennials for all zones. Grows bigger in cold winter areas and has naturalized in the Midwest. It is a popular medicinal plant.

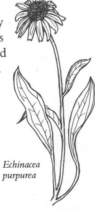

Echinacea purpurea

Echinocactus.　　　　　　✱ *1*
BARREL CACTUS. Big, round, slow-growing cactus for desert areas in zones 9–10.

Echinops exaltatus.　　　　*6*
GLOBE THISTLE. Tall perennial for all zones; used for dry flowers.

Echinopsis.　　　　　　　✱ *2*
EASTER LILY CACTUS. Small cactus to 10 inches. White or red flowers rise above plants.

Echium fastuosum.　　　　　*6*
PRIDE OF MADEIRA. Big, shrubby perennials for zones 9–10. Large spikes of purple or blue flowers are impressive and attractive to bees. The large gray leaves are covered with tiny prickles that may cause contact skin rash, common in those working around these plants.

EDELWEISS.
See *Leontopodium alpinum.*

EEL GRASS.
See *Vallisneria.*

EGGPLANT.
See *Solanum.*

EGLANTINE.
See *Rosa eglanteria.*

Eichhornia crassipes.　　　✱ *2*
WATER HYACINTH. Pond plant with lilac blooms and floating leaves. Needs warmth to grow well.

Elaeagnus.
Group of hardy deciduous and evergreen shrubs or small trees.

E. angustifolia.　　　　　✻ *9*
RUSSIAN OLIVE. Small deciduous tree commonly planted in the Midwest as a wind-

Elaeagnus angustifolia

monly planted in the Midwest as a windbreak. Not a true OLIVE. Small yellow flowers in early summer are the cause of much allergy in some areas.

E. commutata. 8
SILVERBERRY. Deciduous shrub, hardy all zones. Birds relish the small fruits.

E. ebbingei. 7
Thornless evergreen shrub bearing edible red berries.

E. pungens. ✳9
EVERGREEN SILVERBERRY. A large, hardy, thorny shrub often used as hedge plant.

★Variegated species of *Elaeagnus*, with green leaves marked with yellow or white, are sold as *E. marginata* or *E. variegata*. All cause allergies.

Elaeis. 8
Tropical palms.

ELDERBERRY.
See *Sambucus*.

ELEPHANT TREE.
See *Bursera*.

ELEPHANT'S EAR.
See *Alocasia; Colocasia*.

ELEPHANT'S EAR TREE.
See *Enterolobium*.

ELEPHANT'S FOOD.
See *Portulacaria afra*.

ELM.
See *Ulmus*.

ELM, WATER.
See *Planera aquatica*.

Elymus canadensis. 5
WILD RYE. A forage grass widely used across the United States. This useful grass is neither highly allergenic nor a high pollen producer.

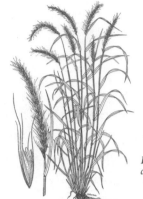

Elymus canadensis

EMERALD LEAF.
See *Peperomia*.

Empetrum. ✳2
ROCKBERRY.

EMPRESS TREE.
See *Paulownia tomentosa*.

Endymion. ✳2
ENGLISH OR SPANISH BLUEBELLS, SCILLA. Hardy bulbs for sun or partial shade. Plant bulbs deeper in colder climates. Many colors, but blue is most common.

ENGLISH DAISY.
See *Bellis perennis*.

ENGLISH IVY.
See *Hedera helix*.

ENGLISH PEAS.
See *Pisum sativum*.

ENGLISH WALNUT.
See *Juglans*.

Enkianthus. *3*
Deciduous shrubs hardy to zone 4. Attractive upright trunk with spreading horizontal branches bearing small bell-shaped white or red flowers in spring.

Ensete. ✱ *2*
ABYSSINIAN BANANA. A native of Ethiopia, where the flowers and seeds are eaten, these large palm-like perennials for zones 9–10 have enormous leaves up to 20 feet long. Plants die after flowering.

Entelea arborescens. *6*
An evergreen shrub or small tree from New Zealand, used in zones 9–10. Relative of the LINDENS.

Enterolobium cycocarpum. *7*
ELEPHANT'S EAR TREE. Large-leafed ornamental for zone 10.

EPAULETTE TREE.
See *Pterostyrax.*

Ephedra. ✱*9*
JOINT FIR. Planted in dry locations as ground cover for its green stems. Source of drug *ephedra.*

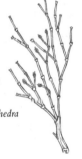
Ephedra

Epidendrum.
See ORCHIDS.

Epigaea repens. *4*
TRAILING ARBUTUS. Very hardy low-growing, pink-flowered sub shrub or ground cover for shady areas. Needs well-drained peaty acid soil and constant moisture to grow well.

Epilobium. *6*
FIREWEED. A tall red or pink flowering annual, known to cause occasional allergy. (See also *Zauschneria.*)

Epimedium. ✱ *1*
BISHOP'S HAT. Low-growing perennial for shady, moist, acid-soil areas to zone 7. Good under trees

or below *Camellias* and *Azaleas.* Tiny white or rose-colored blooms resemble LARKSPUR.

Epipactis gigantea. ✱ *2*
STREAM ORCHID. Hardy terrestrial orchid native to the western United States. Purple, bird-shaped flowers are borne on 10-inch stalks. It needs moist soil in partial shade to thrive.

Epiphyllum. ✱ *2*
ORCHID CACTUS. Shade-house cactus for zones 8–10 or houseplant elsewhere. These are jungle, not desert cactus, and their culture reflects this. Spring-blooming with large showy flowers in many colors.

Epipremnum aureum (Rhapidophora). ✱ *2*
DEVIL'S IVY, POTHOS. Formerly called *Pothos aureus* or *Scindapsus aureus.* Easy-to-grow houseplants, propagated from cuttings. The sap of these plants may cause skin rash in nursery workers making many cuttings. POTHOS is one of the better plants at cleaning up indoor air pollution; however, the broad leaves collect dust and may harbor dust mites. Give plants an occasional lukewarm rinse in the shower.

Episcia. ✱ *2*
CARPET PLANT, FLAME VIOLETS, LOVEJOY. House-plants for hanging baskets; easy to grow in good light and with ample water. Small flowers resemble AFRICAN VIOLETS. They spread by runners.

Equisetum hyemale. *5*
HORSETAIL RUSH. Spore-bearing fern relative for garden wet spots. Hardy in all zones.

Eranthemum pulchellum. ✱ *2*
Evergreen shrub for shady, moist areas of zone 10 or greenhouse plant elsewhere. Tubular blue flowers in late winter to early spring.

Eranthis hyemalis. *4*
BUTTERCUPS, WINTER ACONITE. Early spring-blooming tuberous perennials, hardy in all zones. Thrives in partial shade and moist soil. Plant tubers

deeper in coldest climates. All parts are very poisonous if eaten.

Eremocarpus setigerus. ✷9
TURKEY MULLEIN. Not a true MULLEIN (*Verbascum*). TURKEY MULLEIN is a common low-growing, very strongly-scented California native, rarely used in landscapes. The smell of the crushed leaves affects some; the sap is poisonous and may cause rash.

Eremochloa. ✷9
CENTIPEDE GRASS. A lawn grass for southern areas, often escaped to vacant lots, where it grows rampantly and produces copious amounts of pollen.

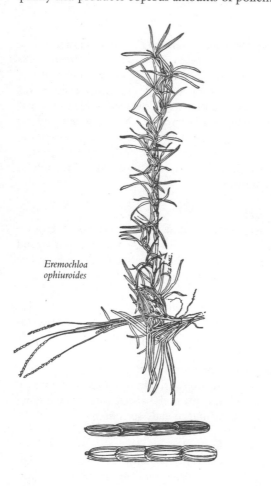

*Eremochloa
ophiuroides*

Eremurus. 5
DESERT CANDLE, FOXTAIL LILY. Hardy perennial with tall spires of flowers to 6 feet.

Erica. 6
HEATH, HEATHER. A very large group of evergreen shrubs or small trees, with small, needle-like leaves, mostly from Europe and South Africa. No species of *Erica* are hardy below 28°. Used as greenhouse flowering plants in all zones. Needs good light, acid soil, fast drainage, good soil moisture to grow well. HEATHER blooms profusely with many small, often fragrant, flowers in many colors. Poisonous.

Erigeron. 6
FLEABANE, BEACH ASTER. Low-growing perennials for full sun in zones 5–10. Small daisylike flowers on spreading, occasionally invasive plants. Easy to grow.

Eriobotrya. 📷 3
LOQUAT. Tall (to about 30 feet) evergreen trees for zones 7–10. Large, handsome leaves and small, yellow, slightly fragrant flowers followed by round, sweet yellow fruits with large brown shiny seeds. These trees are easy, but slow, to grow from seed; budded varieties produce larger fruit, but are hard to find. Leaves and seeds are poisonous.

Eriogonum. 7
WILD BUCKWHEAT. Annuals and perennials native to the West. Very drought tolerant; full sun.

Erodium chamaedryoides. 4
CRANESBILL. Low-growing evergreen perennials hardy in zones 8–10. Small pink or white flowers for full sun or partial shade. Member of the *Geranium* family.

Eryngium. 4
SEA HOLLY. Hardy perennial for all zones. Erect plants resemble flowering THISTLE.

Erysimum. 4
BLISTER CRESS. Hardy drought-tolerant perennials with orange or yellow flowers, which thrive in full sun. Related to WALLFLOWERS.

Erythea.
See *Brahea*.

Erythrina. *6*
CORAL TREE. Evergreen or deciduous flowering trees for zones 9–10. The COCKSPUR CORAL TREE, *E. crista-galli*, is the hardiest of the group. Some species are thorny. All have large leaves and heavy blooms of bright coral-red or orange flowers followed by long beanlike seed pods. Seeds, flowers, and leaves of most species are poisonous.

Erythronium. ✽ *2*
DOG TOOTH VIOLET, FAWN LILY. Perennial corms native to the West. Plant in moist, shady areas.

Erythroxylum coca. *5*
COCA PLANT. Evergreen shrubs or small trees from tropical America. Plant from which the drug cocaine is derived.

Escallonia. *3*
RED ESCALLONIA. Dense, evergreen shrubs much used for landscaping in zones 8–10. They grow largest and flower best near the coast. Small white flowers (when present) and shiny leaves; good foundation shrubs.

Eschscholzia californica. *4*
CALIFORNIA POPPY. Perennial often grown as annual for full sun, in all zones. Fast from seed. Bright orange to yellow flowers. State flower of California.

Espostoa lanata. ✽ *1*
OLD MAN CACTUS. Erect cactus to 9 feet with small hairlike spines and tubular pink flowers.

Eucalyptus. *6–8*
GUM TREES, IRONBARK, MALLEE, PEPPERMINT WILLOW, SALLY, YATE. A very large group of evergreen shrubs and trees native to Australia and widely planted throughout mild areas of the world. All *Eucalyptus* cause some allergy, but some species cause far more problems than others. The odor of fresh or dried *Eucalyptus* leaves and flowers is offensive to certain individuals and may cause an allergic odor response.

There are over 500 species of *Eucalyptus* in Australia, and well over 100 species are grown in the United States. Overplanted in California, Arizona, and Florida, *Eucalyptus* shed profuse amounts of pollen. *Eucalyptus* flowers are pollinated by insects but imperfectly so, and each flower has an unusually high number of pollen-producing stamens.

Several species, such as the FUCHSIA GUM, the SQUARE-FRUITED MALLEE, and the CORAL GUM pose a constant problem because they flower throughout the year. In areas directly below large BLUE GUM trees, the fall of pollen goes on for weeks and covers everything with a persistent dust. Some of the *Eucalyptus*, such as *E. ficifolia*, the RED-FLOWERED GUM, have sticky pollen mixed with nectar, and these do not cause nearly as much allergy. (Some claim that they have gained a measure of allergy protection by eating *Eucalyptus* honey.)

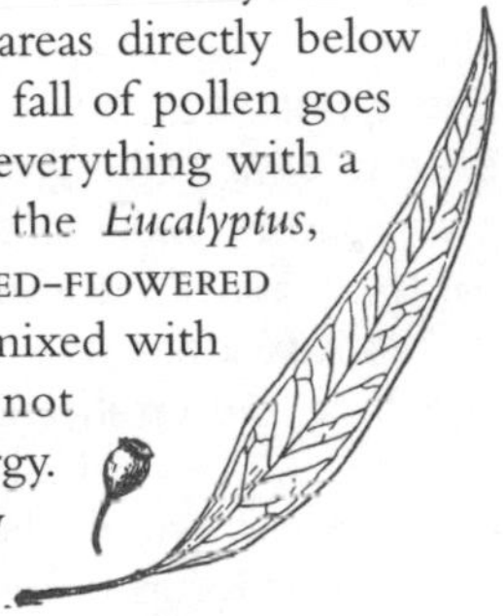

Eucalyptus sideroxylon

Eucomis. *3*
PINEAPPLE FLOWER. Bulb for zones 7–10. A LILY family member that produces a central flower that resembles a PINEAPPLE, *Eucomis* is easily grown from seed.

Eucommia ulmoides. *males 8, females* ✽ *1*
CHINESE RUKKIS TREE, CHINESE THREAD TREE, GUTTA PERCHA TREE, HARDY RUBBER TREE, STONE COTTON TREE. Large deciduous trees from China, hardy in zones 5–7. Leaves resemble ELM. Sap is a rubber-forming latex which can cause contact allergies. Separate-sexed trees, they are not usually sold sexed. The females are a good choice for the allergy-free garden. Usually flowering in mid-spring, the winged seeds resemble those of the ASH.

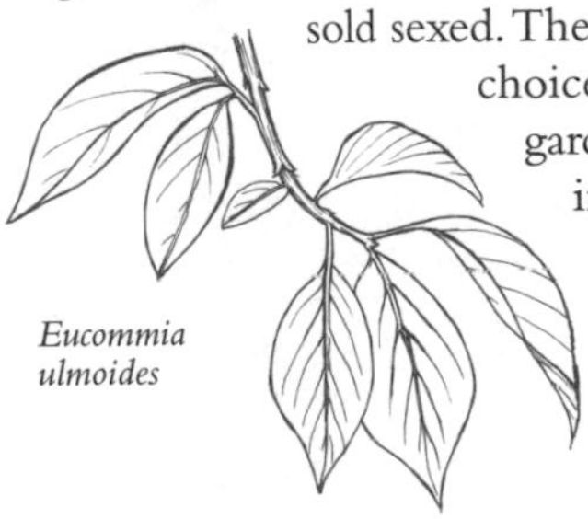

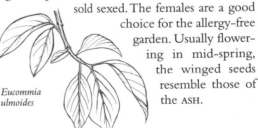

Eucommia ulmoides

Eucryphia. 📷 4

Evergreen shrub or tree for zones 7–10. Not commonly used, the shiny-leafed, white-flowered *Eucryphias* thrive in full sun to partial shade and moist, acidic soil.

Eugenia (Pitanga). 📷 5

Very common landscape evergreen shrub, tree, or hedge plant in zone 10. Small edible fruit ripens from yellow to orange to dark red. (See also *Syzygium paniculatum*.)

Euonymus. 📷 7

SPINDLE TREE. Large group of deciduous and evergreen shrubs and vines. Deciduous *Euonymus* is hardy to zone 3. Although all members of this species have a potential for allergy, as a group they pose little threat if sheared hard annually to prevent flowering. *E. alata*, the BURNING BUSH OR WINGED EUONYMUS, is one of the hardiest deciduous varieties, prized for its intense red autumn color.

E. fortunei is the hardiest of the evergreen *Euonymus* and is occasionally used as a ground cover. *E. japonica*, the JAPANESE EVERGREEN EUONYMUS, has many variegated forms, some of which never bloom.

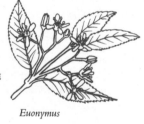

Euonymus

All parts of the plant are poisonous if eaten.

Eupatorium. 7

BONESET, BLUE BONESET, JOE-PYE WEED, MIST FLOWER. Upright flowering perennials for sun or partial shade, hardy all zones. The tubular flowers are pink, purple, rose, or white. One species, *E. rugosum*, called WHITE SNAKEROOT, grows wild in much of the southeastern United States and causes an illness called "the trembles" in milk cows.

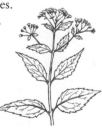

Eupatorium

The toxicity of the leaves passes into the milk and, when consumed by humans, causes "milk sickness," which is characterized by vomiting, delirium, and death. Milk sickness was the cause of death of Abraham Lincoln's mother when he was 7 years old. It was not until 1928 that the relationship between SNAKEROOT and milk sickness was understood.

Euphorbia. 📷 *Rating varies by species*

BASEBALL PLANT, CROWN-OF-THORNS, GOPHER PLANT, MILK BARREL, MILKBUSH, PENCIL TREE, POINSETTIA, SNOW-ON-THE-MOUNTAIN, SPURGE. Very large group of evergreen shrubs, perennials, biennials, vines, succulents, and annuals. With well over 1,000 different species, *Euphorbia* is a complex genus, all members of which have potential for allergy. The milky sap or latex from many is often poisonous and usually has potential to cause skin rash. The white sap of the annual ground cover SNOW-ON-THE-MOUNTAIN (*E. marginata*), can cause severe skin burns even on people who are not allergic. This same highly caustic sap was once used to brand cattle.

Certain of the succulent, leafless *Euphorbias* release a potent gas when cut that may be carcinogenic. Take care when making cuttings; a worker at the University of California, Davis, became violently ill while making *Euphorbia* cuttings in a small enclosed greenhouse.

Pollen from various *Euphorbias* is suspect because none have complete flowers, and all may bear separate male (pollen-producing) flowers. Many Euphorbias are "short day" plants and only bloom in the autumn when the days are short.

The most famous and popular of all *Euphorbias* is the POINSETTIA. Native to Mexico, POINSETTIAS may reach 10 feet when planted outdoors. The red "flowers," which often appear around the Christmas holiday season, are composed not of petals but of colored leaf-like structures called *bracts*. The actual flowers are inconspicuous yellow structures near the center of the rosette of bracts. These flowers are unisexual and shed pollen, especially at midday, although it is not normally airborne. Given their many noxious relatives, it would not be wise to inhale this pollen. Anyone with allergy to rubber would be wise not to get the white latex milky sap of POINSETTIA on their skin.

The many *Euphorbias* that are completely separate-sexed plants can be counted on to contribute to inhalant allergy. (See also *Hevea brasilensis*.)

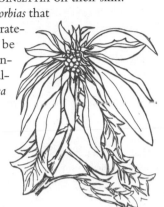

Poinsettia

EUROPEAN CRANBERRY BUSH.
See *Viburnum opulus*.

EUROPEAN MOUNTAIN ASH.
See *Sorbus*.

EUROPEAN SPINDLE TREE.
See *Euonymus*.

EUROPEAN WHITE HELLEBORE.
See *Veratrum*.

Eurya emarginata. ✺9
Ferny-leafed evergreen shrub from Japan, hardy to zone 6, in partial shade and moist acid soil. These are separate-sexed plants; males produce a malodorous scent that may cause allergy. Not sold unsexed, so best to avoid use.

Euryops. 📷 7
GREENLEAF DAISY. Shrubby evergreen perennials, very common in zones 9 and 10. Fast-growing and easy to maintain, *Euryops* produces its yellow flowers almost year round.

Eustoma grandiflorum. 3
GENTIAN, LISIANTHUS, TEXAS BLUEBELLS. Short-lived perennial for sunny areas in all zones. The colorful blooms make long-lasting cut flowers.

Euterpe. 8
A group of tropical and subtropical palm trees.

EVENING LYCHNIS.
See *Silene*.

EVENING PRIMROSE.
See *Oenothera*.

EVENING STAR.
See *Mentzelia*.

EVERGLADES PALM.
See *Acoelorrhaphe wrightii*.

EVERGREEN GRAPE.
See *Rhoicissus capensis*.

EVERGREEN MAPLE.
See *Acer oblongum*.

EVERGREEN PEAR.
See *Pyrus*.

EVERGREEN SILVERBERRY.
See *Elaeagnus pungens*.

EVERLASTING.
See *Helichrysum*.

Exacum. ✳ 2
GERMAN VIOLET. Houseplants requiring good light and warmth. Plants are sensitive to touch and don't do well if handled often.

Exbucklandia. 6
Evergreen trees from the Himalayas, related to *Liquidambar*.

Exochorda. 3
PEARLBUSH. Deciduous shrubs, native to China and hardy to zone 5. Pearl-like buds open to white flowers. Thrives in full sun.

F

Allergy Index Scale: *1* is **Best**, *10* is **Worst**.

✻ for *1* and *2*   ✱ for *9* and *10*

📷 See insert for photograph

Fagus. 📷   7

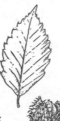

BEECH. Large, hardy, deciduous trees, several species are native to the eastern United States. Fast grow- ing with attractive foliage, some varieties have purple or bronze leaves. The trees produce small edible nuts. BEECH TREES are related to OAKS, and like the OAKS, they cause allergies, although BEECH pollen is rarely as potent an allergen as OAK. Leaves and bark are poisonous.

Fagus grandiflora

FAIRY LILY.
See *Zephyranthes.*

FALSE ACACIA.
See *Robinia.*

FALSE ARALIA.
See *Dizygotheca.*

FALSE ARBORVITAE.
See *Thujopsis.*

FALSE BIRD-OF-PARADISE.
See *Heliconia.*

FALSE BUCKEYE.
See *Ungnadia.*

FALSE CYPRESS.
See *Chamaecyparis.*

FALSE HELLEBORE.
See *Veratrum.*

FALSE SAFFRON.
See *Carthamus tinctorius.*

FALSE SNAPDRAGON.
See *Chaenorrhinum.*

FALSE SOLOMON'S SEAL.
See *Smilacina.*

FALSE SPIREA.
See *Sorbaria sorbifolia.*

FALSE SYCAMORE.
See *Melia.*

FAN PALM.
See *Washingtonia.*

FAREWELL-TO-SPRING.
See *Clarkia.*

Farfugium.
See *Ligularia.*

Fatshedera lizei. 📷   7

FATSHEDERA. Evergreen sub-shrub, vine, or ground cover, hardy in zones 9–10. A naturally occurring hybrid between *Fatsia japonica* and *Hedera helix.* All *Fatshedera* are *mules,* or sterile hybrids, that bear flowers and produce pollen but set no viable seeds. The plants are propagated by cuttings.

Fatsia japonica.   5

JAPANESE ARALIA. Evergreen sub shrubs for zones 7–10, in partial shade.

FAWN LILY.
See *Erythronium.*

FEATHER BUSH.
See *Lysiloma thornberi.*

FEATHER-DUSTER PALM.
See *Rhopalostylis.*

Feijoa sellowiana. 📷 3

PINEAPPLE GUAVA. Attractive evergreen shrub or small (to 18 feet), multi-trunked tree native to Brazil. Hardy to 15 degrees, in full sun or partial shade. Flowers are large, red and white, and followed by egg-sized, oblong green fruit. Reputed to have very high vitamin C content, *Feijoa* fruit has a pleasantly sweet citrus taste. The trees drop a large quantity of fruit, so placement near sidewalks should be avoided.

Most *Feijoas* are seedling grown, and the fruit may vary greatly in size and quantity; grafted varieties are available but are difficult to find. In California *Feijoa* are often pollinated by mockingbirds, which pull off the sweet, edible white petals and, in doing so, distribute the pollen.

Felicia amelloides (Diplopappus). 5

BLUE MARGUERITE. Small evergreen perennial for zones 7–10 that grows best in full sun with average care. Covered with small, blue daisy-like flowers with yellow centers.

FELT FERN, JAPANESE.
See *Pyrrosia lingua.*

FEMALE LINDEN.
See *Tilia.*

FENNEL.
See *Foeniculum vulgare.*

FENUGREEK.
See *Trigonella.*

FERN. 4–7

A very large group of spore-bearing plants. Most grow best in moist, shady situations and they vary greatly by species in ability to withstand cold and frost. All FERNS produce spores on the undersides of the leaves, and because these spores are airborne, can cause allergy. People who are already allergic to molds (or more precisely, to the spores of molds) may well find themselves allergic to FERNS. CLUB MOSS (*Lycopodium*) is a related species that also bears spores; allergy to CLUB MOSS spores is common and often severe, and cross-allergic reactions between FERNS and CLUB MOSS is also common.

In the garden, and if not overused, most small FERNS do not present a great allergy problem. Hanging FERNS and large TREE FERNS, however, may drop spores on tables, chairs, pets, and people below them and should be used with care.

FERN PINE.
See *Podocarpus.*

Ferocactus. ❄ 1

BARREL CACTUS. Native to deserts from Texas to New Mexico, Arizona, and Mexico and hardy to 0 degrees. It thrives with full sun and little water.

Festuca.

FESCUE. Many species of FESCUE are used for pasture, ornamental, or lawn grass.

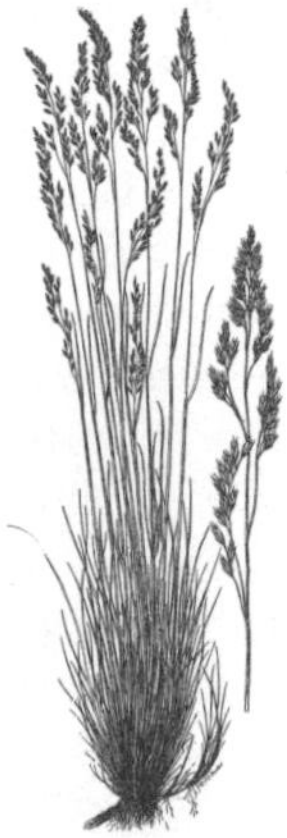

F. elatior. 3

TALL FESCUE. A common sod grass for lawns. It is a good choice because it does not flower when mowed regularly. *F. rubra*, RED FESCUE, is also a good choice for the well-kept lawn.

Festuca elatior

F. glauca. ✸ 9
BLUE FESCUE. An ornamental variety that blooms for an extended period and produces abundant pollen.

FETTERBUSH.
See *Pieris; Leucothoe.*

FEVERFEW.
See *Chrysanthemum parthenium.*

Ficus. 📷 ✿ 2
FIG. Evergreen or deciduous vines, shrubs, houseplants, or trees, hardy to zone 6. Although related to MULBERRY, a known allergen producer, most *Ficus* are relatively benign, although all are capable of provoking skin rash from their milky sap.

F. benjamina is a common indoor tree that normally never flowers and so presents few problems.

The edible FIG, *F. carica*, has its flowers inside the fruits and presents little problem, except that the fuzzy, slightly hairy leaves of edible fig can cause a contact rash in people with sensitive skin. The milky sap from fresh domestic figs also can cause contact skin rash.

The huge evergreen tree, the MORTON BAY FIG, with great spreading heavy branches and large, leathery leaves, also makes tiny figs, and does not pose an allergy problem. A MORTON BAY FIG, one of the largest FIG trees in the United States, grows beside the freeway on the west side of United States 101 in the heart of Santa Barbara, California, near the train station. Local lore has it that a sailor gave the seedling to a Santa Barbara girl and she planted it in 1876.

Ficus elastica

F. microcarpa, the INDIAN LAUREL FIG, is a common street tree in California and Florida. It presents a low allergy risk, but its roots are famous for breaking up sidewalks.

The RUBBER PLANT, *F. elastica decora*, also makes tiny figs and as a houseplant almost never blooms. The same can be said for the huge-leaved *F. lyrata*, the FIDDLELEAF FIG.

Although once used for rubber production, *F. elastica*, the common RUBBER TREE is no longer commercially grown. Rubber is commercially produced from *Hevea brasiliensis*.

FIDDLEWOOD.
See *Citharexylum fruticosum.*

FILBERT.
See *Corylus.*

Filipendula. 4
MEADOWSWEET. Hardy perennial herbs and flowers, some native to the United States.

FINGER GRASS.
See *Chloris.*

FINOCCHIO.
See *Foeniculum vulgare.*

FIR.
See *Abies.*

FIRE LILY.
See *Cyrtanthus mackenii.*

FIREBUSH.
See *Streptosolen jamesonii.*

FIRECRACKER LILY.
See *Dichelostemma.*

FIRETHORN.
See *Pyracantha.*

FIREWEED.
See *Epilobium; Zauschneria.*

FIREWHEEL TREE.
See *Stenocarpus sinuatus.*

Firmiana simplex. 7
CHINESE BOTTLE TREE, CHINESE PARASOL TREE, JAPANESE VARNISH TREE, PHOENIX TREE. Small evergreen or deciduous tree native to Japan and China, for zones 8–10. Large three-lobed tropical looking leaves and greenish white flower clusters.

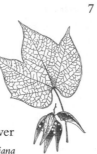

Firmiana platanifolia

FISH POISON PEA.
See *Tephrosia.*

FISHTAIL PALM.
See *Caryota.*

Fittonia. ✳ 1
NERVE PLANT. Houseplant for warm, moist conditions and filtered light.

FIVE-FINGERS.
See *Neopanax.*

FIVE-LEAF AKEBIA.
See *Akebia quinata.*

Flacourtia. 7
MADAGASCAR PLUM, RAMONTCHI. Frost-tender small evergreen trees grown in mildest parts of zone 10. One-inch round fruits are edible.

FLAME FREESIA.
See *Tritonia.*

FLAME TREE.
See *Brachychiton acerifolius; Derris.*

FLAME VINE.
See *Pyrostegia venusta; Senecio.*

FLAME VIOLET.
See *Episcia.*

FLANNEL BUSH.
See *Fremontodendron.*

FLANNEL PLANT.
See *Verbascum.*

FLAX.
See *Linum.*

FLAX, YELLOW.
See *Reinwardtia indica.*

FLEABANE.
See *Erigeron.*

FLEECEFLOWER.
See *Polygonum.*

FLORIDA ARROWWOOD.
See *Zamia.*

FLORIDA FUDDLEWOOD.
See *Citharexylum fruticosum.*

FLORIDA THATCH PALM.
See *Thrinax.*

FLORIDA TORREYA.
See *Torreya.*

FLOSS SILK TREE.
See *Chorisia.*

FLOWER-OF-THE-INCAS.
See *Cantua buxifolia.*

FLOWERING DOGWOOD.
See *Cornus.*

FLOWERING GARLIC.
See *Allium.*

FLOWERING MAPLE.
See *Abutilon.*

FLOWERING OAK.
See *Crinodendron patagua.*

FLOWERING ONION.
See *Allium*.

FLOWERING QUINCE.
See *Chaenomeles*.

FLOWERING SNEEZEWEED.
See *Helenium autumnale*.

FLOWERING STONES.
See *Lithops*.

FLOWERING TOBACCO.
See *Nicotiana*.

Foeniculum.   5
ANISE, FENNEL. Perennial herbs grown as annuals. Odor can bother a few people. ANISE oil occasionally causes skin rashes, so it is reasonable to suspect that the leaves may also.

Fontanesia.   8
Two species of deciduous shrubs, resembling PRIVET, hardy to zone 5.

Forestiera.   *males* ✳ *9, females* ✻ *1*
DESERT OLIVE, SWAMP PRIVET. Twenty species of shrubs and small deciduous or evergreen trees for zones 5–10, related to OLIVE. Separate-sexed.

Forestiera

FORGET-ME-NOT.
See *Cynoglossum; Mertensia*.

FORMOSAN REDWOOD.
See *Taiwania cryptomerioides*.

Forsythia.   8
GOLDEN BELLS. Several species of deciduous, hardy shrubs grown for their early, bright yellow flowers. Related to OLIVES.

FORTNIGHT LILY.
See *Dietes*.

Fortunella.   ✻ 2
KUMQUAT. KUMQUATS have smaller flowers than oranges or lemons, are less fragrant, and are somewhat hardier. They need high summer heat to bear their small fruit, which resemble ORANGES. These sharp and sweet tasting fruits are often eaten whole, rind and all. KUMQUAT trees are usually much smaller than most other *Citrus*.

Fortuneria.   7
Deciduous shrub from China occasionally grown in United States in zones 6–9.

Fothergilla.   7
Native deciduous shrubs hardy in zones 5 to 10. Good fall color, and easy to grow in wet soil.

FOUNTAIN GRASS.
See *Pennisetum setaceum*.

Fouquieria splendens.   ✻ 1
OCOTILLO. Tall (to 10 feet), thorny, mostly leafless deciduous shrubs native to hot, dry desert areas of the Southwest. Very drought-tolerant; needs light soil and full sun. Bright red flowers. Easily propagated by cuttings.

FOUR O'CLOCKS.
See *Mirabilis jalapa*.

FOXBERRY.
See *Vaccinium*.

FOXGLOVE.
See *Digitalis*.

FOXTAIL GRASS.
See *Alopecurus*.

FOXTAIL LILY.
See *Eremurus*.

FOXTAIL MILLET.
See *Setaria*.

Fragaria. 📷 ✳ 1
STRAWBERRY. Hardy perennial fruiting plants; also *F. chiloensis*, a good ground cover for small areas, sun or shade. STRAWBERRIES grow best on sandy loam soils.

FRAGRANT SNOWBALL.
See *Viburnum*.

FRAGRANT SNOWBELL.
See *Styrax*.

FRAGRANT SUMAC.
See *Rhus*.

FRANCESCHI PALM.
See *Brahea elegans*.

Francoa ramosa. ✳ 2
MAIDEN'S WREATH. Evergreen, spreading perennial, native to Chile, bearing spikes of small pink or white flowers. It grows well in filtered shade.

FRANGIPANI.
See *Plumeria*.

Franklinia alatamaha (Gordonia). 3
Deciduous tree, once native to eastern United States but now only known in cultivation. Small- to medium-sized; has large, unusual white flowers and smooth, tan, very attractive bark. Large leaves turn orange-red in fall. They do best in well-drained, moist acid soil under conditions similar to *Camellias*, to which they are related.

FRAXINELLA.
See *Dictamnus albus*.

Fraxinus.
ASH, BLACK ASH, FLOWERING ASH, WHITE ASH. Related to the OLIVES, ASH are large, native, deciduous trees that produce copious amounts of potent pollen. In some countries, ASH is a primary allergy plant. Various ASH species are hardy in almost any zone.

Luckily, most ASH are separate-sexed trees; females are easy to identify by their drooping clusters of winged seeds. Commercial budded or grafted varieties sold as SEEDLESS ASH are male trees that produce pollen. The inconspicuous flowers appear early in the year, often before the leaves. ASH are handsome, large, fast-growing shade trees and their strong wood makes good firewood and fine lumber. WHITE ASH is used to make professional baseball bats.

F. americana. ✳ 9

WHITE ASH. Common named male varieties are 'Autumn Applause', 'Autumn Purple', 'Blue Mountain', 'Cimmaron', 'Rosehill', or 'Rose Hill', and 'Skyline'.

Fraxinus americana

F. angustifolia. ✳ 1
NARROWLEAF ASH. Common named female varieties are 'Flame', 'Moraine', and 'Raywood'.

F. anomala. 6
SINGLELEAF ASH.

F. bungeana. ✳ 2
CHINESE DWARF ASH.

F. dipetala. 4
CALIFORNIA SHRUB ASH.

F. excelsior. males ✳ 9, females ✳ 1
ENGLISH ASH. Common named male varieties are 'Gold Cloud', 'Hessei', 'Juglandifolia', and 'Kimberly'. The WEEPING ASH, *F. excelsior* 'Pendula', is an excellent tree for the allergy-free landscape.

F. nigra. ✳ 10
BLACK ASH. 'Fallgold' is a common named variety.

F. ornus. males 7, females ✳ 1
FLOWERING ASH, MANNA ASH. 'Emerald Elegance' and 'Victoria' are pollen-producing trees that may cause some allergy. 'Aire Peters', however, is an excellent choice for allergy-free landscapes.

F. pennsylvanica.   males ✳ *9, females* ✳ *1*

GREEN ASH. Common named male varieties of this heavy pollen producer are 'Aerial', 'Bergeson', 'Cardan', 'Dakota Centennial', 'Emerald', 'Honeyshade', 'King Richard', 'Mahle', 'Marshall Seedless', 'Newport', 'Patmore', 'Prairie Dome' or 'Prairie Spire', 'Robinhood', and 'Select'.

Several named varieties, 'Jewel', 'Niobara', 'Summit' or 'Summit Ash', and 'Tornado', are excellent female pollen-free trees for the allergy-free landscape.

F. uhdei.   males ✳ *9, females* ✳ *1*

EVERGREEN ASH, FRESNO ASH, MEXICAN ASH, SHAMEL ASH. 'Majestic Beauty' is a male cultivar. 'Tomlinson' is a good female.

> *F. uhdei* 'Majestic Beauty'.   ✳ *9*

> *F. uhdei* 'Tomlinson'.   ✳ *1*

F. velutina.   ✳ *9*

ARIZONA ASH, DESERT ASH, VELVET ASH. Some common named male varieties are 'Fan West', 'Modesto', 'Stribling', 'Sunbelt', and 'Von Ormy'.

Freesia.   4

Low-growing flowers with wispy stems and grasslike leaves. The corms are fully hardy only in zones 7–10; elsewhere they must lifted and overwintered indoors. Many colors, all strongly fragrant. The fragrance may cause allergy in odor-sensitive individuals.

Fremontodendron.   6

FLANNEL BUSH. Very large evergreen shrubs with gray hairy leaves and large, bright yellow flowers, for zones 8–10. This plant was named for John Frémont, the first governor of California. Very drought-tolerant, it grows well

Fremontodendron

on sunny, dry hillsides. Leaves and seed pods have sharp hairs that cause rash. Handle and prune with care.

FRENCH TARRAGON.
See *Artemisia.*

FRINGE BELLS.
See *Shortia.*

FRINGE CUP.
See *Tellima grandiflora.*

FRINGE HYACINTH.
See *Muscari.*

FRINGE TREE.
See *Chionanthus.*

FRINGED GALAX.
See *Shortia.*

FRINGED WORMWOOD.
See *Artemisia.*

Fritillaria.   ✳ *2*

FRITILLARY. Hardy bulbs for zones 3–10. Tall plants with bell-shaped red, yellow, or orange flowers grow well in partial shade with good moisture. The flowers and plants are attractive but malodorous.

Fuchsia. 📷   3

Evergreen in zones 9 and 10, and houseplants or summer annuals elsewhere. Hanging, tubular flowers with brightly colored petals and sepals. Easily grown from cuttings, *Fuchsia* flowers attract hummingbirds. They grow best in filtered sunlight with good soil, plenty of moisture, and regular feeding. Plants are occasionally bothered by aphids or whiteflies; these can be controlled with a soap spray.

In California, a tiny insect called the *fuchsia gall mite* has infested many *Fuchsia*, causing distorted leaves and branches. Cut off diseased portions well below the affected parts and dispose of them.

F. magellanica is hardier than other species and can be grown outside into zones 4 or 5 if the roots are heavily mulched. Tops die back in autumn and resprout from crowns in spring. (See also *Correa*.)

FUCHSIA GUM.
See *Eucalyptus.*

FUDDLEWOOD.
See *Citharexylum fruticosum*.

FUNKIA.
See *Hosta*

G

Allergy Index Scale: *1* **is Best,** *10* **is Worst.**

❊ for *1* and *2* ✸ for *9* and *10*

📷 See insert for photograph

Gaillardia. 📷 *6*
BLANKET FLOWER. Annuals and perennials for full sun in all zones. Easy to grow and fast from seed; many varieties and different species.

Galanthus. ❊ *2*
SNOWDROPS. Hardy bulbs for all zones but grow best in cool climates. Need moist, rich soil. White flowers bloom very early in spring. Bulbs are very poisonous.

Galax urceolata. ❊ *1*
COLTSFOOT, WAND FLOWER. A perennial hardy in all zones, the WAND FLOWER makes a good ground cover for shady, moist areas with acidic humus-rich soil. White flowers are borne on short, erect, spikes. Slow-growing but worth the effort. Large, shiny, heart-shaped leaves are often used in flower arrangements.

Galium odoratum (Asperula). ❊ *2*
SWEET WOODRUFF. Hardy perennial that thrives in cool climates, *Galium* makes a good ground cover in shady, moist areas.

Galtonia candicans. ❊ *2*
SUMMER HYACINTH. Bulbs for shady, moist areas in zones 8–10. Fragrant white flowers on 3-foot-tall stems.

Galvezia speciosa. ❊ *2*
ISLAND BUSH SNAPDRAGON. Native to the California Coastal Islands, and hardy to zone 8, this evergreen shrub has red flowers that resemble SNAPDRAGONS. It grows best in full sun near the coast or in partial shade further inland.

GAMMA GRASS.
See *Tripsacum*.

Gamolepis chrysanthemoides. *6*
Fast-growing evergreen subshrub with many bright yellow daisy-like flowers. Similar in many respects to *Euryops* but more winter hardy. Very easy to grow and somewhat drought resistant.

Garcia. *8*
Two species of shrubs or small trees native to Mexico. Both species can cause allergy.

Garcinia mangostana. *4*
MANGOSTEEN. An evergreen fruit tree from the tropics, very popular in Indonesia and the Philippines. Many claim that a fresh MANGOSTEEN is the best-tasting fruit in the world. A handsome tree, growing to 30 feet, with thick, leathery, glossy-green leaves. Unfortunately, trees fail to fruit outside of the tropics.

Gardenia. *4*
Evergreen shrubs with shiny, dark-green leaves and large, highly fragrant white flowers. An extremely attractive plant when well grown. *Gardenia* is hardy to zone 8 and is often grown as a greenhouse or container plant in all zones. They thrive in rich, acid, moist soil with fast drainage and plenty of humus, in full sun close to the coast or partial shade further inland. Heavy feeders, requiring an acid based fertilizers, *Gardenias* may become chlorotic in soil that is too alkaline. Low-growing *G.* 'Radicans' is occasionally as a ground cover for a small area. The heavy fragrance of *Gardenia*, so pleasant to many, may be too much for some who are odor-sensitive.

GARDEN VERBENA.
See *Verbena*.

GARLIC, FLOWERING GARLIC.
See *Allium*.

Garrya.   males 7, females ✱ 1

SILK TASSEL. Evergreen shrubs native to western coastal ranges. Hardy to zone 7 and very drought tolerant The plants are separate-sexed and the males have the showiest flowers, hence most selected varieties are male. Females are perfect allergy-free choices; males are not.

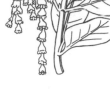

Garrya

GAS PLANT.
See *Dictamnus albus*.

Gaultheria.   ✱ 1

CHECKERBERRY, SALAL, TEABERRY, WINTERGREEN. Evergreen shrubs for zones 7–10 that require partial shade and moist, acid soil. Small white flowers resemble the blossoms of BLUEBERRY and are sometimes followed by small edible but tasteless black or red fruits. *G. procumbens* is hardy to zone 4 and can be used as a ground cover under deciduous trees.

Gaura lindheimeri.   ✱ 2

GAURA. Hardy perennial for full sun in all zones. Drought-tolerant natives of the Southwest, plants grow 3 feet tall and have pink buds and white flowers. Easy to grow and long-lived.

Gaussia.   7

Several species of palms from Puerto Rico and Cuba, sometimes grown in Florida.

GAYFEATHER.
See *Liatris*.

Gazania.   5

Ground cover perennials in zones 9–10. Easy-to-grow plants come in a wide selection of hybrid colors. May naturalize in mild winter areas.

Geijera parviflora.   6

AUSTRALIAN WILLOW, WILGA. Common evergreen landscape tree in California, covered with tiny white flowers when in bloom. Not a true willow,

Gelsemium sempervirens.   4

CAROLINA JESSAMINE. Evergreen vine with tubular yellow flowers. All parts of this JESSAMINE are extremely poisonous.

Genipe.
See *Melicoccus*.

Genista.   4

BROOM, SPANISH BROOM. Deciduous sub shrubs with green stems and yellow flowers. Poisonous.

GENTIAN.
See *Eustoma; Gentiana*.

Gentiana.   ✱ 1

GENTIAN. Low-growing, spreading perennial for all zones. Thrives in full sun or partial shade, in moist, fast-draining, acidic soil. A good rock-garden plant, with bright blue flowers held upright above foilage.

GERALDTON WAXFLOWER.
See *Chamelaucium uncinatum*.

Geranium.   3

CRANESBILL, TRUE GERANIUMS. Low-growing, spreading perennials hardy into zone 3. Not to be confused with the showier related pot-plant or greenhouse GERANIUM (*Pelargonium*), TRUE GERANIUMS produce many small flowers in shades of rose, purple, white, red, or blue, and their leaves lack the strong scent of the *Pelargonium*. Fine plants for the perennial border or rock garden, *Geraniums* require constant moisture and do best in cool summer climates.

GERANIUM, CALIFORNIA.
See *Senecio.*

Gerbera jamesonii. 📷 *6*
TRANSVAAL DAISY. Perennial hardy in zones 9–10, grown as annuals elsewhere. Very large, fancy daisy flowers that make long-lasting cut flowers. Full sun with good soil; needs heat to thrive.

GERMAN IVY.
See *Senecio.*

GERMAN VIOLETS.
See *Exacum.*

GERMANDER.
See *Teucrium.*

Geum. ❇ *2*
Perennials hardy in all zones. Sun or part shade, needs good drainage. Flowers are yellow, copper, or orange; 'Mrs. Bradshaw' is a popular double red variety.

GIANT HYSSOP.
See *Agastache.*

GIANT REED.
See *Arundo donax.*

GIANT SEQUOIA.
See *Sequoiadendron giganteum.*

Gilia. *3*
BIRD'S EYES, BLUE THIMBLE FLOWER, YARROW GILIA. Tall western native annual for full sun.

GINGER.
See *Alpinia; Asarum; Zingiber officinale.*

GINGER LILY.
See *Hedychium.*

GINGERBREAD PALM.
See *Hyphaene.*

Ginkgo biloba. 📷 *males 7, females* ❇ *2*
CHINESE MAIDENHAIR TREE. Deciduous trees hardy into zone 4. *Ginkgos* are separate-sexed trees; mature female trees produce large, malodorous fruits which contain an edible pit. Oil from these seeds can cause skin rash, as can handling the ripe fruit. Because most find the fruit objectionable, male trees are commonly used in landscaping.

The female *Ginkgo* trees grow broader than the males and are often more handsome. A good tree for large landscapes where it can be planted far from the house. There are at least three female cultivars sold: 'Golden Girl' has outstanding bright yellow fall color, 'Liberty Splendor' is a tall, wide tree of perfect form, and 'Santa Cruz' is a low spreading tree.

Ginkgo extract is used to improve memory and also for certain heart conditions.

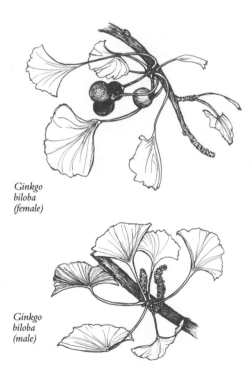

Ginkgo biloba (female)

Ginkgo biloba (male)

GINNALA MAPLE.
See *Acer ginnala.*

GINSENG.
See *Panax.*

Gladiolus. 3
GLADS. Corms that are hardy only to zone 7; else-where they must be lifted and stored for winter. They do best in full sun and well-drained soil. Tall, colorful stalks of lily-like flowers make these pop-ular as cut flowers.

Glaucium. 3
HORNED POPPY, SEA POPPY. Perennials or annuals for full sun. Red or orange flowers on gray-leafed, shrubby plants.

Glechoma hederacea. ✳ 2
GROUND IVY. A member of the MINT family, this low-growing perennial is hardy in all zones. Its small blue flowers and bright green round leaves make it a good ground cover for small areas in full sun to partial shade. Uncontained, it may become an invasive weed.

Gleditsia triacanthos.
males 7, females ✳ *1, bisexual 4*
HONEY LOCUST. Fast growing, thorny, deciduous trees hardy for all zones; tolerant of desert condi-tions. Pendant clusters of small yel-low or white flowers followed by long messy seed pods. Grafted vari-eties are thornless and produce fewer seed pods. Some of these "seedless" trees are males; however *Gleditsia* trees may be bisexual, monoecious, or dioecious.

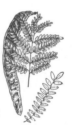
Gleditsia triacanthos

GLOBE AMARANTH.
See *Gomphrena globosa.*

GLOBE FLOWER.
See *Trollius.*

GLOBE THISTLE.
See *Echinops exaltatus.*

GLORIOSA DAISY.
See *Rudbeckia.*

Gloriosa rothschildiana. 3
CLIMBING LILY, GLORY LILY. Tuberous perennial hardy only in the mildest areas of zone 10. This African native climbs to 6 feet, with tendrils on the tips of the leaves, and covers itself with bold red and yellow flowers. Poisonous.

GLORY BUSH.
See *Tibouchina urvilleana.*

GLORY LILY.
See *Gloriosa rothschildiana.*

GLORY-OF-THE-SNOW.
See *Chionodoxa.*

GLORYBOWER.
See *Clerodendrum.*

GLOXINIA.
See *Sinningia.*

Glyptostrobus lineatus. 6
CHINESE SWAMP CYPRESS, CHINESE WATER PINE. De-ciduous conifer hardy to zone 9. Tolerant of wet soils.

GOATNUT.
See *Simmondsia.*

GODETIA.
See *Clarkia.*

GOLD DUST PLANT.
See *Aucuba japonica.*

GOLD MEDALLION TREE.
See *Cassia.*

GOLD VINE.
See *Hibbertia; Stigmaphyllon.*

GOLDBACK FERN.
See *Pityrogramma.*

GOLDEN BELLS.
See *Forsythia*.

GOLDEN CANDLES.
See *Pachystachys lutea*.

GOLDEN CREEPER.
See *Stigmaphyllon*.

GOLDEN CUP.
See *Hunnemannia*.

GOLDEN DROPS.
See *Onosma tauricum*.

GOLDEN EAR-DROPS.
See *Dicentra*.

GOLDEN FLEECE.
See *Dyssodia tenuiloba*.

GOLDEN HEATHER.
See *Hudsonia*.

GOLDEN LARCH.
See *Pseudolarix kaempferi*.

GOLDEN RAGWORT.
See *Senecio*.

GOLDEN TRUMPET TREE.
See *Tabebuia*.

GOLDEN WATTLE.
See *Acacia*.

GOLDENCHAIN TREE.
See *Laburnum*.

GOLDENRAIN TREE.
See *Koelreuteria paniculata*.

GOLDENROD.
See *Solidago*.

GOLDFISH PLANT.
See *Alloplectus nummularia*.

Gomphrena globosa.   4
GLOBE AMARANTH.   Small annual for full sun. The globe-shaped pink, white, or violet flowers resemble CLOVER blooms. Don't use these as cut flowers.

GOOSE PLANT.
See *Asclepias*.

GOOSEBERRY.
See *Ribes*.

GOOSEFOOT.
See *Chenopodium*.

GOPHER PLANT.
See *Euphorbia*.

Gordonia.
See *Franklinia*.

Gossypium hirsutum.   3
COTTON.   Annual or perennial subshrub. This is the cotton plant of commerce. Grown as a garden curiosity, cotton is easy to grow in full sun with plenty of fertilizer and water.   Flowers resemble those of HOLLYHOCK and are followed by pods containing seeds and cotton.   The cotton plant poses no real allergy potential; the fields in which it is grown, however, are among the most heavily fertilized and chemically sprayed of all land.   For this reason, refrain from using cottonseed meal fertilizer on your vegetable garden. Leaves are poisonous.

GOUTWEED.
See *Aegopodium*.

GRAIN SORGHUM.
See *Sorghum*.

GRAMA GRASS.
See *Bouteloua gracilis*.

GRAND FIR.
See *Abies.*

GRAPE HYACINTH.
See *Muscari.*

GRAPE IVY.
See *Cissus.*

GRAPEFRUIT.
See *Citrus.*

GRAPES.
See *Vitis.*

Graptopetalum.   ✳ 1
Succulent for zones 9–10.

GRASS NUT.
See *Triteleia.*

GRASS PALM.
See *Cordyline.*

GRASS TREE.
See *Xanthorrhoea.*

GRAY SANTOLINA.
See *Santolina.*

GREASEWOOD.
See *Salvia; Senecio.*

GRECIAN LAUREL.
See *Laurus nobilis.*

GREEN CARPET.
See *Herniaria glabra.*

GREEN SANTOLINA.
See *Santolina.*

GREENBRIER.
See *Smilax.*

GREENLEAF DAISY.
See *Euryops.*

Grevillea. 📷   6
SILK TREE. *G. noellii* is an evergreen shrub; *G. robusta* is a large,
fast-growing evergreen tree from
Australia. Both are hardy in zones
9 and 10.   *Grevillea robusta*

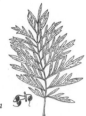

Grewia occidentalis.   5
LAVENDER STARFLOWER. A fast-growing, easy, evergreen shrub for zones 9–10. The small lavender
flowers with yellow centers do not drop cleanly,
leaving the bush looking dirty.

Griselinia. 📷   8
Evergreen shrub for zones 9–10, popular in Cali-
fornia. The round leaves are sometimes variegated.
Griselinia are separate-sexed, but not sold sexed.

GROUND CEDAR.
See *Lycopodium.*

GROUND CHERRY.
See *Physalis.*

GROUND IVY.
See *Glechoma hederacea.*

GROUND PINE.
See *Lycopodium.*

GROUSEBERRY.
See *Viburnum.*

GRU-GRU PALM.
See *Acrocomia.*

GUADALUPE FAN PALM.
See *Brahea edulis.*

Guaiacum sanctum.   3
LIGNUM-VITAE. Evergreen shrub or tree used in
zones 9–10. This tree has some of the hardest and
heaviest wood of any tree in the world. Attractive

leaves and flowers, the plant is good for seaside plantings. Flowers are usually purple or blue.

GUATEMALAN HOLLY.
See *Olmediella betschlerana*.

GUAVA.
See *Feijoa; Psidium*.

GUAYULE.
See *Hevea; Parthenium argentatum*.

GUELDER ROSE.
See *Viburnum*.

GUINEA GOLD VINE.
See *Hibbertia*.

GUM MYRTLE.
See *Angophora costata*.

GUM TREES.
See *Eucalyptus; Liquidambar*.

GUMBO–LIMBO TREE.
See *Bursera*.

GUMMY ACACIA.
See *Robinia*.

Gunnera.   5
Large perennial with giant leaves, up to 8 feet across; they thrive in moist, rich, well-drained soil.

GUTTA PERCHA TREE.
See *Eucommia ulmoides*.

Guzmania.
See *Bromelia*.

Gymnocladus dioica.   *males* ✹ *9, females* ✿ *1*
KENTUCKY COFFEE TREE. Deciduous tree, hardy to zone 5. Interesting large compound leaves. These are separate-sexed trees; the grafted cultivars are male. Female trees produce large, poisonous seed pods and do not cause allergy, although they can

be very messy. 'Expresso' is a male *Gymnocladus* sold as a "seedless" landscape tree.

Gynura aurantiaca. 📷   7
PURPLE VELVET PLANT. Houseplant with soft, hairy leaves and large clusters of malodorous yellow flowers in early summer. Poisonous.

GYP CORN.
See *Sorghum*.

Gypsophila.   6
BABY'S BREATH. Annuals or perennials for all zones. Small white or pink flowers. Florists often develop allergy to BABY'S BREATH.

H

Allergy Index Scale: *1 is Best, 10 is Worst.*

❋ for *1* and *2*   ✸ for *9* and *10*

📷 See insert for photograph

HACKBERRY.
See *Celtis.*

Haemanthus.
See *Hippeastrum.*

HAIRY LYCHEE.
See *Nephelium lappaceum.*

Hakea.   5
PINCUSHION TREE, SEA URCHIN, SWEET HAKEA.
Evergreen shrubs or small trees from Australia. Stiff leaves and fluffy, fragrant red or white flower clusters. Used for hedges and screens in zones 9–10.

Halesia.   3
OPPOSSUMWOOD, SILVERBELL TREE, SNOWDROP TREE. Several species of deciduous shrubs and trees native to the eastern United States and China. Attractive trees reach 50–60 feet, but grow slowly. Good show of flowers in late spring.

Halimiocistus sahucii.   3
Dense small evergreen shrub hardy to zone 7. Covered with small yellow flowers; drought-tolerant.

Halimium.   ❋ 2
Small, low-growing, spreading shrublets with bright yellow flowers resembling SUNROSE (*Helianthemum*). Thrive in full sun with good drainage.

Hamamelis.   5
WINTERBLOOM, WITCH HAZEL. Very early flowering deciduous trees or shrubs. Common WITCH HAZEL is hardy into zone 2. Bare branches are often brought inside in late winter where they will soon flower; when used in flower arrangements they may cause allergy.

Hamamelis

Hardenbergia.   3
Easy-to-grow evergreen vines for zones 9–10. They bear purple flowers in long loose clusters.

HARDTACK.
See *Ostrya.*

HARDY RUBBER TREE.
See *Eucommia ulmoides.*

Harpephyllum caffrum. 📷
males ✸ 9, females 4
KAFFIR PLUM. Separate-sexed evergreen tree for zones 9–10. Related to POISON IVY, the female trees bear small edible red fruits. Male trees resemble BRAZILIAN PEPPER TREES and shed allergenic pollen in late summer. Not sold sexed. Contact with leaves and sap may cause skin rash.

Harpullia.   8
Group of 35 species of trees and shrubs native to tropical Asia, Australia, and Madagascar, all with high potential for causing allergy.

HART'S-TONGUE FERN.
See *Phyllitis scolopendrium.*

HAT PALM.
See *Sabal.*

HAT TREE.
See *Brachychiton discolor*.

HAW.
See *Viburnum*.

HAWTHORN.
See *Crataegus*.

HAWTHORN-LEAF MAPLE.
See *Acer crataegifolium*.

HAZELNUT.
See *Corylus*.

HEAL-ALL.
See *Prunella*.

HEATH.
See *Erica; Daboecia*.

HEATHER.
See *Calluna; Erica*.

HEAVENLY BAMBOO.
See *Nandina domestica*.

Hebe.   ✷ 2
VERONICA. Evergreen shrubs, some hardy to zone 7. *Hebes* grow best near the coast and do not thrive in hot, dry areas. The many small flowers are blue, purple, lavender, or white. Easy to grow under right conditions and with ample moisture.

Hedera.

H. canariensis. 📷   8
ALGERIAN IVY. Big-leaved subtropical vine, occasionally appearing in a variegated form. Much used in zones 9–10 as a ground cover. May be invasive and difficult to remove.

H. colchica.   8
PERSIAN IVY. Hardy in zones 8–10. Has larger leaves than *H. canariensis*.

H. helix. 📷   7
ENGLISH IVY. The hardiest, most common, and most popular of the IVIES, used as a ground cover, houseplant, or hanging basket plant. *H. helix* 'Baltica' is the hardiest of all small-leafed ENGLISH IVIES.

All *Hedera* pose serious allergy potential unless kept small and grown in containers. The sap is known to cause occasional severe skin rash and the pollen can bring on sudden, intense allergic reactions. Ivy usually blooms only on old wood, so that if it is pruned hard each year there is much less chance of exposure to the pollen. Occasionally, IVY grows up the trunks of trees, eventually killing them and in rare cases, forming an "ivy tree." The leaves are poisonous if eaten and the black seed heads are especially toxic. Birds, however, especially robins, will eat IVY fruit in early spring when there is little else to consume. A good substitute for *Hedera* is perennial *Vinca*.

HEDGE APPLE.
See *Maclura pomifera*.

HEDGE FERN.
See *Polystichum*.

HEDGE MAPLE.
See *Acer campestre*.

Hedycarya arborea.   8
Evergreen tree from New Zealand occasionally grown in California, with 5-inch-long, leathery, toothed leaves and small red olive-shaped fruits. Separate sexed, but not sold sexed. Males pose allergy problem.

Hedychium.   5
GINGER LILY. Very tall perennials for zone 10. Big leaves and large flower spikes.

Hedyscepe canterburyana.   8
UMBRELLA PALM. Medium-sized palm tree hardy only in zone 10.

HE HUCKLEBERRY.
See *Cyrilla racemosa*.

Helenium autumnale. ✹9
FLOWERING SNEEZEWEED. A tall perennial hardy in all zones. The name says it all! The leaves and flowers of *Helenium* may cause skin rashes, and all parts of the plant are poisonous if eaten.

Helianthemum nummularium. *3*
SUNROSE. Slow-growing, sun-loving perennial hardy to zone 4. Attractive small flowers in many bright colors cover this small, spreading rock garden plant. Will not take overwatering.

Helianthus. *5*
SUNFLOWER. Annuals and perennials. Big, bold, handsome flowers in many sizes and colors. Unfortunately, SUNFLOWERS are closely related to RAGWEEDS, and cross-allergenic reactions are not uncommon.

Helichrysum. *5*
EVERLASTINGS, STRAWFLOWERS. Annuals used as dried flowers. Easy from seed.

Heliconia. ❇ *2*
FALSE BIRD-OF-PARADISE, LOBSTER-CLAW. Large group of tropical evergreens grown as greenhouse plants for their big leaves and showy flowers.

Heliopsis helianthoides scabra. 7
OX-EYE DAISY. Hardy perennial for cooler zones.

HELIOTROPE, GARDEN.
See *Valeriana officinalis*.

HELIOTROPE, WILD.
See *Phacelia distans*.

Heliotropium arborescens. *5*
COMMON HELIOTROPE. Perennial that may form a shrubby evergreen in zone 10. Grown as annual in colder climates. Big clusters of strongly fragrant flowers are usually purple, occasionally white. Intense Fragrance. Poisonous.

Helipterum roseum. 7
Annual daisy for full sun; easy from seed. Used as dried flower.

Helleborus. 7
CHRISTMAS ROSE, HELLEBORE, LENTEN ROSE. Perennials hardy in all zones. With their unusually colored small fragrant flowers, the HELLEBORES grow best in moist, shady areas. The scent of HELLEBORES can cause allergy in certain individuals. The sap can cause severe skin rash and all parts of this plant are extremely poisonous. For another very poisonous plant known as HELLEBORE or FALSE HELLEBORE, see *Veratrum*.

Hemerocallis. *3*
DAYLILY. Hardy, easy-to-grow perennial. Many possible flower colors. Thrives in sun or partial shade, with ample moisture. Poisonous.

Hemigraphis. ❇ *1*
WAFFLE PLANT. Houseplants grown for their attractive, heart-shaped leaves.

Hemiptelea davidii. *males* ✹*10, females* ❇ *1*
A hardy deciduous tree from Korea, eastern Mongolia, Manchuria, and China, occasionally used in zones 5–8 as a small landscape tree or as a fast growing, thorny hedge. An ELM relative, the separate-sexed male flowers are tiny but numerous and produce abundant pollen.

HEMLOCK, HEMLOCK SPRUCE.
See *Tsuga*.

HEMP TREE.
See *Vitex*.

HENS-AND-CHICKS.
See *Echeveria; Sempervivum*.

Hepatica. ❇ *2*
LIVERLEAF. Very hardy small perennial for all zones, but best in cool summer areas. Large, pretty, three-lobed leaves and violet or pink flowers on early spring-blooming plants for shady, moist spots. Whole plant is poisonous.

HERALD'S TRUMPET.
See *Beaumontia grandiflora*.

HERCULES' CLUB.
See *Zanthoxylum*.

Heritiera. 8
A group of about 30 trees from Australia or the tropics, all with high allergy potential.

Hermannia verticillata (Mahernia). ✻ 2
HONEY BELLS. Evergreen perennial often sold in hanging baskets. Yellow, bell-shaped flowers. Poisonous.

Hernandia ovigera. 8
Evergreen tree from subtropics occasionally grown in zone 10. Large rounded leaves, 8 inches long. Tree has high allergy potential.

Herniaria. ✻ 2
GREEN CARPET, RUPTURE WORT. Very hardy evergreen spreading ground cover. Will stand some light traffic.

Hesperaloe parviflora. ✻ 1
Perennial native of Texas and Mexico. Tall spikes of pink flowers emerge from rosette of leaves. Drought-tolerant desert plant.

Hesperis matronalis. 4
DAME'S ROCKET, SWEET ROCKET. Perennial or hardy annual for all zones, bearing panicles of lavender or white flowers on 3-foot stems. Fast growing from seed.

Heterocentron elegans (Schizocentron). ✻ 2
SPANISH SHAWL. Trailing perennial for hanging baskets or as ground cover in shady areas of zones 9–10. Reddish leaves and red flowers.

Heteromeles arbutifolia. 3
CALIFORNIA HOLLY, CHRISTMAS BERRY, TOYON. Evergreen native tree of west coastal areas, hardy to zone 7. Small leaves; white flowers followed by clusters of small red berries. Drought tolerant. Can be pruned into large shrub. Often used along freeways in California.

Heterospathe. 7
SAGISI PALM. Subtropical palm common in southern Florida.

Heuchera. ✻ 1
CORAL BELLS. Low-growing perennials, some species hardy in all zones. Easy to grow in sun or partial shade with plenty of water. Red flowers rise up from low basal foliage. Good rock garden plants.

Hevea brasiliensis. ⧉ ✳10
RUBBER TREE. A large tropical tree grown commercially for the production of rubber. Both the pollen and the sap are highly allergenic for many people. *Hevea* is a member of the SPURGE or *Euphorbia* family, a large group infamous for causing many serious contact allergies, including swelling, rash, itching, burning, and in some cases, death.

Allergy to rubber (also called PARA RUBBER), or latex, is on the rise, because of the increased use of latex gloves by medical personnel, food service personnel, police, and emergency workers. The allergy often takes months or years of repeated exposure to emerge. Reaction can then be swift and often severe; there are reported cases of fatalities occuring when rubber dental implements, catheters, and other medical devices have been placed in contact with sensitive individuals. Severe rashes and other allergic responses to the wearing of latex gloves, or from inhaling the powdery dust found on gloves, are also possible.

In addition to *Hevea, Parthenium argentatum,* or GUAYULE, is occasionally used in the production of natural rubber. This desert shrub is related to RAGWEED, and it is quite possible that cross-allergic reactions will occur with increased use of GUAYULE-based natural rubber. This is especially true because GUAYULE rubber is being touted as a safe alternative to rubber from *Hevea brasiliensis*.

HIBA ARBORVITAE.
See *Thujopsis dolabrata*.

HIBA CEDAR.
See *Thujopsis dolabrata*.

Hibbertia (Candollea cuneiformis).   *3*
GUINEA GOLD VINE. Yellow-flowered evergreen shrubs and vines for zone 9–10.

Hibiscus. 📷   *4*
ALTHEA, MALLOW, ROSE-OF-SHARON. A large group of over 200 species of annuals, perennials, herbs, shrubs, and trees mostly grown as ornamentals. Common *Hibiscus* relatives are HOLLYHOCKS and COTTON. Most members of this group have large, highly-colored flower petals that are well-designed by nature for pollen transfer by insects; thus, although most *Hibiscus* flowers have exposed pollen, few if any members of this group cause allergy. *H. syriacus*, ROSE-OF-SHARON or SHRUB ALTHEA, is a tall, hardy shrub. *H. moscheutos*, the ROSE MALLOW, is a large-flowered perennial that dies back in winter but regrows from a fleshy hardy rootstock. *H. rosa-sinensis*, the CHINESE HIBISCUS, is a popular shrub in zone 10, with many beautiful hybrids in a wide array of colors. All *Hibiscus* are easy-to-grow plants in good sun with average soil and ample water.

HICKORY.
See *Carya*.

HIMALAYAN POPPY.
See *Meconopsis betonicifolia*.

HINDU-ROPE PLANT.
See *Hoya*.

Hippeastrum.   *3*
AMARYLLIS. South American native bulb for zone 10; in colder zones the bulbs are dug and stored over winter. Very large, showy trumpet-shaped flowers on sturdy stalks, arising from a base of strap-shaped leaves. Many fine hybrid varieties available in dozens of color combinations. Often grown in pots, AMARYLLIS are popular flowering pot plants for sunny windows. They do best when fed lightly every few weeks during the bloom period.

Hippocrepis comosa.   ✳ *2*
Perennial leguminous ground cover for zones 9 and 10, resembling VETCH. Thrives in full sun; drought tolerant but benefits from regular watering. May be mowed after the pea-like yellow flowers bloom. Tolerates light foot traffic—a good lawn substitute in smaller areas.

Hippophae.   ✳*9*
BUCKTHORN, SEA BUCKTHORN. Several species of small-leafed, thorny European deciduous shrubs or small trees. Many species bear small, vitamin-rich, orange fruits or berries in later summer; these are occasionally eaten but may be poisonous in large quantities. These same berries have possible value as anti-cancer agents. Many BUCKTHORNS are separate-sexed, but are rarely sold sexed; male plants contribute to allergy; females (fruiting) plants do not.

HOG PLUM.
See *Pleiogynium*.

Hoheria.   *3*
LACEBARK, MOUNTAIN RIBBONWOOD. Evergreen trees and deciduous shrubs and trees from New Zealand for zones 9–10. Thrive in full sun with ample moisture.

Holcus.   ✳*10*
VELVET GRASS. A European species used in the western United States. An important allergy grass.

HOLLY FERN.
See *Cyrtomium; Polystichum*.

HOLLY, MOUNTAIN.
See *Nemopanthus*.

HOLLYHOCK.
See *Alcea*.

HOLLYLEAF CHERRY.
See *Prunus ilicifolia*.

HOLLYLEAF REDBERRY.
See *Rhamnus.*

HOLLYLEAF SWEETSPIRE.
See *Itea ilicifolia.*

Holodiscus.   6
CREAM BUSH, OCEAN SPRAY.
Deciduous shrubs related to
and resembling *Spiraea.* Hardy
to zone 4, *Holodiscus* grow best
in dry, sunny spots. The native CREAM
BUSH produces long clusters of small
creamy white flowers which birds
like to eat.   *Holodiscus*

Holoptelea.   ✳ 9
Two species of deciduous trees, one from India
and the other from Africa, both ELM relatives.

HOLY THISTLE.
See *Silybum.*

HOLY TREE.
See *Melia.*

Homalanthus.   ✳ 10
About 40 species of shrubs and trees with allergenic milky sap, native to tropical Asia and Africa.
None are frost-hardy, but some species are grown
in the United States in zone 10 or in greenhouses
as ornamentals. One species, *H. populifolius,* the
QUEENSLAND POPLAR, is used to make a commercial black dye that is probably a potent allergen.
Many species of *Homalanthus* are separate-sexed;
the male plants can be depended on to release extremely toxic pollen.

H. populifolius.   ✳ 9
QUEENSLAND POPLAR. Evergreen trees from Pacific
islands to Ceylon.

Homalocladium platycladum.   5
CENTIPEDE PLANT, RIBBON BUSH. Odd-looking
novelty plant usually grown in pots, or outdoors in
zones 9 and 10. Leafless with small red berries.

HONESTY.
See *Lunaria annua.*

HONEY BELLS.
See *Hermannia verticillata.*

HONEY LOCUST.
See *Gleditsia triacanthos.*

HONEY MYRTLE.
See *Melaleuca.*

HONEY PALM.
See *Jubaea.*

HONEY TREE.
See *Hovenia dulcis.*

HONEYBERRY.
See *Melicoccus.*

HONEYBUSH.
See *Melianthus.*

HONEYSUCKLE.
See *Lonicera.*

HOP BUSH.
See *Dodonaea viscosa.*

HOP HORNBEAM.
See *Ostrya.*

HOP TREE.
See *Ptelea.*

HOPS.
See *Humulus.*

HOPSEED.
See *Dodonaea viscosa.*

Hordeum.   4, ✳ 9
BARLEY. Pollen from BARLEY is heavier than that
of most grasses and poses less of an allergy problem. Pollen from the weedy varieties like *H. juba-*

tum or FOXTAIL BARLEY provoke allergy. *(Domestic variety 4, weed species 9.)*

HOREHOUND.
See *Marrubium vulgare.*

HORNBEAM.
See *Carpinus.*

HORNBEAM MAPLE.
See *Acer carpinifolium.*

HORNED MAPLE.
See *Acer diabolicum.*

HORNED POPPY.
See *Glaucium.*

HORSE CHESTNUT.
See *Aesculus.*

HORSEMINT.
See *Monarda.*

HORSERADISH.
See *Armoracia rusticana.*

HORSETAIL RUSH.
See *Equisetum hyemale.*

HORSETAIL TREE.
See *Casuarina.*

HOSEDOUP.
See *Mespilus.*

Hosta. 📷 ✳ *1*
PLANTAIN LILY. Very hardy perennials, members of the LILY family, grown for their large, ornamental leaves. *Hostas* grow best in rich, moist soil in partial shade, and are especially beautiful when planted under trees. The large leaves are frequently damaged by snails and slugs. Many hybrid varieties are available. White, pink, or pale lavender, sometimes fragrant flowers are held up above foliage on long, slender stalks.

HOT-DOG-CACTUS.
See *Senecio.*

HOTTENTOT FIG.
See *Carpobrotus.*

HOUSELEEK.
See *Sempervivum.*

Hovenia dulcis. 📷 *males 8, females* ✳ *1*
HONEY TREE, JAPANESE RAISIN TREE. Asian native shade tree with small, edible raisin-like fruit. Separate-sexed but not usually sold sexed. A member of the BUCKTHORN family.

Howea. 7
KENTIA PALM, PARADISE PALM, SENTRY PALM. Houseplant palms used outside in zone 10. As houseplants they are frequent hosts to spider mites, which can cause allergy. When used outdoors, the pollen can also cause allergy.

Hoya. 3
WAX FLOWER, WAX PLANT. Houseplants for sunny rooms, with thick leaves and clusters of pink flowers that look as though they're made of wax. The flowers are very fragrant and last for months. Not a pollen problem, but some may find the heavy, sweet fragrance intolerable.

HUCKLEBERRY.
See *Vaccinium.*

HUCKLEBERRY, HE.
See *Cyrilla racemiflora.*

Hudsonia. 6
GOLDEN HEATHER, POVERTY GRASS. Three species of small, evergreen shrubby plants, native to the northeastern United States, used in some landscapes in cold winter areas. Hardy to zone 2. May cause occasional allergy.

Humata tyermannii. 4
BEAR'S FOOT FERN. Slow-growing, Chinese native fern for partial shade in frost-free zones.

HUMMINGBIRD FLOWER.
See *Zauschneria*.

Humulus. *males 5, females* ✳ *1*
HOPS. Annual and perennial, hardy, fast-growing vines. *H. lupulus* is used to flavor beer. HOP vines are separate-sexed; male vines infrequently are the cause of allergy. Commercial HOPS fields use only female plants because these make larger flowers, which are preferred for brewing beer. As a result, these large HOP growing areas present no pollen problems at all.

Hunnemannia. 4
GOLDEN CUP, MEXICAN TULIP POPPY. Short-lived perennial poppy for bright, sunny areas. Fast from seed; long-lasting flowers. Poisonous.

Hura. ✸*9*
MONKEY PISTOL, SANDBOX TREE. Two species of tropical trees from Central America occasionally used in zone 10. Sap from either can cause severe rash.

HYACINTH.
See *Hyacinthus; Galtonia*.

HYACINTH BEAN.
See *Dolichos*.

HYACINTH, WILD.
See *Dichelostemma*.

Hyacinthus. 3
HYACINTH. Hardy bulbs for all zones. Very fragrant flowers may cause odor challenges when planted en masse. Bulbs are poisonous.

Hybophrynium braunianum. ✳ *1*
Tall houseplant grown for its unusual foliage. Grows best with regular fertilizer and water, in partial shade.

Hydnocarpus. 8
Many species of tropical trees. The seeds of *H. kurzii*, a large tree, yield *chaulmoogra oil*, which is used in the treatment of leprosy.

Hydrangea.
Many species of deciduous shrubs or vines, many hardy into zone 3. All *Hydrangeas* grow best in good soil with ample moisture, and none are drought-tolerant. In cooler climates, they thrive in full sun, but in hot summer areas, appreciate partial shade. The large floral panicles, in white, pink, red, or blue, are formed of many small flowers clustered together. *Hydrangea* leaves contain a natural sweetener, but because the leaves also contain toxic compounds, they should not be eaten. Allergy potential varies by species.

H. anomale. 4

H. macrophylla. 📷 3
BIG-LEAF HYDRANGEA. May reach 12 feet outdoors in mild climates. Most often sold as a potted plant. Broad leaves and large, flat flower heads in pink, blue, or white.

H. paniculata. 6
PEE-GEE HYDRANGEA. Among the hardiest of the *Hydrangeas*, the PEE-GEE can withstand winters in zone 3. Large panicles of white flowers are borne in midsummer.

H. quercifolia. 📷 7
OAK-LEAF HYDRANGEA. Large, deeply lobed leaves characterize the OAK-LEAF HYDRANGEA. Forms a fairly large shrub in areas of adequate moisture.

*Hydrangea flowers are pH sensitive—rather like a natural litmus paper. Blue flowers can be changed to pink with the addition of limestone to sweeten or raise the pH of the soil. Conversely, pink flowers can be changed to blue by lowering the pH or acidifying the soil with sulfur.

Hymenanthera. 8
Several species of evergreen trees and shrubs native to New Zealand and Australia. Some are grown outside in California. All are separate-sexed and cause allergy.

Hymenocallis (Ismene). *3*

SPIDER LILY, BASKET FLOWER. Frost-tender native bulbs, producing lily-like flowers in midsummer. Poisonous.

Hymenosporum flavum. *3*

SWEETSHADE. Small evergreen tree from Australia for zones 9–10. A nice tree with few bad habits.

Hypericum. 📷 *5*

SAINT JOHN'S-WORT. Hardy perennial that is often used as a drought-tolerant ground cover that will grow in either sun or shade. In the Pacific Northwest this plant has naturalized and is known as KLAMATHWEED. It is the bane of livestock who eat it, because it causes photosensitivity; many cattle die from the resulting sunburn. SAINT JOHN's-WORT also contains natural calmative compounds and is used in herbal medicine as a mood enhancer.

Hyphaene. *7*

DOUM PALM, GINGERBREAD PALM. Several species of separate-sexed palms occasionally grown in Hawaii and Florida.

Hypocyrta nummularia.

See *Alloplectus nummularia*.

Hypoestes phyllostachya. ❋ *1*

PINK POLKA-DOT PLANT. With its dark green leaves splashed in pink, *Hypoestes* makes a good plant for shade in zone 10, and is a popular houseplant in colder zones. Easy to grow and propagate from seeds or cuttings, it is kept compact through constant pinching back.

HYSSOP.

See *Agastache; Hyssopus officinalis*.

Hyssopus officinalis. *3*

HYSSOP. Hardy ornamental herb for sun or shade in all zones with handsome large leaves and white, rose, or red flowers. A member of the MINT family.

I

Allergy Index Scale: *1* **is Best,** *10* **is Worst.**

❋ for *1* and *2* ✸ for *9* and *10*

📷 See insert for photograph

Iberis. ❋ *2*

CANDYTUFT. Annuals and perennials. Annual CANDYTUFT is usually grown from direct seedings. Perennial *Iberis* is a small, frost-hardy, low-growing, evergreen plant with a good show of very bright white flowers in spring.

ICEPLANT.

See *Carpobrotus; Cephalophyllum; Delosperma; Drosanthemum.*

Idesia polycarpa. 📷 *males 7, females* ❋ *1*

WONDER TREE. Large heart-shaped leaves on this small deciduous Asian native, hardy to zone 7. Separate-sexed, the female trees produce small, ornamental orange fruits. The males pose an allergy problem.

Ilex. 📷 *males 7, females* ❋ *1*

HOLLY. Many species; most are hardy evergreen shrubs or small trees, although some are deciduous. All HOLLIES are separate-sexed, and the male plants present potential for some airborne allergy. A great number of named, sexed cultivars are available for sale. To produce their characteristic red, white, yellow, or black berries, female HOLLIES must be pollinated; one male plant can pollinate many females.

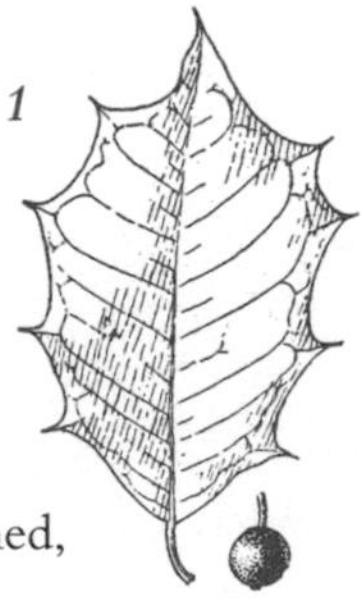

Ilex opaca

Landscapers frequently use all-male varieties as hedge plants, and in this situation they pose serious allergy potential. Allergy from HOLLY pollen is not well documented, but is worthy of further research. Fruit is poisonous but not fatal.

Illicium anisatum. *3*

JAPANESE ANISE TREE, ANISE TREE. Broadleaf evergreen tree with fragrant leaves, small white flowers, and star-shaped seed cluster capsules, for zones 8–10. Poisonous seed.

IMMORTELLE.

See *Xeranthemum annuum.*

Impatiens. 📷 ❋ *1*

BALSAM, BUSY LIZZY, TOUCH-ME-NOTS. A tender annual for all zones, with shade and ample moisture. All *Impatiens* were once tall and white-flowered, but through selective breeding, there are hundreds of compact, dwarf, multiflowered, and multicolored varieties available at almost any nursery. *Impatiens* are easy to root from cuttings stuck in small pots of potting soil and kept well watered in the shade for a few weeks. As an annual for shady areas *Impatiens* are the top bedding plant used in the United States, easy to grow and dependable.

From an allergy point of view *Impatiens* is one of our best annual flowers. The petals are large and highly colored, and the pollen-producing parts are few and deeply hidden well inside the flower. They are not known to cause any rashes nor do they have any close allergenic relatives.

The yellow- and orange-flowered wild *Impatiens* grows along the margins of woodlands in much of North America. The juice from its soft stems is a time-honored remedy for rashes caused by stinging nettle and poison ivy, which usually thrive under similar cultural conditions.

Both the Latin name *Impatiens* and the common name of TOUCH-ME-NOT refer to the fact that the ripe, oval-shaped seed pods eject their seeds forcefully when even lightly touched or slightly squeezed.

Incarvillea delavayi. ✽ 2
Large perennial hardy to zone 6. The fleshy roots may be dug and stored over winter north of zone 6. Needs good drainage and sun or part shade to produce bold, trumpet-shaped purple flowers with yellow throats.

INCENSE CEDAR.
See *Austrocedrus; Calocedrus decurrens.*

INCHWORM.
See *Senecio.*

INDIA HAWTHORN.
See *Rhaphiolepis indica.*

INDIAN BEAN TREE.
See *Catalpa.*

INDIAN CHERRY.
See *Rhamnus.*

INDIAN CURRANT.
See *Symphoricarpos.*

INDIAN MOCK STRAWBERRY.
See *Duchesnea indica.*

INDIAN PINK.
See *Silene.*

INDIAN PLUM.
See *Oemleria cerasiformus.*

INDIAN POKE.
See *Veratrum.*

INDIGO, WILD.
See *Baptisia australis.*

INSIDE-OUT FLOWER.
See *Vancouveria.*

Iochroma cyaneum. 3
Tall evergreen shrub for full sun in zones 9–10. Produces clusters of long tubular purple flowers.

Ipheion uniflorum. ✽ 2
SPRING STAR FLOWER. Bulb for zones 7–10. Easy to grow; frequently naturalizes.

Ipomoea (Calonyction, Quamoclit). 📷 4
MORNING GLORY. Perennial or annual vines for full sun or partial shade. Very fast-growing when well adapted. In zones 9 and 10, MORNING GLORY can become rampant and overgrow fences, shrubs, and sheds. Annual varieties reseed readily. Flowers come in many colors, but perhaps the most impressive is the very large flowered annual 'Heavenly Blue'. All MORNING GLORY leaves are capable of causing skin rash in sensitive individuals.

The individual flowers of the MORNING GLORY have little exposed pollen and do not present much problem as an inhalant allergen. However, when growing strongly, the sheer mass of blooms may present an overwhelming fragrance for perfume-sensitive individuals; will often reseed and can indeed become weedy.

The seeds of *Ipomoea* contain a powerful hallucinogen similar to the drug LSD.

Ipomopsis. 3
SCARLET GILIA. Short-lived perennials or annuals for any zone. Slender plants are several feet tall and do best in groups. Direct seed in full sun. Long, tubular red or red-and-yellow flowers. One species is native to the southern United States and can grow to 6 feet.

Iresine herbstii. males 8, females ✽ 1
BEEF PLANT, BLOOD-LEAF. Shade plant in zone 10 or houseplant in other zones. Frost-tender foliage plant with large green leaves with deep red veins. Fast-growing from cuttings. Separate-sexed.

Iris. 📷 4
A large group of rhizomatous or bulbous perennials. The rhizomatous varieties are very hardy and easy to grow, given full sun and well-drained soil. Bulbous varieties perfer moist soil and may even be grown as bog plants. In the mild winter areas, large BEARDED or GERMAN IRIS are grown in clay pots that can be set aside when the short bloom

period is over. *Orris root*, a fixative for perfumes, powders, and potpourris is made from *Iris* roots. Allergy to orris root is very common, and skin rash from handling *Iris* roots is also not uncommon. Odor-sensitive individuals may be allergic to the fragrance of the *Iris*.

IRISH MOSS.
See *Sagina subulata*.

IRONBARK.
See *Eucalyptus*.

IRONWEED.
See *Verbesina; Vernonia*

IRONWEED, YELLOW.
See *Verbesina*.

IRONWOOD.
See *Cyrilla racemiflora; Lyonothamnus floribundus; Olneya tesota; Parrotia*.

ISLAND BUSH SNAPDRAGON.
See *Galvezia speciosa*.

Ismene.
See *Hymenocallis*.

Isotoma fluviatilis.
See *Laurentia*.

ITALIAN MAPLE.
See *Acer opalus*.

ITCHWEED.
See *Veratrum*.

Itea ilicifolia. 5
HOLLYLEAF SWEETSPIRE. Evergreen shrub with long drooping clusters of small white fragrant flowers, for zones 6–9. Needs plenty of soil moisture.

ITHURIEL'S SPEAR.
See *Triteleia*.

Iva. ✺ 10
A group of common tall allergenic weeds usually growing in wet areas in most zones. A dwarf form of *Iva* is now being used in some "native" landscapes, a trend that should be discouraged.

IVY.
See *Hedera*.

IVY-LEAFED MAPLE.
See *Acer cissifolium*.

IVY, WATER.
See *Senecio*.

Ixia. 3
AFRICAN CORN LILY. Corm hardy in zones 8–10.

Ixiolirion. 3
An Asian native bulb hardy in zones 8–10. Blue flowers in spring.

J

Allergy Index Scale: *1* **is Best**, *10* **is Worst.**

❋ for *1* and *2*   ✸ for *9* and *10*

📷 See insert for photograph

Jacaranda mimosifolia. 📷   *4*
JACARANDA. A large deciduous tree from Brazil
which puts on a glorious display of small, tubular,
sky-blue flowers. Cold-hardy only to about 20 degrees, *Jacaranda* is grown in mild winter areas
around the world.

Jacobaea.
See *Senecio.*

Jacobinia.
See *Justicia.*

JACOB'S LADDER.
See *Polemonium; Smilax.*

Jacquemontia.   *4*
Large group of mostly tropical vines with blue
flowers, occasionally grown in zone 10.

Jacquinia.   *6*
BARBASCO. Tropical shrubs and trees with small
red, white, or yellow flowers followed by small orange fruits used by South American natives to poison fish. Several species of *Jacquinia* are grown in
Florida.

JADE PLANT.
See *Crassula.*

JAMBU.
See *Syzygium.*

JAPAN PEPPER.
See *Zanthoxylum.*

JAPANESE ANISE TREE.
See *Illicium anisatum.*

JAPANESE ARALIA.
See *Fatsia japonica.*

JAPANESE CARPET.
See *Zoysia.*

JAPANESE CEDAR.
See *Cryptomeria japonica.*

JAPANESE EUONYMUS.
See *Euonymus.*

JAPANESE FELT FERN.
See *Pyrrosia lingua.*

JAPANESE MAPLE.
See *Acer japonicum.*

JAPANESE NUTMEG TREE.
See *Torreya.*

JAPANESE POINSETTIA.
See *Pedilanthus tithymaloides.*

JAPANESE RAISIN TREE.
See *Hovenia dulcis.*

JAPANESE SNOWBELL.
See *Styrax.*

JAPANESE SPURGE.
See *Pachysandra.*

JAPANESE VARNISH TREE.
See *Firmiana simplex*.

JAPANESE ZELKOVA.
See *Zelkova*.

JASMINE BOX.
See *Phillyrea decora*.

Jasminum.   7
JASMINE. Several hundred species of evergreen or deciduous flowering vines and shrubs. Members of the OLIVE family. Flowers, usually strongly fragrant, are white, yellow, or pink. The flowers present allergy potential both from their intense fragrance and for their pollen, which is similar to that of OLIVES, a well-known and potent allergen.

Jatropha.   ✳9
AUSTRALIAN BOTTLE PLANT, BARBADOS NUT, CORAL PLANT, PEREGRINA, PHYSIC NUT. Large group of subtropical plants occasionally planted in zone 10 and in greenhouses. All plants in this group present numerous allergy potentials. Several species have attractive yellow fruit, which is poisonous if eaten.

JAVA APPLE, JAVA PLUM.
See *Syzygium*.

JAVAN GRAPE.
See *Tetrastigma*.

JELLY PALM.
See *Butia capitata*.

JERUSALEM ARTICHOKE.
See *Helianthus*.

JERUSALEM CHERRY.
See *Solanum*.

JERUSALEM SAGE.
See *Phlomis fruticosa; Pulmonaria*.

JERUSALEM THORN.
See *Parkinsonia aculeata*.

JESSOP.
See *Ledebouria socialis*.

JEWEL VINE.
See *Derris*.

JEWISH MYRTLE.
See *Ruscus*.

JIMSON WEED.
See *Datura*.

Joannesia.   ✳10
Several species of large trees from Brazil, occasionally used in zones 9–10.

JOB'S TEARS.
See *Coix lacryma-jobi*.

JOE-PYE WEED.
See *Eupatorium*.

Johannesteijsmannia.   ✳ 1
Four species of small palm trees from Borneo and Sumatra, occasionally grown in Florida.

JOHNNY-JUMP-UP.
See *Viola*.

JOHNSON GRASS.
See *Sorghum*.

JOINT FIR.
See *Ephedra*.

JOJOBA.
See *Simmondsia*.

JONQUIL.
See *Narcissus*.

JOSHUA TREE.
See *Yucca*.

JOVE'S FRUIT.
See *Lindera*.

Juania.   8
Tall palm trees from Chile.

Jubaea.   7
COQUITO PALM, HONEY PALM. A large palm tree
from Chile, hardy to 20 degrees.

Jubaeopsis caffra.   7
Palm tree used in California and Florida.

Juglans. 📷   8– ✳ 9
BLACK WALNUT, BUTTERNUT, ENGLISH WALNUT,
MADEIRA NUT, WALNUT. Large deciduous nut-
bearing trees, some species hardy in all zones. All
WALNUTS produce airborne pollen and allergy, but
some are worse than others. By
far the most problematic in
number and intensity of attack is
the CALIFORNIA BLACK WALNUT,
a large native tree. The BUT-
TERNUT and English walnut
are slightly less potent allergens. Allergy is also reportedly
triggered by the odor of rotting husks that surround the
nuts. On some occasions this
odor-allergy is more severe than
that to the pollen.

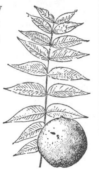

Juglans nigra

JUJUBE.
See *Ziziphus.*

JUNEBERRY.
See *Amelanchier.*

Juniperus.
males ✳ *10, females* ✣ *1, monoecious plants* ✳ *9*
CEDAR, HABBEL, JUNIPER, MOUNTAIN CEDAR, OZARK
WHITE CEDAR, RED CEDAR, WHITE CEDAR. Hardy,
drought-tolerant, easy-to-grow, common coniferous evergreen shrubs and trees, which are related
to CYPRESS, not CEDAR. JUNIPER is the cause of allergies in many parts of the world. In certain areas
of the United States, JUNIPER is the primary cause
of asthma and hay fever. Cross-allergenic reactions
are common between JUNIPER and CYPRESS.

The different species bloom in different ways:
the very worst are the males of the separate-sexed
species (dioecious); monoecious species always
present allergy problems as well; the female plants
of separate-sexed species, however, are fine for allergy-free landscapes.

Most JUNIPERS bloom from early winter into
late spring, sometimes releasing so much pollen
that the shrubs appear to smoke. A few species of
mostly western JUNIPERS bloom from September
to November. Other species bloom sporadically
throughout the year, creating an almost constant
level of airborne pollen in many areas. In zones
8–10 in particular, JUNIPERS, especially male plants,
may bloom several times each year.

In Arkansas, Missouri, Oklahoma, Texas, and
parts of Mexico the most common JUNIPER is
J. Ashei, the OZARK WHITE CEDAR, which is a JUNIPER,
despite its name. All of these are separate-sexed.

In New Mexico, Arizona, parts of Texas, and
into Mexico the most common species is the AL-
LIGATOR JUNIPER, *J. Deppeana,* also separate-sexed.

In the Eastern United States the most common
species is the RED CEDAR, *J. virginiana,* again a separate-
sexed species.

In much of the Rocky Mountain area the pre-
dominant JUNIPER is the COLORADO RED CEDAR,
J. scopulorum, another separate-sexed species.

In parts of California, there is a common monoecious JUNIPER, the CALIFORNIA JUNIPER, *J. occidentalis.* This species is sometimes separate-sexed. Other
JUNIPERS native to California are all separate-sexed.

In separate-sexed JUNIPER species, only the
pollen-free female plants produce the round JUNIPER
berries. Plants without berries are male.

Each male JUNIPER bush or tree produces
enough pollen to fertilize thousands of female
plants. In some areas of the United States, during
the early spring or fall months of the JUNIPER
bloom, there is so much male pollen in the air that
every person living there is inhaling hundreds of
JUNIPER pollen grains with every breath.

The relative humidity of an area has much to do with the actual amount of allergy to JUNIPER pollen. In humid areas there is less allergy but in warm, dry areas, typical of much of the western United States, JUNIPER pollen floats easily in the air, causing a great deal of allergy. JUNIPER pollen can also irritate the skin and is capable of causing contact dermatitis as well as severe inhalant allergy.

In certain geographical locations where cities are surrounded by hills full of wild JUNIPERS, the only effective measure may be to selectively remove many of the wild male JUNIPERS growing close to the urban areas; males are easy to identify since they are the ones with no berries.

Throughout America there are many millions of imported JUNIPER trees, shrubs, and ground covers, most of which are separate-sexed; the female plants of these species can be used in allergy-free landscapes. One notable exception is the HIMALAYAN JUNIPER (*J. recurva*), which is monoecious and, like all plants bearing flowers of both sexes on the same tree, sheds allergenic pollen.

Over the years landscapers have preferred to plant JUNIPERS without berries to reduce the amount of litter produced by each plant, and wholesale nurseries have propagated many millions of these pollen-producing male selections, all of which cause allergy. The net result has been a steady increase in urban *Juniperus* pollen and related allergic reactions. The answer is to identify and use female-only JUNIPERS in all future landscaping applications. Listed below are sexed JUNIPERS, of which many are female clones.

J. chinensis.

CHINESE JUNIPER. Female CHINESE JUNIPER cultivars include 'Foemina', 'Blue Point', 'Excelsior', 'Femina', 'Iowa', 'Keteleeri Beissn', 'Mountbatten', 'Obelisk', 'Oblonga', 'Olympia', and 'Pyramidis Variegata'.

Male named varieties include 'Armstrong', 'Aurea', 'Blue Pfitzer', 'Columnaris Glauca', 'Leena', 'Pendula', 'Pfitzerana glauca', 'Pyramidalis', and 'Story'.

Some cultivars are monoecious, bearing flowers of both sexes on one plant. Avoid using 'Hornibrook', 'Robusta Green', and 'Sphoerica'.

J. c. 'Torulosa', the HOLLYWOOD JUNIPER, is a very common tall, twisted JUNIPER. The plants are usually female (identified by their berries), although some cultivars of this variety are male and should be avoided.

J. communis.

COMMON JUNIPER, ENGLISH JUNIPER, POLISH JUNIPER, SWEDISH JUNIPER. All plants of this species are separate-sexed. Use only female plants, which are identifiable by their berries. 'Hornibrookii' is a female shrub and is a good choice for allergy-free landscapes.

J. davurica.

'Expansa' is a named male cultivar.

J. deppeana.

ALLIGATOR JUNIPER. Separate-sexed; look for berries indicating female plants.

Juniperus deppeana

J. drupacea.

All known cultivars of this species are males.

J. flaccida.

This variety bears flowers of both sexes, each on separate branches. Do not use.

J. horizontalis.

CREEPING JUNIPER, PROSTRATE JUNIPER. 'Admirabilis' is a male plant and should be avoided.

Good female cultivars for allergy-free landscapes include 'Bar Harbor', 'Emerson', 'Filicina', 'Glenmore', and 'Viridis'.

J. × media.

'Globosa' and 'Hetzii' are female plants and good allergy-free choices; 'Pfitzeriana' and 'Plumosa' are male.

J. occidentalis.

CALIFORNIA JUNIPER. A monoecious species that should be avoided.

J. oxycedrus.
A separate-sexed species. Look for berries that indicate safe female plants.

J. phoenicea.
A monoecious species that should be avoided.

J. recurva.
HIMALAYAN JUNIPER. A monoecious species that should be avoided.

J. rigida.
A separate-sexed species. Look for berries that indicate allergy-free female plants.

J. sabina 'Cupressa.'
The named cultivar 'Femina' is an allergy-free female. 'Arcadia', 'Blue Danube', 'Broadmore', 'Buffalo', 'Savin', 'Scandia', and 'Tamariscifolia' are all male and should be avoided.

J. silicicola.
SOUTHERN JUNIPER. A separate-sexed species. Look for berries that indicate allergy-free female plants.

J. scopulorum. 📷
COLORADO RED CEDAR. A separate-sexed species. Allergy-free cultivars include 'Admiral', 'Blue Heaven', 'Blue Moon', 'Cologreen', 'Gracilis', 'Platinum', 'Spearmint', 'Sutherland', and 'Welchii.' Male cultivars include 'Emerald' or 'Emerald Green', 'Gray Gleam', 'Skyrocket', 'Steel Blue', and 'Wichita Blue'. *J. s.* 'Moonglow' can be either a male or a female. Don't buy 'Moonglow' unless it has the berries that indicate a female plant.

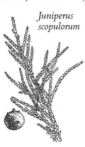

Juniperus scopulorum

J. squamata.
'Meyeri' is an allergy-free female cultivar.

J. virginiana. 📷
EASTERN RED CEDAR. A separate-sexed species; safe, allergy-free named female cultivars include 'Canaertii', 'Chamberlaynii', 'Pendula Chamberlaynii', and 'Pendula Virdis'. Male cultivars to be avoided include 'Burkii', 'Cupressifolia', 'Filifera', 'Hillspire', 'Prostrata Silver', 'Silver', and 'Tripartita'.

Some *J. virginiana* may be of either sex; look for berries indicating female plants on these named varieties: 'Glauca', 'Manhattan Blue', 'Pendula', and 'Reptans' or 'Pendula reptans.'

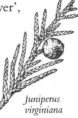

Juniperus virginiana

J. wallichiana.
BLACK JUNIPER. A separate-sexed species. Look for berries indicating allergy-free female plants. Juniper berries are used to flavor gin, and are also used in herbal medicine as a natural diuretic and decongestant; large doses may be poisonous.

JUPITER'S BEARD.
See *Centranthus ruber.*

Jurinea.   6
Large group of daisy-like annuals and perennials often grown from seed.

Justicia (Beloperone, Jacobinia). 📷   ❋ 1
A very large group of herbs and shrubs from the subtropics into temperate North America. The most commonly used is *J. brandegeana*, the SHRIMP PLANT. This unusual-looking flowering shrub grows best in sunny locations in zone 10, and produces drooping yellow or reddish flowers that look like large shrimps.

K

Allergy Index Scale: *1* **is Best,** *10* **is Worst.**

❁ for *1* and *2*   ✳ for *9* and *10*

📷 See insert for photograph

Kadsura japonica.   7
Evergreen vine for zones 9–10.

KAFFIR LILY.
See *Clivia.*

KAFFIR PLUM.
See *Harpephyllum caffrum.*

Kalanchoe.   ❁ *2*
Succulents used as houseplants.

Kalmia.   8
MOUNTAIN LAUREL. Hardy evergreen shrubs or small trees with large clusters of showy flowers in many colors. Hardy to zone 5, *Kalmia* grows best in moist, well-drained, acid soil in the partial shade of large deciduous trees. *Kalmia* produces a large amount of pollen and allergy to it is common. All parts are highly poisonous, including the pollen.

Kalmiopsis leachiana.   4
Oregon native evergreen shrub, hardy to zone 7, producing quantities of small pink flowers in spring. Thrives only where soil is moist, shady, and acidic.

Kalopanax septemlobus. 📷   4
CASTOR OIL TREE. Large deciduous tree, hardy into zone 5, which produces small white flowers in spring. Native of China. Needs moist soil to thrive.

KANGAROO PAW.
See *Anigozanthos.*

KAPOK.
See *Chorisia.*

KARO.
See *Pittosporum.*

KATSURA TREE.
See *Cercidiphyllum japonicum.*

KAVA-KAVA.
See *Piper.*

KAWA-KAWA.
See *Macropiper.*

KEI APPLE.
See *Dovyalis hebecarpa.*

KENTIA PALM.
See *Howea.*

KENTUCKY COFFEE TREE.
See *Gymnocladus dioica.*

KENYA IVY.
See *Senecio.*

Kerria japonica.   ❁ *2*
Deciduous shrub for partial shade to zone 3. An easy-to-grow member of the ROSE family, its flowers resemble little double yellow roses.

Keteleeria.   3
Several species of tall, evergreen trees, hardy to zone 8. Native to Asia and related to PINES, *Keteleeria* are often grown in California. In the wild, they may reach 160 feet.

KEY PALM.
See *Thrinax.*

KHAT.
See *Catha edulis.*

KIKUYUGRASS.
See *Pennisetum clandestinum.*

KING PALM.
See *Archontophoenix.*

KINNIKINNICK.
See *Arctostaphylos.*

KIWI.
See *Actinidia.*

KLAMATHWEED.
See *Hypericum.*

Kleinia.
See *Senecio.*

Kniphofia uvaria (Tritoma). 4
RED-HOT POKER, TORCH LILY. Perennial hardy to zone 4 and easy to grow. Tall spikes of red-orange-yellow flowers.

KNOTWEED.
See *Polygonum.*

Kochia. 8
BURNING BUSH, SUMMER CYPRESS. Annuals grown in all zones.

Koeleria. ✳9
WESTERN JUNE GRASS. A forage grass in the western United States.

Koelreuteria paniculata. 4
GOLDENRAIN TREE, VARNISH TREE. Large deciduous tree native to Asia, grown for its pendant fragrant yellow flowers, followed by long-lasting clusters of seed pods shaped like

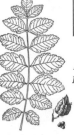
Koelreuteria paniculata

Chinese lanterns. Common in California and hardy to zone 7.

KOHUHU.
See *Pittosporum.*

Kolkwitzia amabilis. 3
BEAUTY BUSH. Deciduous shrub hardy to zone 4. Pink HONEYSUCKLE-like flowers with yellow throats bloom in early summer; the flowers are followed by bristly pink fruits.

KOREAN VELVET GRASS.
See *Zoysia.*

KOWHAI.
See *Sophora.*

KUDSU.
See *Pueraria lobata.*

KUMQUAT.
See *Citrus; Fortunella.*

L

Allergy Index Scale: *1* is **Best**, *10* is **Worst**.

✻ for *1* and *2*   ✺ for *9* and *10*

📷 See insert for photograph

Laburnum.   7
GOLDENCHAIN TREE. Deciduous tree, hardy to
zone 4. Produces long chains of pea-like yellow
flowers. The three-lobed leaflets resemble CLOVER
leaves. Often confused with another yellow flowering deciduous tree, *Koelreuteria paniculata*, the
GOLDENRAIN TREE. The trees produce a quantity of
seeds and pods, and this seed is very poisonous if
eaten. All parts of the *Laburnum* are highly toxic.
Children have been poisoned from simply sucking
on the fresh Laburnum flowers.

LACEBARK.
See *Hoheria*.

LACEBARK, QUEENSLAND.
See *Brachychiton discolor*.

Lachenalia.   ✻ 2
CAPE COWSLIP. Bulb for zone 10.

LADIES'-TOBACCO.
See *Antennaria*.

LADY FERN.
See *Athyrium*.

LADY PALM.
See *Rhapis*.

LADY SLIPPER.
See *Cypripedium*.

Laelia.
See ORCHIDS.

Lagerstroemia indica. 📷   5
CRAPE MYRTLE. Hardy into zone 6, CRAPE MYRTLE
does best where summer days are bright and hot.
In cooler areas it blooms, but is susceptible to
mildew, which may in itself contribute to allergy.
CRAPE MYRTLE is not related to the true MYRTLES,
and allergy to their flowers is not well documented, despite the fact that it produces a huge
number of small flowers, each bearing an unusually high number (up to 200) of stamens (the male
pollen parts).

Lagunaria patersonii. 📷   ✺ 9
COW ITCH TREE, PATERSON PLUM, PRIMROSE TREE.
An upright evergreen tree, hardy to zone 9. It
bears attractive purple primrose-like flowers,
which are followed by seed pods filled with incredibly itchy tiny hair-like fibers. Just opening
one of these pods spreads the irritating hairs to
hands, face, neck, and eyes, producing sudden, severe contact irritation. Not a tree to spread the
picnic blanket under.

LAMB'S EAR.
See *Stachys byzantina*.

Lamium maculatum.   3
DEAD NETTLE. Perennial hardy to zone 3, occasionally used as hanging basket plant or ground cover.
May become weedy. Thrives in moist soil and partial shade.

Lampranthus. 📷   3
ICEPLANT.

LANCEPOD.
See *Lonchocarpus*.

LANCEWOOD.
See *Pseudopanax.*

Lantana. 7
Evergreen or deciduous shrubs or ground covers, hardy only in warm winter areas. The prickly leaves may cause skin rash in some individuals. The odd scent of the flowers or crushed leaves also may make some people nauseous. The green berries are highly poisonous.

Lapageria rosea. ✽ 2
CHILEAN BELLFLOWER. Evergreen vine hardy to zone 8. National flower of Chile, with large, rosy-red flowers. Needs shade and ample water to thrive.

LARCH.
See *Larix.*

Larix. 📷 ✱ 2
LARCH, TAMARACK. Deciduous conifer that loses its needles in winter. Hardy to coldest zones 1 and 2, LARCH do not tolerate warm climates. Slow-growing and very long-lived, it will thrive in damp, poorly drained areas. The golden autumn color and attractive soft green of the emerging springtime foliage make the LARCH an attractive tree for most of the year.

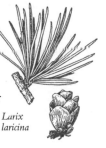

Larix laricina

LARKSPUR.
See *Consolida ambigua; Delphinium.*

Larrea tridentata. 8
CREOSOTE BUSH. Evergreen shrub native to hot, desert areas. It produces small yellow flowers. The odd smell of these shrubs will bother some and the pollen affects others. Skin rash is possible from contact with the sap.

Latania. 7
LATAN PALMS. Three species of palms common to Florida. Separate-sexed; males cause allergy.

Lathyrus. 3
SWEET PEA. *Lathyrus* is fast-growing from seed planted very early in the season and does best in cool summer areas. In warmer zones, the best stands of SWEET PEA are had by planting the seed in September, in loose soil in a sunny spot next to a fence or other support structure. *L. odoratus* is the common annual SWEET PEA. *L. littoralis* is a perennial vine that grows profusely all along the coast from Northern California to Washington.

SWEET PEAS are not to be confused with garden peas—all parts of Lathyrus are poisonous. As a cut flower, the intense fragrance of some SWEET PEAS may bother odor-sensitive individuals.

LAUREL.
See *Antidesma; Laurus; Prunus; Umbellularia.*

LAUREL SUMAC.
See *Rhus.*

Laurelia. 8
Two species of tall evergreen trees from Chile grown in California. The 3-inch-long, rounded leaves are very glossy. Neither species is a good choice for the allergy-free garden.

Laurentia (Isotoma) fluviatilis. ✽ 1
BLUE STAR CREEPER, ISOTOMA. Very low-growing perennial for zones 7–10. Related to *Lobelia*, its tiny leaves and blue, star-shaped flowers make a beautiful ground cover for fall. Requires regular feeding and ample water to thrive.

Laurophyllus. ✱ 10
Small evergreen tree or shrub from South Africa. Dioecious but not sold sexed.

Laurus nobilis. males ✱ 9, females ✽ 2
BAY, GRECIAN LAUREL, ROMAN LAUREL, ROYAL BAY, SWEET BAY, SWEET LAUREL. A large, slow-growing evergreen tree with aromatic leaves that are used in cooking. Hardy into zone 6, the SWEET BAY is a popular large container plant. The males of these separate-sexed trees produce abundant allergenic pollen. Allergy to the pollen is fairly common, and

cross-reaction allergies caused by eating foods flavored with the leaves are also not uncommon. *Laurus* is not usually sold sexed except for the cultivar 'Saratoga', which is a male and should not be used.

LAURUSTINUS.
See *Viburnum*.

Lavandula. 📷   6
LAVENDER. Several species of evergreen, gray-leafed shrubby plants with fragrant leaves and flowers used in sachets and for perfumes. Although the pollen is rarely allergenic, LAVENDERS are a common cause of allergy in those who are sensitive to perfumes and other strong odors. *Oil of lavender*, made from the fresh flowers and leaves, is known to cause skin rash.

Lavatera.   3
TREE MALLOW. Annuals and sub shrubs grown as perennials in zones 9 and 10, and as fast-growing annuals or pot plants elsewhere. The rosy pink or lavender flowers resemble HOLLYHOCK and are attractive to hummingbirds. All MALLOWS are easy to grow and not fussy about soil or water.

LAVENDER.
See *Lavandula*.

LAVENDER COTTON.
See *Santolina*.

LAVENDER MIST.
See *Thalictrum*.

LAVENDER STARFLOWER.
See *Grewia occidentalis*.

LAWNS.
Lawns are a leading factor in allergy in the United States, because of the pollen that they produce when flowering, the airborne mildew and mold spores that often thrive in turf, and the host of pollen-producing weeds that are often part of the average lawn.

When selecting grass for a lawn, choose slow-growing, disease-resistant varieties that do not flower when kept mowed short. TALL FESCUES are good choices for many areas because they do not bloom while short. Ordinary BERMUDA GRASS lawns, on the other hand, flower at almost any length and are constant, year-round sources of potent allergenic pollen. HYBRID BERMUDA GRASS, however, grows more slowly, flowers less, and is a far better choice.

To keep a lawn in good shape it is necessary to fertilize it regularly with high-nitrogen fertilizer, water it frequently, and keep it mowed weekly during the growing season. With some lawns (BENT GRASS or BERMUDA, for instance), it may be necessary to mow every two or three days. Keeping the blades on the lawnmower sharp is always a good idea, too. (A note about lawn fertilizer: Some lawns in warm areas may benefit from as much as eight pounds of actual nitrogen per year per 1,000 square feet. To simplify this, with a common high-nitrogen fertilizer like ammonium sulfate (21-0-0), these lawns could use up to forty pounds annually on a section of lawn that measures about 35 by 30 feet.)

Most lawn grasses release their pollen in the early morning, and it is best to mow later in the day to reduce the amount of pollen scattered by the mower blades. Do not mow grass when it is still damp from dew or rain because this can cause fungus diseases to spread. Many people who are allergic to grass pollen will also be allergic to the gases given off (VOCs) during mowing. If you are highly allergic to grass, get someone else to cut it for you, or consider planting a low-allergy ground cover.

Spraying or spreading chemical insecticides on your lawn is not recommended, because in many cases these lawn chemicals cause allergies themselves. Likewise, the products that fertilize grass and kill dandelions at the same time are not safe either. They have been implicated as causing leukemia in cats and dogs that play on treated lawns. If these can cause cancer in cats and dogs, they can't be all that good for kids or adults either.

If bald spots occur in a good lawn they should be worked up and new sod placed, or seed, fertilizer, and mulch should be sprinkled on the problem spot. When trying to grow a lawn from seed it is good policy to cover the seed with at least a quarter-inch of manure or similar mulch. If bare spots are left in a lawn, they are usually quickly filled with broadleaf weeds or with ANNUAL BLUEGRASS (*Poa annua*), which blooms at almost any height and causes allergy.

The development of all-female and low pollen-producing lawn grass cultivars offers much promise for allergy-free lawns of the future. For further information on lawn grasses, see *Agropyron* (QUACKGRASS); *Arrhenatherum elatius* (TALL OATGRASS); *Bromus* (BROME GRASS); *Buchloe dactyloides* (BUFFALO GRASS); and *Pennisetum clandestinum* (KIKUYUGRASS).

LAWSON CYPRESS.
See *Chamaecyparis*.

Layia platyglossa. *4*
TIDYTIPS. California native flowering annual. Fast-growing in sunny areas.

LEATHERLEAF.
See *Viburnum*.

LEATHERLEAF FERN.
See *Rumohra adiantiformis*.

Lechea. *5*
A wildflower native to the northeastern United States and related to the ROCKROSE, the seed is occasionally used in wildflower mixes. Suspected of causing limited allergy, *Lechea* grows best in dry, sandy soils.

Ledebouria socialis. ❋ *2*
JESSOP. Bulbous, succulent-leafed houseplants that need bright light to grow well.

Ledum. *5*
Hardy shrubs for cold, damp areas. Related to HEATHER.

Leitneria floridana. *males ✹9, females ❋ 1*
CORKWOOD. Small separate-sexed, deciduous trees or shrubs, native to wet forest areas of the southeast United States.

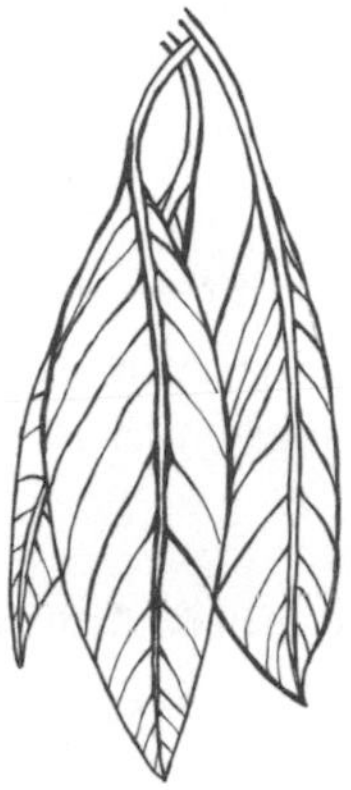

Leitneria floridana

Lemaireocereus thurberi.
See CACTUS.

LEMON.
See *Citrus*.

LEMON VERBENA.
See *Aloysia triphylla*.

LEMONADE BERRY.
See *Rhus integrifolia*.

LENTEN ROSE.
See *Helleborus*.

Leonotis. *5*
LION'S EAR, LION'S TAIL. Orange flower spikes on tall, erect, frost-tender perennials. Odd-smelling (but not unpleasant) leaves. A member of the MINT family.

Leontopodium alpinum. *8*
EDELWEISS. Low-growing woolly-leafed hardy perennial, usually with white flowers.

LEOPARD FLOWER.
See *Belamcanda chinensis*.

LEOPARD PLANT.
See *Ligularia.*

LEOPARD'S BANE.
See *Doronicum; Senecio.*

Lepidorrhachis. 7
Subtropical palms trees common in Florida.

Lepidozamia. 8
Palm-like plants from Australia, grown in zone 10. Dioecious, but not sold sexed.

Leptospermum. 4
TEA TREE. Small native Australian trees bearing many tiny flowers.

Leucodendron. males 8, females ✳ 1
SILVER TREE. Large group of evergreen shrubs and trees from South Africa, used as landscape plants in California. These are separate-sexed, but not usually sold sexed.

Leucojum. ✳ 2
SNOWFLAKE. Hardy spring-blooming bulbs.

Leucophyllum frutescens. ✳ 2
TEXAS RANGERS. Native Texas tall desert shrub with gray leaves and rosy-purple bell-shaped flowers. Drought tolerant.

Leucospermum. 4
PINCUSHION. Shrubby *Protea* relative with long clusters of showy tubular flowers; difficult to grow outside of zone 10.

Leucothoe. 4
FETTERBUSH. Evergreen shrubs native to southeast United States, hardy to zone 5. Need moist, acid soil with good drainage and partial shade to thrive. Produces tall spikes of white flowers. All parts of plant are extremely poisonous.

Levisticum officinale. 3
LOVAGE. Hardy perennial herb grows to 6 feet. Aromatic seeds.

Lewisia. ✳ 1
BITTERROOT. Hardy perennials with succulent-like leaves and clusters of white, pink, or red flowers; good choice for rock gardens. Plants need perfect drainage.

Liatris. 4
GAYFEATHER. Tall, showy perennials with spikes of white- or rose-colored flowers.

Libocedrus.
See *Calocedrus.*

LICHI NUT.
See *Litchi chinensis.*

Licuala. ✳ 1
A large group of small palm trees, some hardy into zone 9. They are good in containers and occasionally used as houseplants.

LICURI PALM.
See *Syagrus.*

LIGNUM-VITAE.
See *Guaiacum sanctum.*

Ligularia (Farfugium). 6
LEOPARD PLANT. Foliage plant hardy in zones 6–10; elsewhere a houseplant grown for its long, leathery, thick leaves.

Ligustrum. 📷 8
PRIVET. Deciduous or evergreen shrubs or small trees, often used as hedges in all parts of the United States. PRIVET is among our most common landscape shrubs, but as members of the OLIVE family, they present several allergy problems. The fragrance of the many small white flowers may cause allergy in odor-sensitive people, and the pollen from the flowers also causes an often severe reaction, especially in people already allergic to OLIVE pollen. Keep PRIVET hedges low and well-pruned to discourage blooming. Plants and seeds are poisonous.

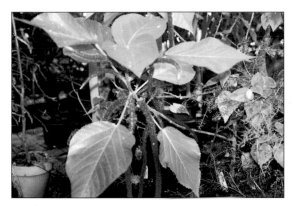

Acalypha hispida
CHENILLE PLANT
Female
1   Page 30

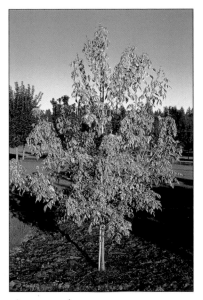

Acer negundo
'Variegata'
BOX ELDER
A female tree
1   Page 31

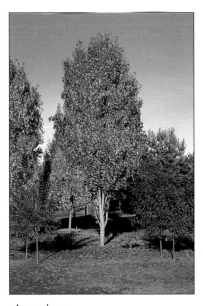

Acer rubrum
'Bowhall'
RED MAPLE
A female tree
1   Page 32

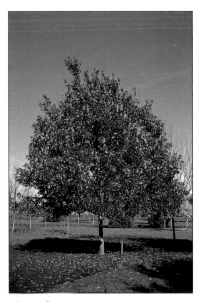

Acer rubrum
'October Glory'
RED MAPLE
A female tree
1   Page 32

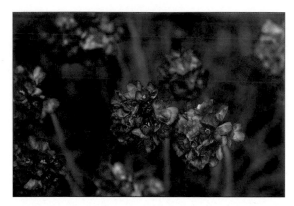

Armeria maritima
THRIFT
1   Page 43

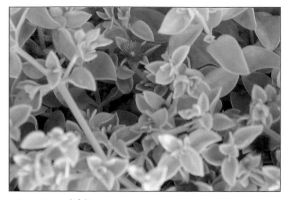

Aptenia cordifolia
RED-APPLE ICEPLANT
1   Page 41

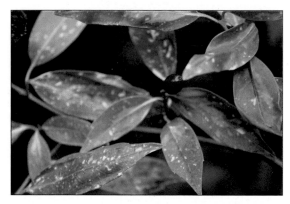

Aucuba japonica
GOLD DUST PLANT
A female shrub
1   Page 45

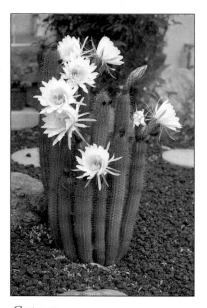

Cactus sp.
1   Page 60

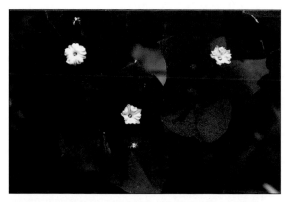

Bougainvillea sp.
'Raspberry Ice'
1   Page 55

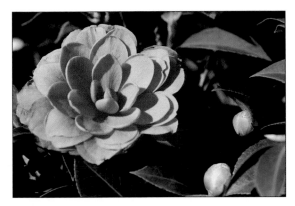

Camellia japonica
TINGLEY
A formal double
1   Page 62

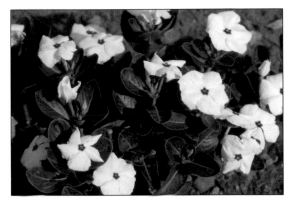

Catharanthus roseus (Vinca rosea)
PERIWINKLE
Annual vinca
1   Page 67

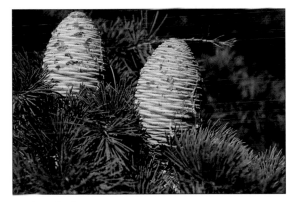

Cedrus deodara
CEDAR DEODARA
1   Page 69

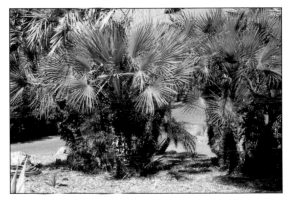

Chamaerops humilis
EUROPEAN FAN PALM
A female tree
1   Page 72

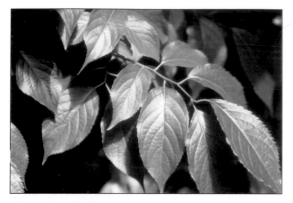

Eucommia ulmoides
HARDY RUBBER TREE
A female tree
1   Page 99

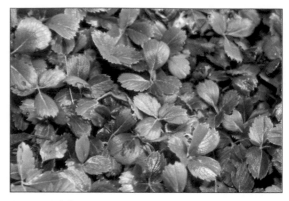

Fragaria chiloensis
WILD STRAWBERRY
Groundcover
1   Page 107

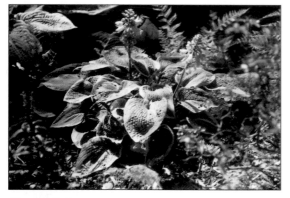

Hosta hybrid
HOSTA
1   Page 123

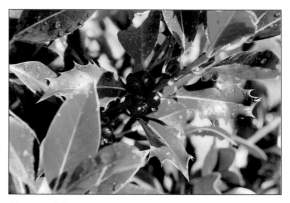

Ilex aquifolium
ENGLISH HOLLY
A female tree
1   Page 126

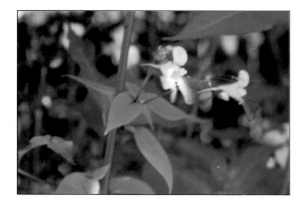

Impatiens sp.
BUSY LIZZY
1   Page 126

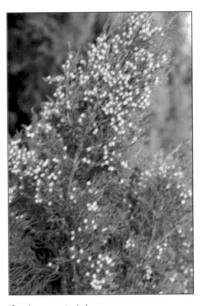

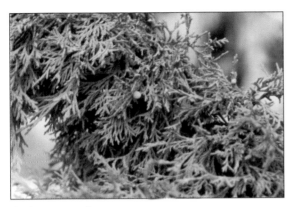

Juniperus scopulorum
'Platinum'
A female shrub
1   Page 133

Juniperus virginiana
'Manhattan Blue'
A female tree
1   Page 133

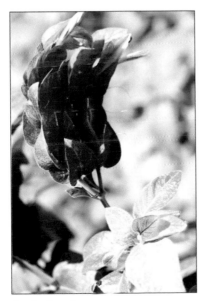

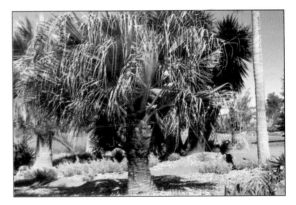

Livistona chinensis
CHINESE FAN PALM
1   Page 143

Justica brandegeana
SHRIMP PLANT
1   Page 133

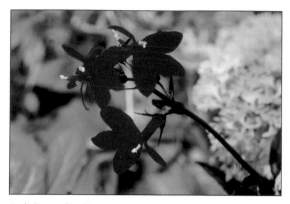

Lobelia cardinalis
PERENNIAL RED LOBELIA
1   Page 143

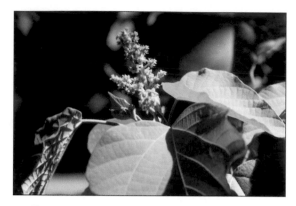

Mallotus japonica
A female tree
1   Page 148

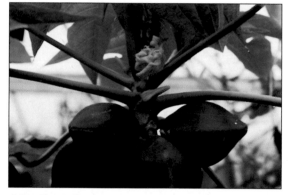

Mangifera indica
MANGO
Female
1   Page 149

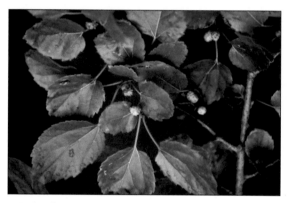

Morus alba
WHITE MULBERRY
Female tree with unripe fruit
1   Page 156

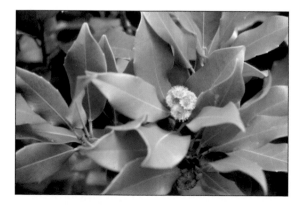

Olmediella betschlerana
GUATEMALAN HOLLY
Female flowers on female tree
1   Page 164

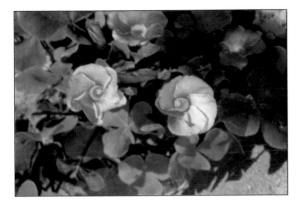

Oxalis hybrid
1   Page 166

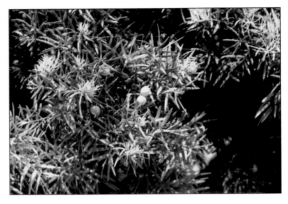

Podocarpus gracilior
FERN PINE
A female tree
1   Page 180

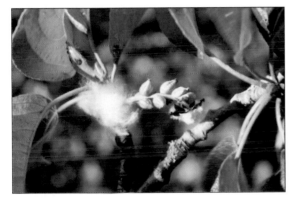

Populus maximowiezii
JAPANESE POPLAR
A female tree
1   Page 182

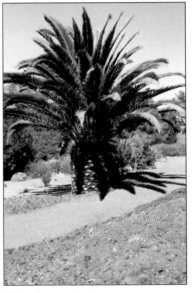

Phoenix canariensis
CANARY ISLAND DATE PALM
A female tree
1   Page 175

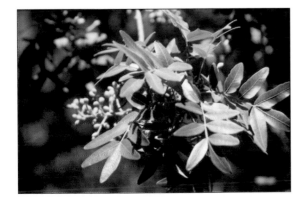

Pistache atlantica
MT. ATLAS PISTACHE
A female tree
1   Page 178

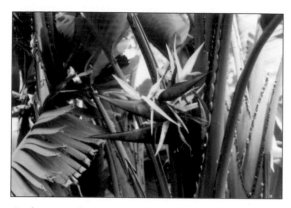

Strelitzia nicolai
GIANT BIRD-OF-PARADISE
1   Page 218

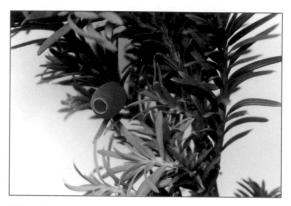

Taxus baccata
ENGLISH YEW
A female shrub
1   Page 224

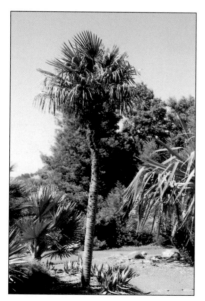

Trachycarpus fortunei
WINDMILL PALM
A female tree
1   Page 229

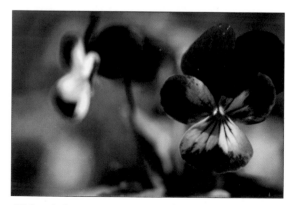

Viola tricolor
JOHNNY-JUMP-UP
1   Page 238

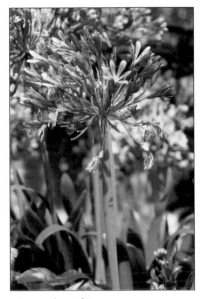

Agapanthus africanus
LILY-OF-THE-NILE
2   Page 34

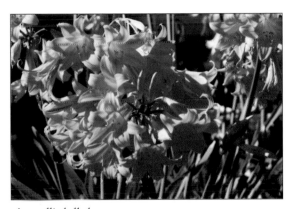

Amaryllis belladonna
NAKED LADY
2   Page 38

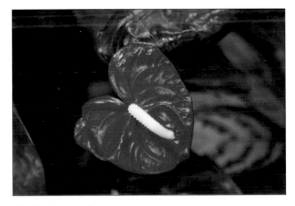

Anthurium andraeanum
ANTHURIUM
2   Page 40

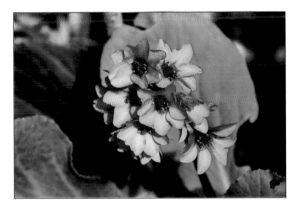

Bergenia crassifolia
2   Page 50

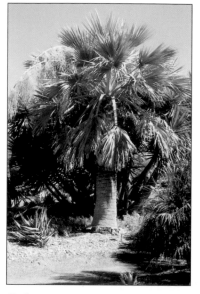

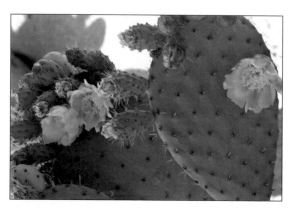

Optunia
PRICKLY CACTUS
2   Page 60

Brahea armata
MEXICAN BLUE PALM
2   Page 56

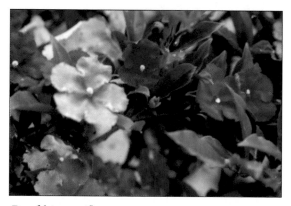

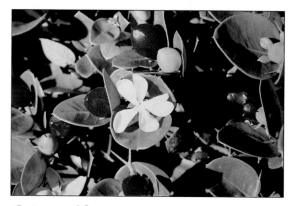

Brunfelsia pauciflora
YESTERDAY-TODAY-AND-TOMORROW
2   Page 57

Carissa grandiflora
NATAL PLUM
2   Page 64

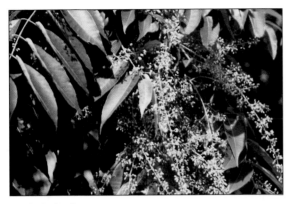

Cedrela fissilis
CIGAR BOX TREE
2   Page 68

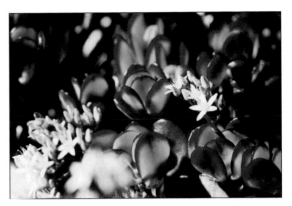

Crassula
JADE PLANT
2   Page 83

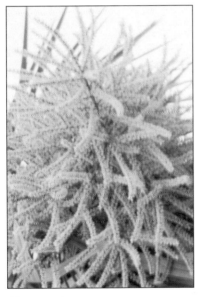

Dracaena draco
DRAGON TREE
2   Page 93

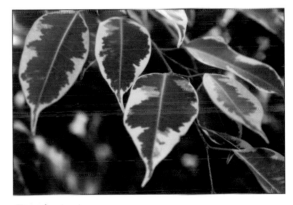

Ficus benjamina
Variegated
2   Page 104

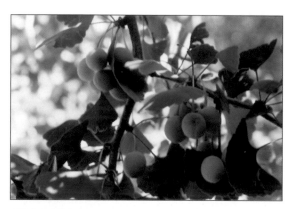

Ginkgo biloba
A female tree
2   Page 112

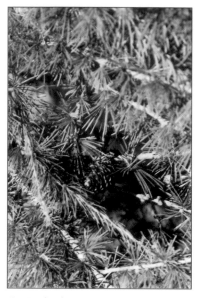

Larix decidua
EUROPEAN LARCH
2   Page 137

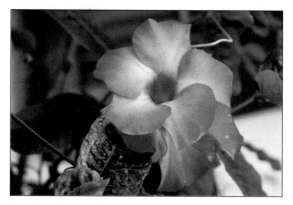

Mandevilla splendens
EVERGREEN MANDEVILLA
2   Page 149

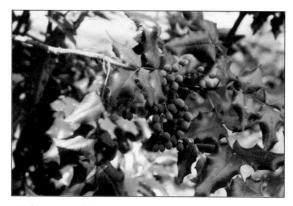

Mahonia aquifolium
OREGON GRAPE
2   Page 148

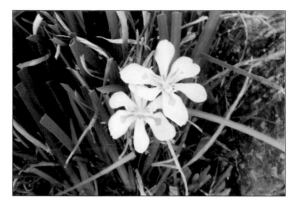

Moraea Dietes
2   Page 91

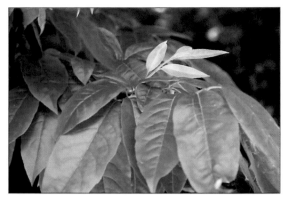

Oxydendrum arboreum
SOURWOOD TREE
2   Page 167

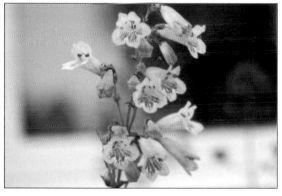

Penstemon heterophyllus
BEARD TONGUE
2   Page 172

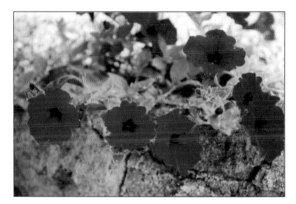

Petunia hybrid
'Purple Wave'
2   Page 173

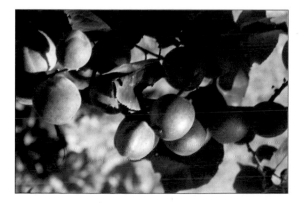

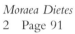

Prunus armeniaca
APRICOT
2   Page 186

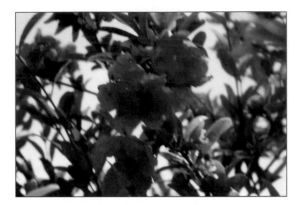

Punica granatum
POMEGRANATE
Double flowered
2   Page 188

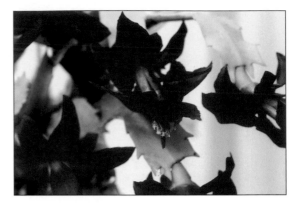

Schlumbergera bridgesii
CHRISTMAS CACTUS
2   Page 206

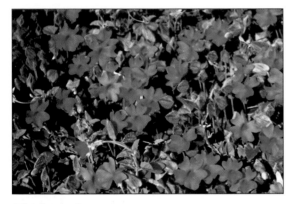

Thunbergia alata
BLACK-EYED SUSAN VINE
2   Page 226

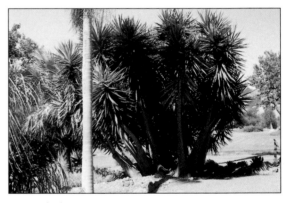

Yucca elephantipes
GIANT YUCCA
2   Page 247

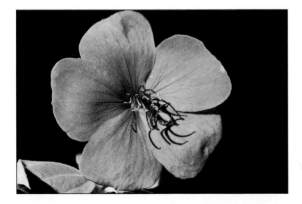

Tibouchina urvilleana
PRINCESS FLOWER
2   Page 227

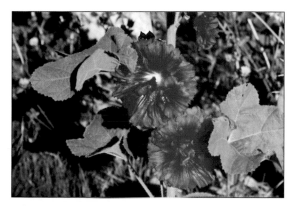

Alcea rosea
HOLLYHOCK
3   Page 36

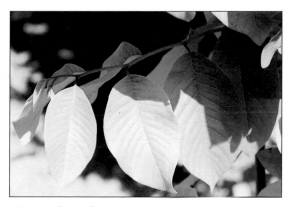

Annona cherimola
CHERIMOYA
3   Page 40

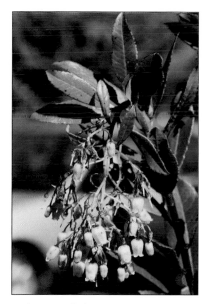

Arbutus undedo
STRAWBERRY TREE
3   Page 42

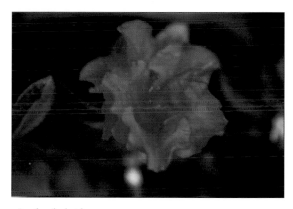

Azalea hybrid
AZALEA
3   Page 194

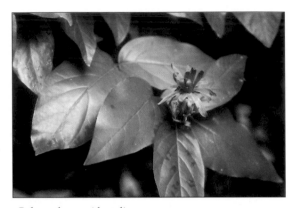

Calycanthus occidentalis
SPICE BUSH
3   Page 62

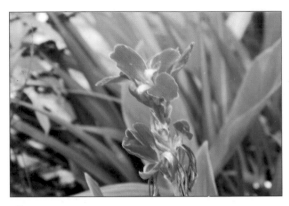

Canna sp.
CANNA LILY
3   Page 63

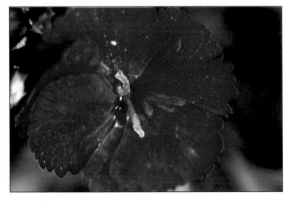

Dianthus sp.
PINKS
3   Page 90

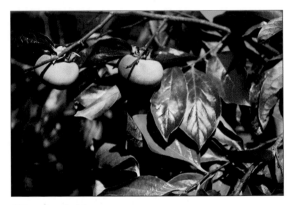

Diospyros kaki
JAPANESE PERSIMMON
'Fuyu'
3   Page 92

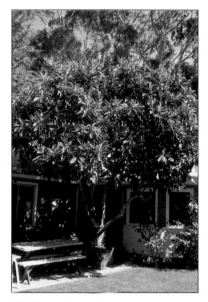

Eriobotrya japonica
LOQUAT TREE
3 Page 98

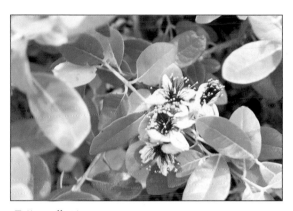

Feijoa sellowiana
PINEAPPLE GUAVA
3   Page 103

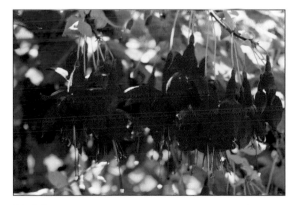

Fuchsia sp.
3   Page 108

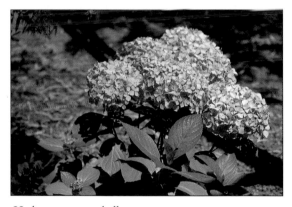

Hydrangea macrophylla
HYDRANGEA
3   Page 124

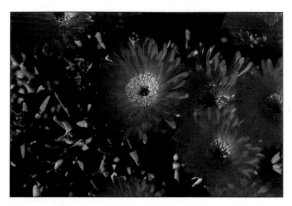

Lampranthus aurantiacus
ICEPLANT
3   Page 136

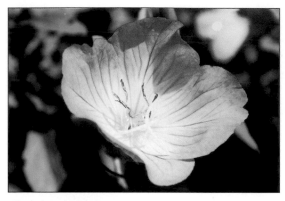

Oenothera berlandii
MEXICAN EVENING PRIMROSE
3   Page 163

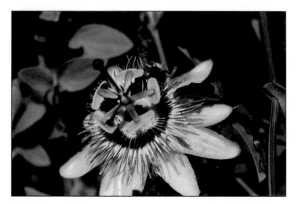

Passiflora edulis
PASSION FLOWER
3   Page 170

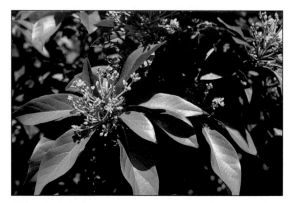

Persea americana
AVOCADO
3   Page 173

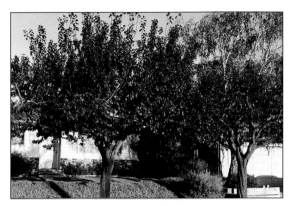

Prunus sp.
RED LEAF PLUMS
3   Page 186

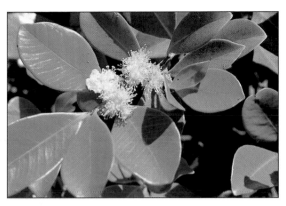

Psidium cattleianum
STRAWBERRY GUAVA
3   Page 187

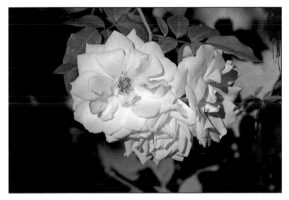

Rosa hybrid
'Iceberg'
3   Page 197

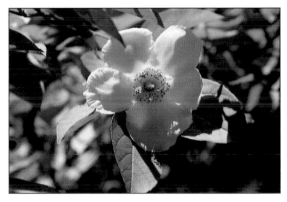

Stewartia Pseudocamellia
'Koreana'
3   Page 217

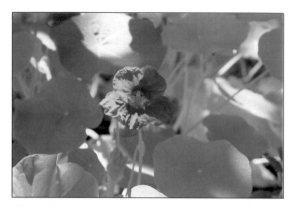

Tropaeolum majus
NASTURTIUM
3   Page 231

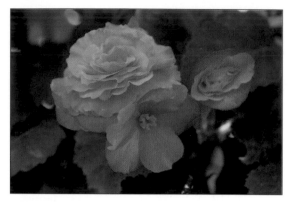

Tuberous begonia
Male flower (top); female flower (bottom)
Male Sterile
1   Page 49

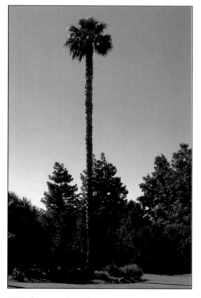

Washingtonia robusta
MEXICAN FAN PALM
3   Page 240

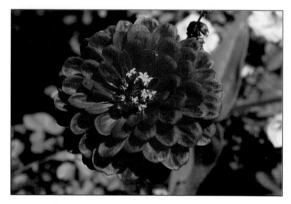

Zinnia elegans
ZINNIA
3   Page 251

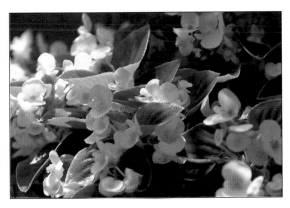

Begonia sp.
Fibrous Begonia
4   Page 49

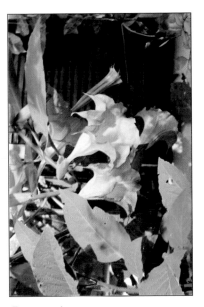

Brugmansia sp.
ANGEL TRUMPET
4   Page 57

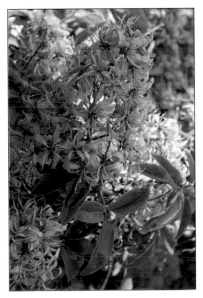

Calodendrum capense
CAPE CHESTNUT TREE
4   Page 62

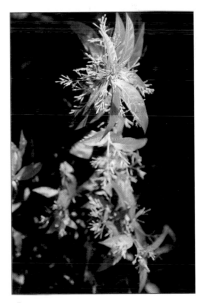

Cestrum nocturnum
NIGHT BLOOMING JASMINE
4   Page 71

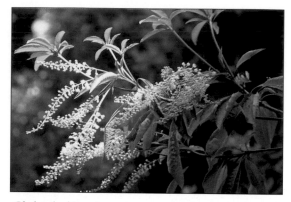

Clethra barbinervis
SUMMERSWEET TREE
4   Page 77

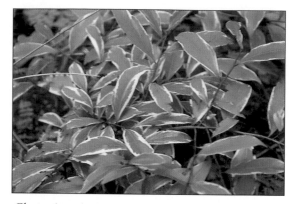

Cleyera japonica
4   Page 77

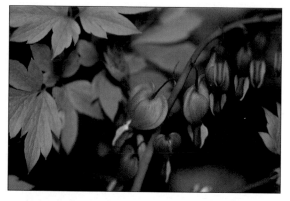

Dicentra spectabilis
BLEEDING HEARTS
4   Page 91

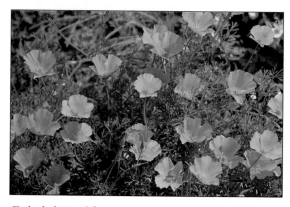

Eschscholzia californica
CALIFORNIA POPPY
4   Page 99

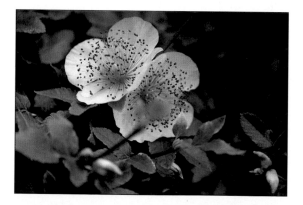

Eucryphia glutinosa
4   Page 100

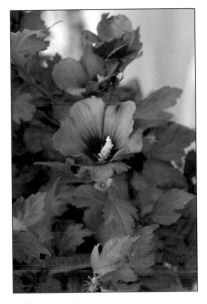

Hibiscus syriacus
ROSE-OF-SHARON
4   Page 121

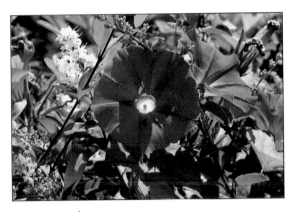

Ipomoea tricolor
MORNING GLORY
4   Page 127

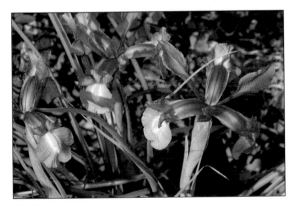

Iris Japonica
IRIS
4   Page 127

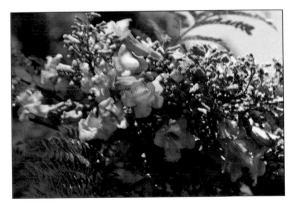

Jacaranda mimosifolia
JACARANDA
4   Page 129

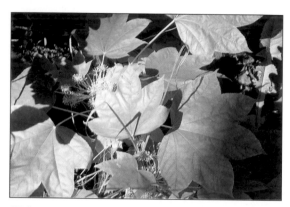

Kalopanax septemlobus
CASTOR OIL TREE
4   Page 134

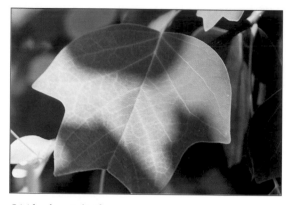

Liridendron tulipifera
TULIP POPLAR
4   Page 142

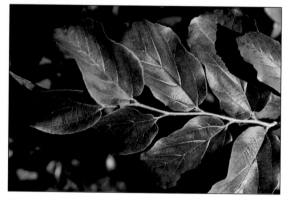

Parrotia persia
PARROT BEAK
4   Page 170

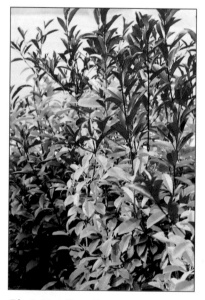

Photinia × Fraseri
PHOTINIA
4   Page 175

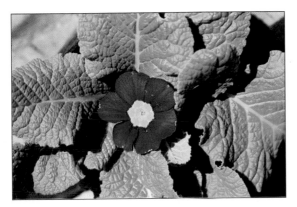

Primula polyantha
PRIMROSE
4   Page 184

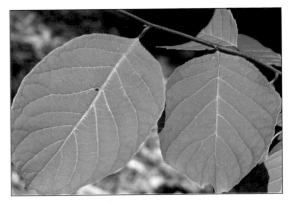

Pterostyrax psilophylia
EPAULETTE TREE
4   Page 188

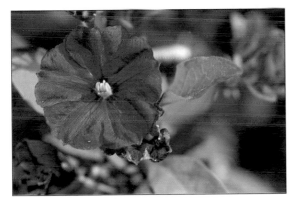

Solanum rantonnetii
BLUE SOLANUM
4   Page 212

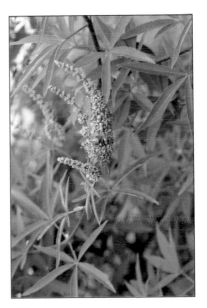

Vitex sp.
CHASTE TREE
4   Page 238

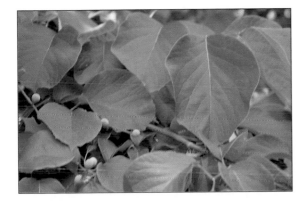

Styrax obassia
FRAGRANT SNOWBELL TREE
4   Page 218

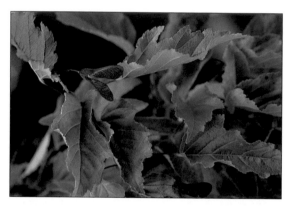

Acer tataricum
TARTARIAN MAPLE
5   Page 33

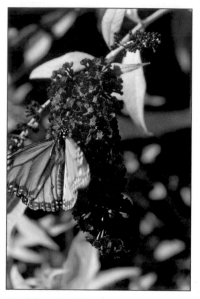

Buddleia davidii
BUTTERFLY BUSH
5   Page 58

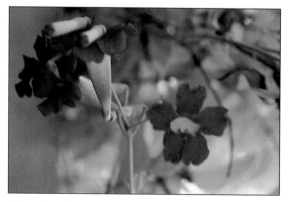

Campsis radicans
SCARLET TRUMPET VINE
5   Page 63

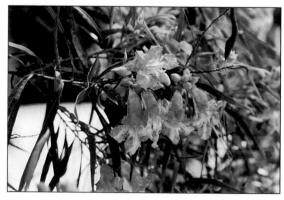

Chilopsis linearis
DESERT WILLOW
5   Page 73

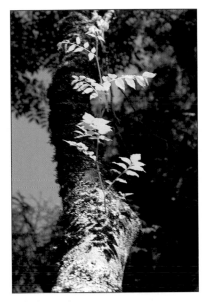

Cladrastis lutea
YELLOWWOOD TREE
5   Page 76

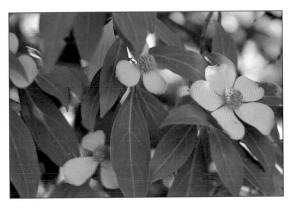

Cornus sp.
DOGWOOD
5   Page 81

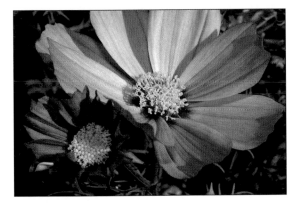

Cosmos bipinnatus
COSMOS
5   Page 82

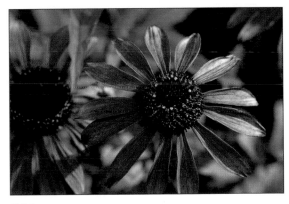

Echinacea purpurea
PURPLE CONEFLOWER
5   Page 95

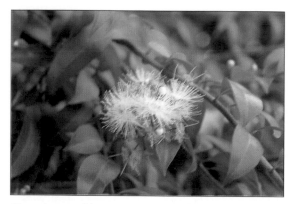

Eugenia myrtifolia
EUGENIA
5   Page 100

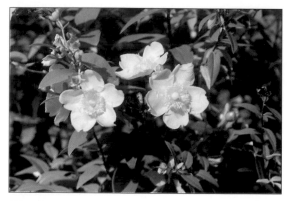

Hypericum sp.
SAINT JOHN'S WORT
5   Page 125

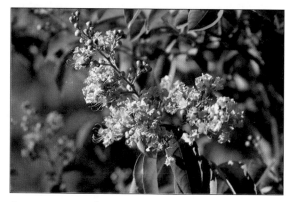

Lagerstroemia indica
CRAPE MYRTLE
5   Page 136

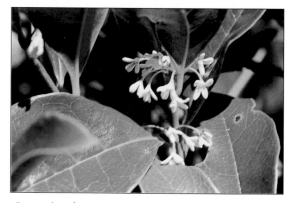

Osmanthus fragrans
SWEET OLIVE
5   Page 166

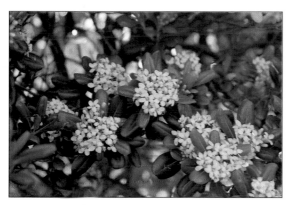

Pittosporum tobira
5   Page 179

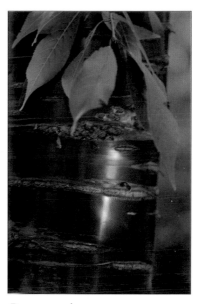

Prunus serrula
BIRCH BARK CHERRY
5   Page 186

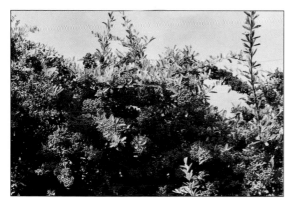

Pyracantha sp.
FIRETHORN
5   Page 189

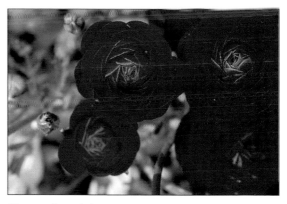

Ranunculus asiaticus
RANUNCULUS
5   Page 192

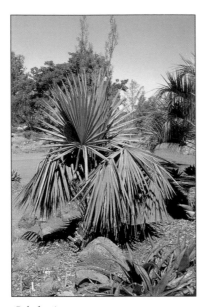

Sabal minor
SABAL PALM
5   Page 200

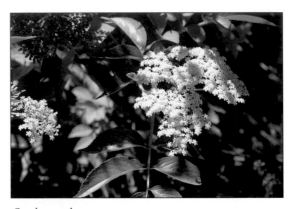

Sambucus glauca
ELDERBERRY
5   Page 203

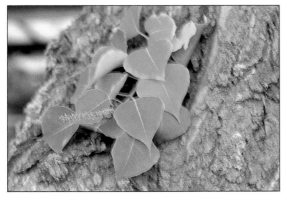

Sapium sebiferum
CHINESE TALLOW TREE
A female tree
5   Page 204

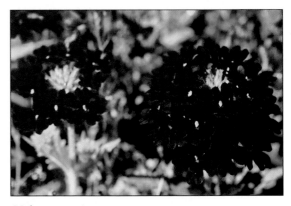

Verbena peruviana
PERENNIAL VERBENA
5   Page 236

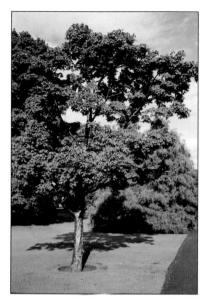

Acer griseum
PAPERBARK MAPLE
6   Page 31

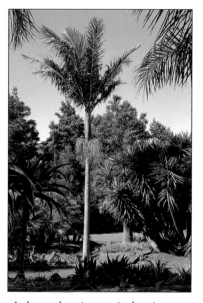

Archontophoenix cunninghamiana
KING PALM
6   Page 42

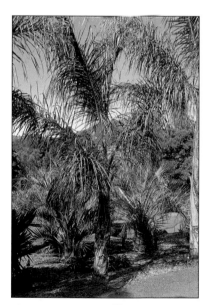

Arecastrum romanzoffianum
QUEEN PALM
6   Page 42

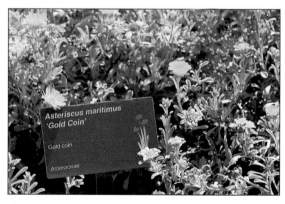

Asteriscus maritmus
'Gold Coin'
6   Page 45

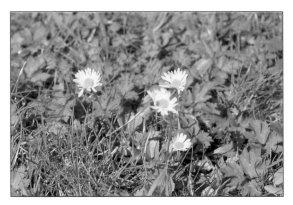

Bellis perennis
ENGLSIH DAISY
6   Page 50

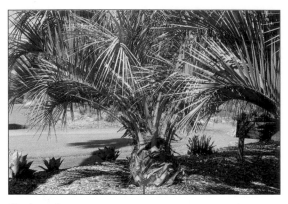

Butia capitate
PINDO PALM
6   Page 59

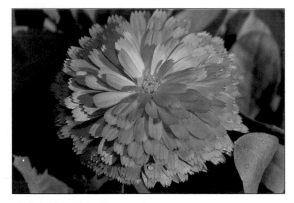

Calendula officinalis
CALENDULA
6   Page 60

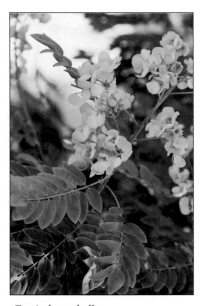

Cassia leptophylla
SENNA
6   Page 66

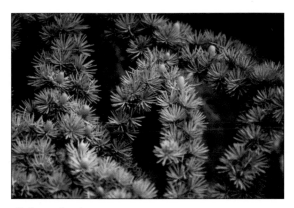

Cedrus atlantica
ATLANTIC CEDAR
A male tree
6   Page 69

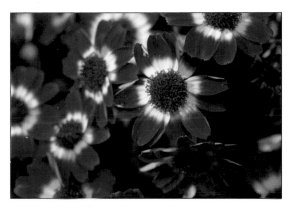

Cineraria hybridus
CINERARIA
6   Page 76

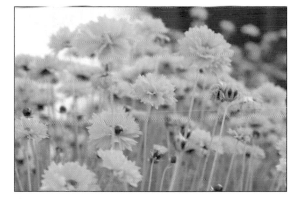

Coreopsis grandiflora
COREOPSIS
6   Page 81

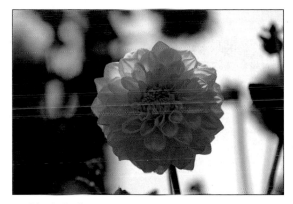

Dahlia hybrid
6   Page 88

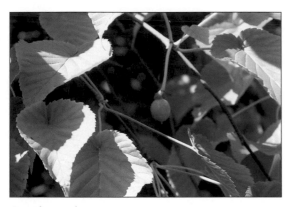

Davidia involucrata
DOVE TREE
6   Page 89

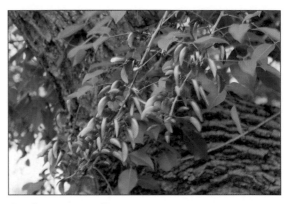

Erythrina crista-galli
COCKSPUR CORAL TREE
6   Page 99

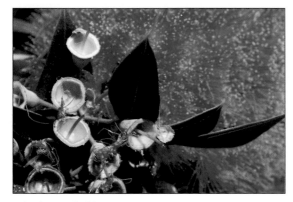

Eucalyptus ficifolia
6   Page 99

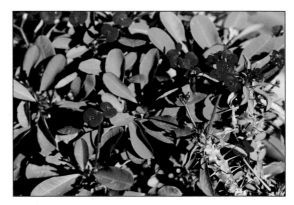

Euphorbia milii
CROWN-OF-THORNS
6   Page 100

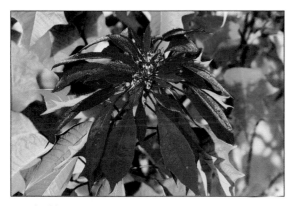

Euphorbia poinsettia
POINSETTIA
6   Page 100

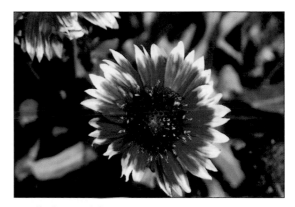

Gaillardia grandiflora
GALLIARDIA
6   Page 110

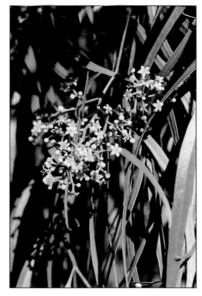

Geijera parvifolia
AUSTRALIAN WILLOW
6   Page 111

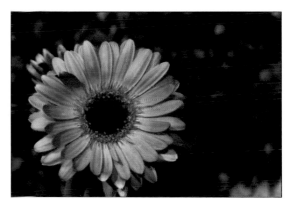

Gerbera jamesonii
TRANSVAAL DAISY
6   Page 112

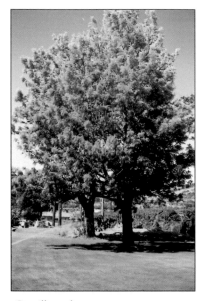

Grevillea robusta
SILK OAK
6   Page 115

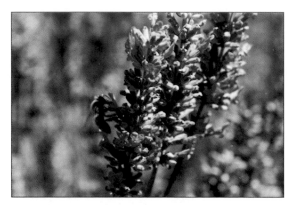

Lavandula angustifolia
ENGLISH LAVENDER
6   Page 138

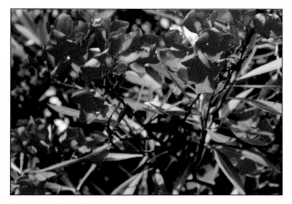

Nerium oleander
OLEANDER
6   Page 160

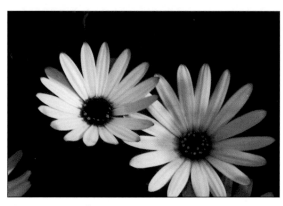

Osteospermum fruticosum
AFRICAN DAISY
6   Page 166

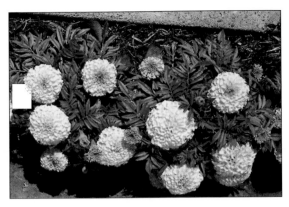

Tagetes patula
MARIGOLDS
6   Page 222

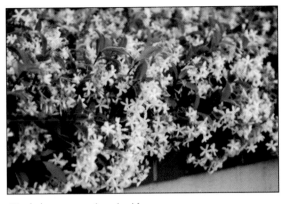

Trachelospermum jasminoides
STAR JASMINE
6   Page 228

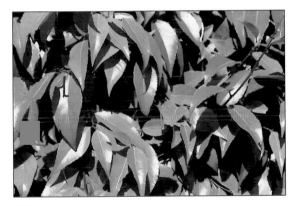

Xylosma congestum
SHINY XYLOSMA
A male shrub
6 Page 246

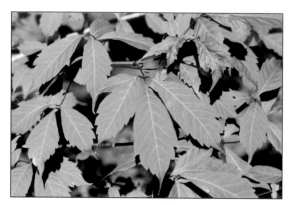

Acer cissifolium
IVY-LEAFED MAPLE
A male tree
7   Page 30

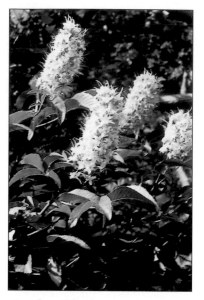

Aesculus californica
CALIFORNIA BUCKEYE
7   Page 34

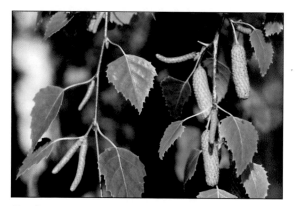

Betula sp.
BIRCH TREE
Male flowers (left); female flowers (right)
7   Page 51

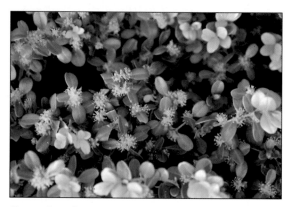

Buxus japonica
BOXWOOD w/ separate male & female flowers
7   Page 59

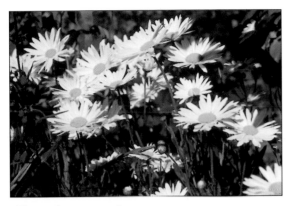

Chrysanthemum maximum
SHASTA DAISY
Single flowered
7   Page 75

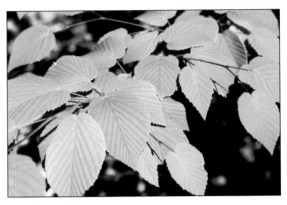

Corylopsis glabrescens
WINTER HAZEL
7   Page 82

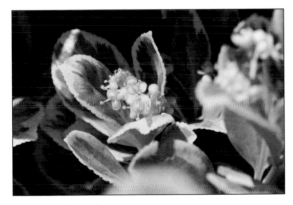

Euonymus japonica
JAPANESE EVERGREEN EUONYMUS
7   Page 100

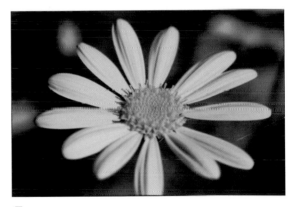

Euryops acraeus
YELLOW DAISY
7   Page 101

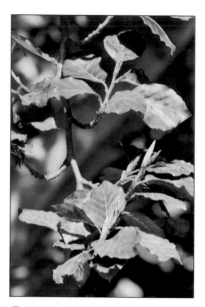

Fagus americana
BEECH TREE
7 Page 102

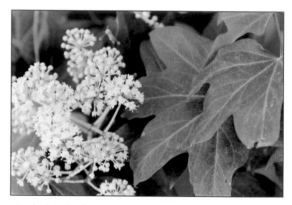

Fatshedera lizei
FATSHEDERA
Note pollen on leaves
7 Page 102

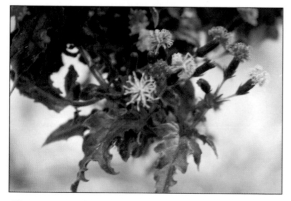

Gynura aurantiaca
PUPRLE VELVET PLANT
7 Page 116

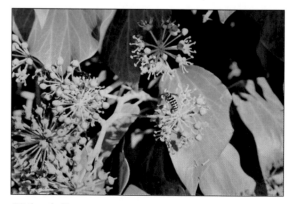

Hedera helix
ENGLISH IVY
7 Page 118

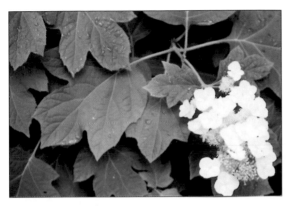

Hydrangea quercifolia
OAKLAEF HYDRANGEA
7   Page 124

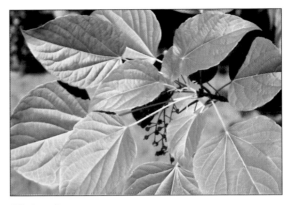

Idesia polycarpa
IGIRI TREE
A male tree
7   Page 126

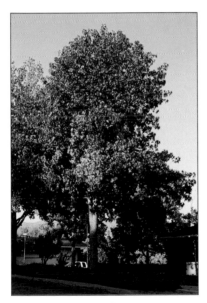

Liquidambar styraciflua
SWEET GUM TREE
7   Page 142

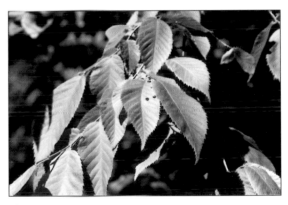

Ostrya virginiana
HOP HORNBEAM
7   Page 166

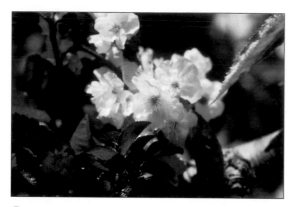

Prunus sp.
SWEET CHERRY
7   Page 185

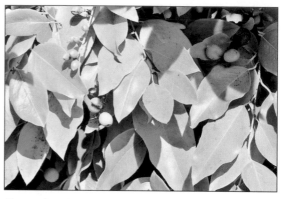

Prunus lyonii
CATALINA CHERRY
7   Page 185

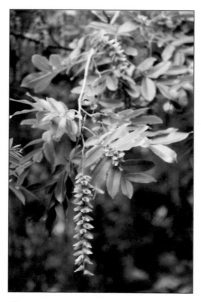

Pterocarya stenoptera
CHINESE WINGNUT TREE
7   Page 188

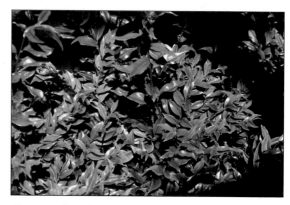

Sarcococca humilis
SWEET BOX
7   Page 204

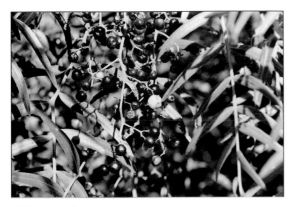

Schinus molle
CALIFORNIA PEPPER TREE
A female tree
7   Page 205

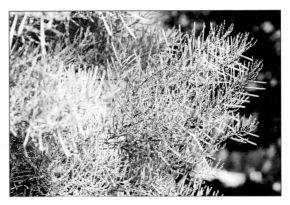

Tamarix sp.
SALT CEDAR
7   Page 223

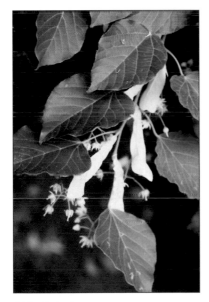

Tilia hybrid
HYBRID BASSWOOD TREE
7   Page 227

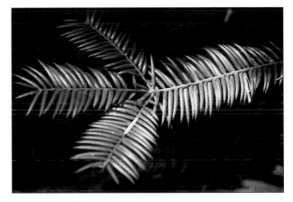

Torreya taxifolia
CALIFORNIA TORREYA
A male tree
7   Page 228

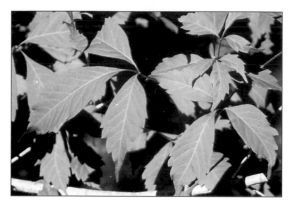

Acer cissifolium
AMAHOGI MAPLE
A male tree
8   Page 30

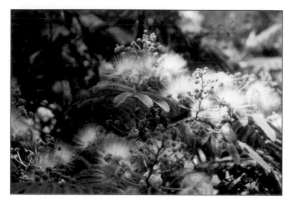

Albizia julibrissin
MIMOSA
8   Page 36

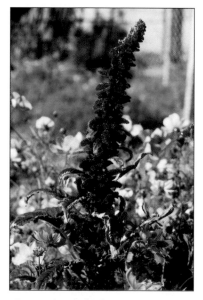

Amaranthus hybrid
AMARANTH
8   Page 37

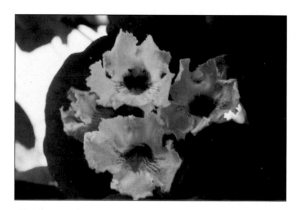

Catalpa speciosa
CATALPA
8   Page 66

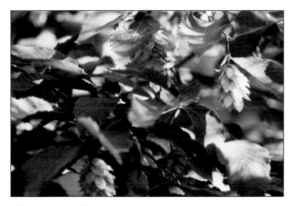

Carpinus betulus
HORNBEAM
8 Page 65

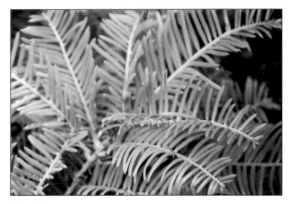

Cephalotaxus sp.
A male shrub
8 Page 70

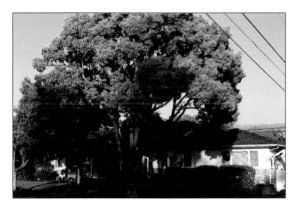

Cinnamomum camphora
CAMPHOR TREE
8 Page 76

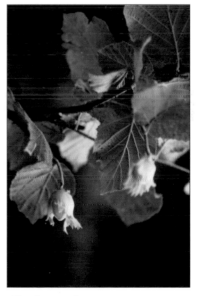

Corylus maxima
FILBERT
8 Page 82

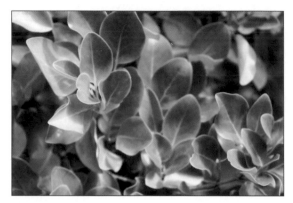

Griselina littoralis
GRISELINA
A male shrub
8   Page 115

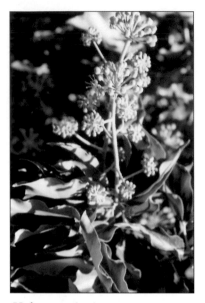

Hedera canariensis
ALGERIAN IVY flowers
8   Page 118

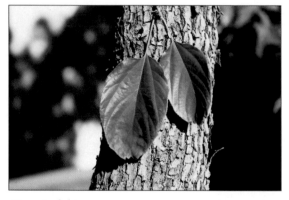

Hovenia dulcis
A male tree
8   Page 123

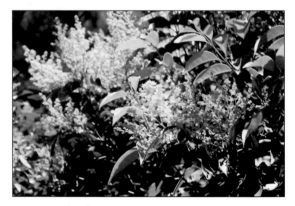

Ligustrum lucidum
GLOSSY PRIVET
8   Page 140

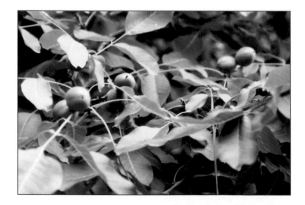

Juglans regia
ENGLISH WALNUT
8   Page 131

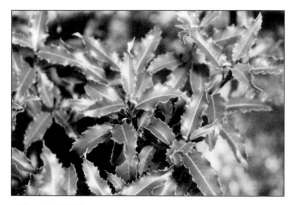

Olearia ilicifolia
HOLLYLEAF OLERIA
8   Page 164

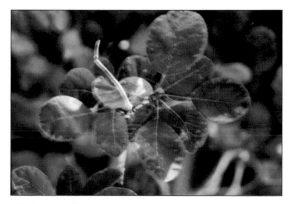

Olearia ilicifolia
HOLLYLEAF OLERIA
8   Page 164

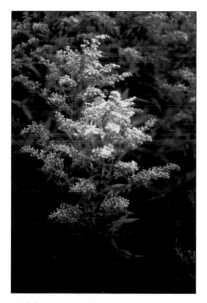

Solidago perennis
GOLDENROD
8   Page 213

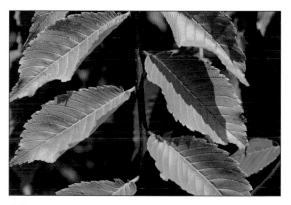

Ulmus americana
AMERICAN ELM
8   Page 233

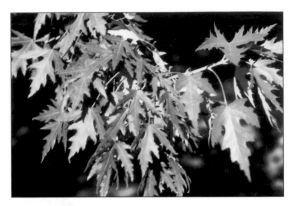

Acer saccharinum
SILVER MAPLE
A male tree
9   Page 32

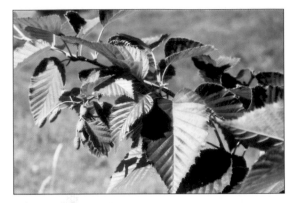

Alnus maximowiczii
JAPANESE SAKHALIN ALDER
9   Page 37

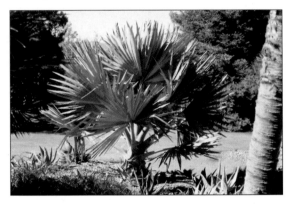

Bismarckia nobilis
A male tree
9   Page 52

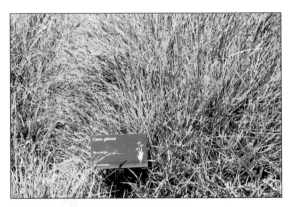

Carex glauca
SEDGE
9   Page 64

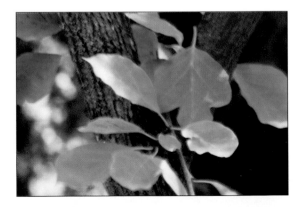

Cudrania tricuspidata
A male tree
9   Page 85

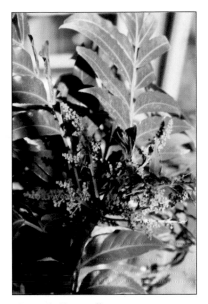

Harpephyllum caffrum
KAFFIR PLUM
A male tree
9   Page 117

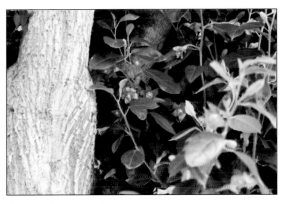

Lagunaria patersonii
COW-ITCH TREE, PRIMROSE TREE
9   Page 136

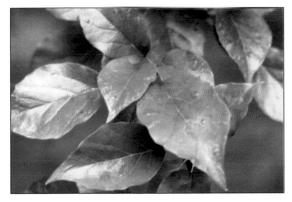

Maclura pomifera
OSAGE ORANGE
A male tree
9   Page 147

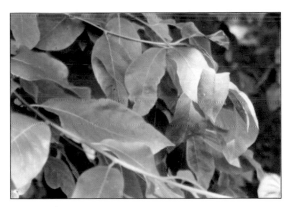

Nyssa sylvatica
SOURWOOD TREE, TUPELO
A male tree
9   Page 162

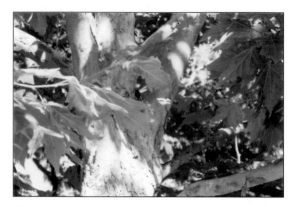

Platanus racemosa
SYCAMORE
9   Page 179

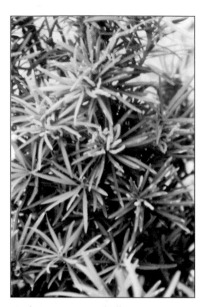

Podocarpus macrophyllus
'Select Spreader'
A male clone
9   Page 180

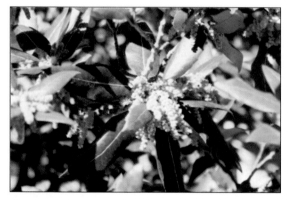

Quercus sp.
LIVE OAK
Male flowers
9   Page 190

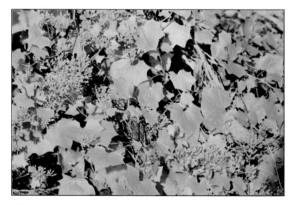

Senecio sp.
GERMAN IVY
9   Page 208

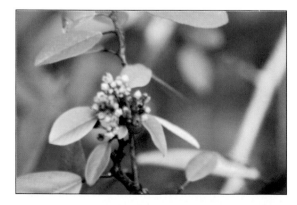

Rhamnus californica
COFFEEBERRY
9   Page 193

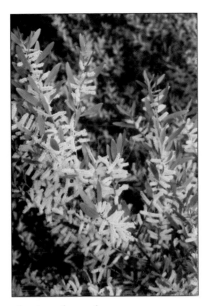

Acacia melanoxylon
BLACK ACACIA
10   Page 29

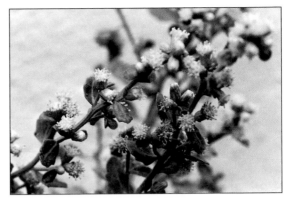

Baccharis sp.
COYOTE BRUSH
A male shrub
10   Page 47

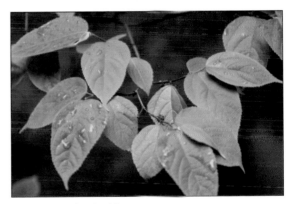

Broussonetia kazinoki
JAPANESE PAPER MULBERRY
A male tree
10   Page 57

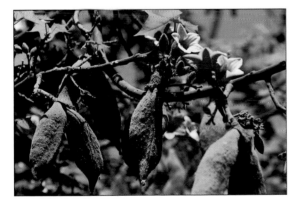

Brachychiton discolor
QUEENSLAND LACEBARK
10   Page 55

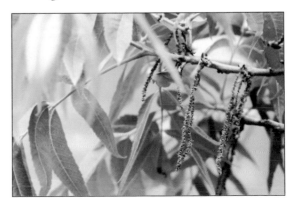

Carya illinoensis
PECAN TREE
Male flowers
10   Page 65

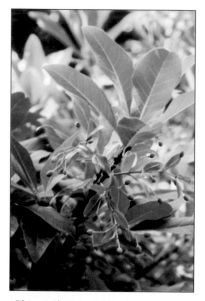

Chionanthus virginicus
FRINGE TREE
A male tree
10   Page 74

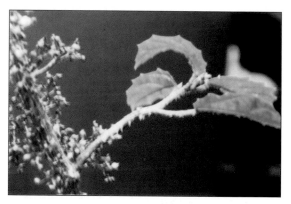

Cnidoscolus urens
TREAD–SOFTLY
A male plant
10   Page 78

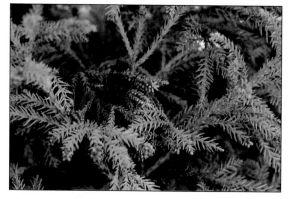

Cryptomeria japonica
JAPANESE CEDAR
10   Page 84

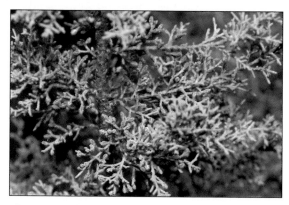

Cupressus arizonica
ARIZONA CYPRESS
Male flowers
10   Page 86

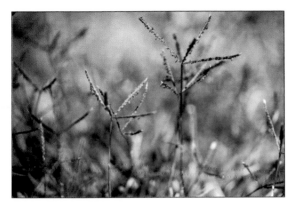

Cynodon dactylon
COMMON BERMUDA GRASS
10   Page 86

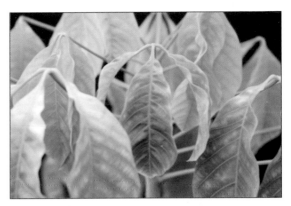

Hevea brasiliensis
PARA RUBBER TREE
10   Page 120

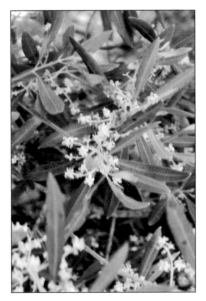

Olea europaea
OLIVE TREE
10   Page 164

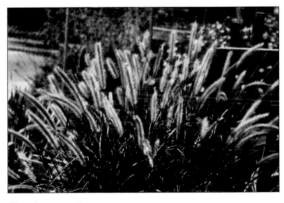

Pennisetum setaceum
FOUNTAIN GRASS
10   Page 172

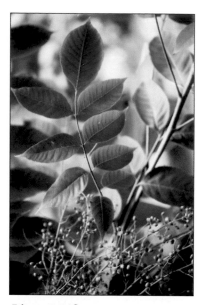

Rhus verniciflua
VARNISH TREE
A male tree
10   Page 194

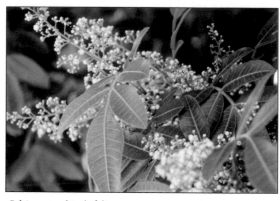

Schinus terebinthifolius
PEPPER TREE
A male tree
10   Page 205

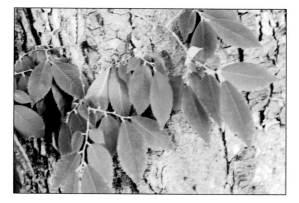

Zelkova serrata
ZELKOVA
10   Page 250

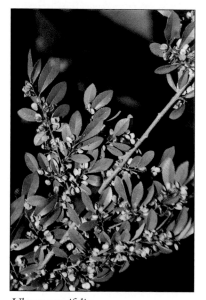

Ulmus parvifolia
CHINESE ELM
10   Page 232

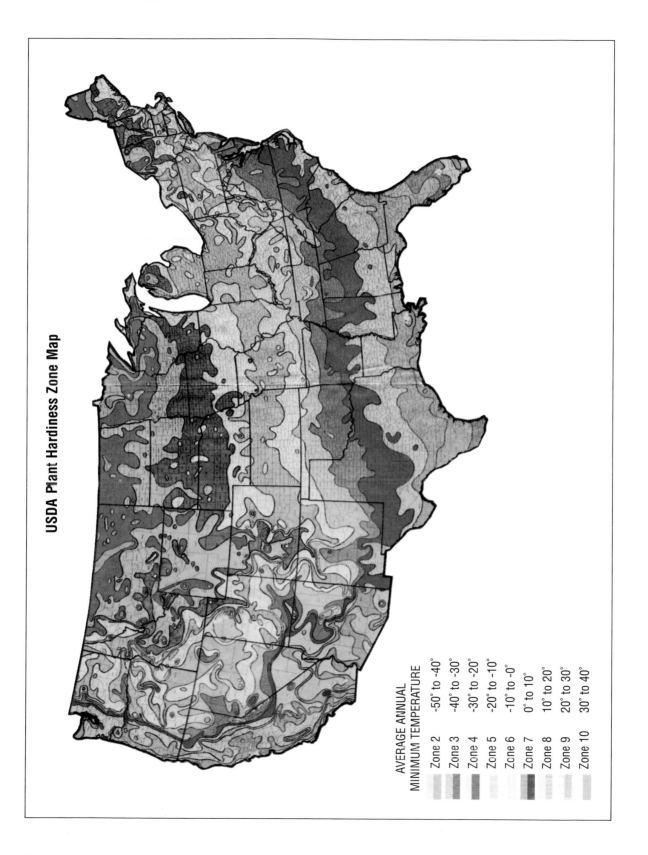

USDA Plant Hardiness Zone Map

AVERAGE ANNUAL
MINIMUM TEMPERATURE

Zone 2   -50° to -40°
Zone 3   -40° to -30°
Zone 4   -30° to -20°
Zone 5   -20° to -10°
Zone 6   -10° to -0°
Zone 7   0° to 10°
Zone 8   10° to 20°
Zone 9   20° to 30°
Zone 10   30° to 40°

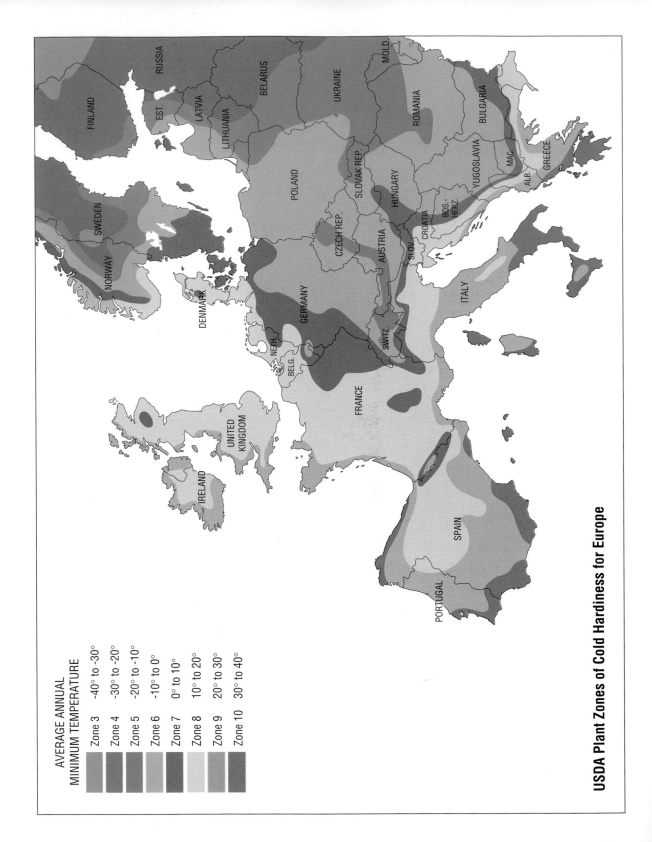

USDA Plant Zones of Cold Hardiness for Europe

AVERAGE ANNUAL
MINIMUM TEMPERATURE

Zone 3   -40° to -30°
Zone 4   -30° to -20°
Zone 5   -20° to -10°
Zone 6   -10° to 0°
Zone 7   0° to 10°
Zone 8   10° to 20°
Zone 9   20° to 30°
Zone 10   30° to 40°

LILAC.
See *Syringa*.

Lilium. 4
LILIES. Numerous varieties of bulbous perennials, hardy in most zones. Like most bulbs, they require fertile, well-drained soil to thrive. Allergy to LILY pollen is not common, despite the fact that it is held on exposed stamens and easily contacted. The pollen is heavy and not designed by nature to travel far in the air, and the petals of all LILIES are large, highly colored, and attractive to insect pollinators. People handling large numbers of LILY bulbs, especially those working in fields or packing houses, frequently develop contact rashes from the bulbs. Many LILIES are poisonous if eaten.

LILLY–PILLY TREE.
See *Acmena smithii; Syzygium*.

LILY.
See *Lilium*.

LILY-OF-THE-NILE.
See *Agapanthus*.

LILY-OF-THE-VALLEY.
See *Convallaria majalis*.

LILY-OF-THE-VALLEY BUSH.
See *Pieris*.

LILY-OF-THE-VALLEY TREE.
See *Clethra arborea; Crinodendron patagua; Liriope; Oxydendrum*.

LILYTURF.
See *Liriope*.

LIME.
See *Citrus*.

LIME TREE.
See *Tilia*.

LIMELEAF MAPLE.
See *Acer distylum*.

Limonium. 3
SEA LAVENDER, STATICE. Annuals and perennials, some hardy to zone 3. Easy to grow, these make good long-lasting dried flowers.

Linanthus. 3
Group of annuals and a few perennials, some California natives.

Linaria. ✳ 1
TOADFLAX. Annuals and perennials, with flowers resembling those of SNAPDRAGON.

LINDEN.
See *Tilia*.

Lindera. *males 8, females* ✳ *1*
BENJAMIN BUSH, JOVE'S FRUIT, SPICEBUSH. Many species of trees and shrubs from Asia, hardy in zones 7–10. Separate-sexed trees, the males cause allergies. Females are identified by the small, black, single-seeded berries which change from green, to red, to black.

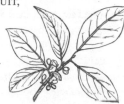
*Lindera
(female)*

LINGONBERRY.
See *Vaccinium*.

Linnaea borealis. ✳ 1
TWINFLOWER. Small evergreen sub shrub hardy to zone 2. Bears small, twinned, tubular rose or white flowers. Thrives in moist, peaty, acidic soil. This is the only plant that the great Swedish botanist Carl Linnaeus, developer of the binomial system of biological nomenclature, named for himself.

Linum. 4
FLAX. Blue-flowered annuals and perennials. These are the field crops grown in cool areas for their oil-producing seed and for the fiber used to produce linen. Allergy to FLAX flowers is usually limited to

those living close to large fields of blooming flax, and even then is uncommon.

LION'S EAR, LION'S TAIL.
See *Leonotis*.

LIPPIA.
See *Phyla nodiflora*.

LIPSTICK PLANT.
See *Aeschynanthus*.

Liquidambar. 📷   7

SWEET GUM. Large, deciduous trees, native to the eastern United States natives and Asia. Very popular street trees in many cities, SWEET GUM is hardy in zones 5–10. They are prized for their brilliant scarlet autumn color, in which they resemble MAPLES; but unlike MAPLES, SWEET GUMS produce a quantity of small, prickly round seed capsules in late summer.

The trees are monoecious, having both sexes on the same tree but not in the same flowers, and thus relying on the wind for pollination. Allergic reaction to *Liquidambar* pollen is usually not severe.

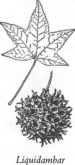

Liquidambar styraciflua

Sap from the Asian SWEET GUM is used to make aromatic *storax*, which is used in incense and perfumes. Allergy to storax itself is not uncommon.

Liriodendron. 📷   4

TULIP POPLAR, TULIP TREE, YELLOW POPLAR. A handsome, large, fast-growing native deciduous tree, hardy in zones 3–10. The TULIP TREE has large, beautiful lyre-shaped leaves, grows to 100 feet, has deep roots, and is tolerant of a very wide array of soil and weather conditions, including city environments. It has good fall color and attractive, large, yellow-orange, tulip-shaped flowers in the

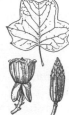

Liriodendron tulipifera

spring. TULIP TREES do not transplant easily and are not as commonly used as they might be.

Liriope.   3

LILYTURF, MONDO GRASS. Grassy evergreen flowering perennials, some hardy into zone 3. Members of the LILY family, and similar to the genus *Ophiopogon*, they produce spikes of small, showy lilac or white flowers and grow best in partial shade.

Lisianthus.

See *Eustoma grandiflorum*.

Litchi chinensis.   5

LICHI NUT, LYCHEE NUT. Evergreen tree only suitable for the warmest, mildest winter areas of zone 10. It grows best in moist, acid soil. The fruit is popular in Asian cuisine and has a sweet, unusual taste.

Lithocarpus densiflorus.   6

TANBARK OAK. Evergreen tree native to the West Coast and not hardy north of zone 7. An OAK relative, the male flowers of *Lithocarpus* are malodorous, although rarely a serious allergen.

Lithodora diffusa (Lithospermum).   ❋ 2

Low, shrubby perennial for partial shade in zones 7–10. Its leaves and stems are covered with fine hairs and the plant bears small, tubular, bright blue flowers.

Lithops.   ❋ 1

FLOWERING STONES, LIVING STONES, STONEFACE. Unusual succulents best grown in pots and kept dry in cool weather. Plants look like small rocks and the flowers are surprisingly large for the size of the plants.

Lithospermum.

See *Lithodora*.

Lithrea.   ❋10

Three species of subtropical trees and shrubs from South America, used in zone 9 and 10, especially in California. Relatives of POISON IVY, *Lithrea* bears creamy yellow lustrous flowers that produce highly allergenic pollen. One species in particular, *L. caustica*, is especially toxic. The flowers and seeds of this plant are poisonous, the pollen becomes airborne and is highly allergenic, and the sap can cause severe and painful skin rashes and swelling.

Litsea. ✳9
A large group of many species of usually deciduous subtropical and tropical trees and shrubs, mostly from Australia and Asia. Popular landscape plants in zones 9–10. Dioecious but not sold sexed.

LITTLELEAF LINDEN.
See *Tilia*.

LIVE FOREVER.
See *Dudleya*.

LIVERLEAF.
See *Hepatica*.

LIVING STONES.
See *Lithops*.

LIVINGSTONE DAISY.
See *Dorotheanthus bellidiformus*.

Livistona. 📷 �֍ 1
Small- to medium-sized Chinese and Australian FAN PALMS, for zones 9–10. They are attractive trees with no allergy problems.

Loasaceae. 8
A large group of herbs used as ornamentals. All members of this species can cause skin irritation.

Lobelia. 📷 ✖ 1
Popular perennials or annual bedding plants for full sun or partial shade in all zones. One species is a tall, red-flowered perennial for shady areas in zones 3–7. The annuals flower in shades of purple or blue. *Lobelia* is poisonous if eaten, but is occasionally used as an aid to quit smoking.

Lobivia; Lobivopsis.
See *Cactus*.

LOBSTER-CLAW.
See *Heliconia*.

Lobularia maritima. 6
SWEET ALYSSUM. A fast-growing annual or short-lived perennial with thousands of tiny white, pink, or purple flowers. Plants will not overwinter outside of zones 9–10 but will often re-seed themselves. ALYSSUM is heavily fragrant in hot weather, and the smell causes allergy in many. The leaves and flowers of SWEET ALYSSUM also are known to sometimes cause skin rash. ALYSSUM may also spread and become weedy in certain locations. A few ALYSSUM in the garden is not much of a problem, but don't overdo this one.

LOCOWEED.
See *Datura; Oxytropis*.

LOCUST.
See *Robinia*.

Lodoicea. 8
DOUBLE COCONUT PALM. A tall palm, rare in cultivation; separate-sexed with males capable of causing allergy.

LOGANBERRY.
See *Rubus*.

Logania. 4
Large group of mostly Australian herbs and shrubs used in zones 8–10.

Lolium. ✳10
DARNEL, RYEGRASS. There are several types of RYEGRASSES: *L. perenne*, or PERENNIAL RYEGRASS, *L. multiflorum,* or ITALIAN RYEGRASS, and a hybrid of the above two species. RYEGRASS pollen is a common, widespread, and often severe allergen in all parts of the United States. Most of this pollen, however, is not coming from lawns: RYEGRASS must usually be over a foot tall before it flowers and most lawns never reach that height. Almost all RYEGRASS allergy comes from plants escaped as weeds or grown in pastures as forage crops. Nonetheless, because al-

lergy to RYEGRASS pollen is so common, cross-allergic reactions to the volatile oils released when ryegrass lawns are mowed are also reported. A great deal of the world's supply of RYEGRASS seed is produced in central Oregon; this seed crop is, of course, allowed to flower, and early summer allergy to RYEGRASS in this area is intense.

In many areas of the southern United States it is common practice to overseed dormant BERMUDA GRASS lawns with ANNUAL RYEGRASS, and the mowing of these lawns contributes to wintertime grass allergy in these areas. (*Note:* RYEGRASS is not the same as RYE (*Secale cerale*), a grain crop.)

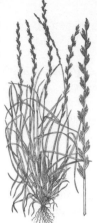

Lolium perenne

Lomaria.
See *Blechnum.*

Lonas annua.   7
Annual for all zones. Umbel-shaped flowers on erect stems resemble YARROW.

Lonchocarpus.   4
LANCEPOD. Evergreen tropical trees from which the botanical insecticide *Rotenone* is derived. One species, *L. violaceus*, has long leaves covered in translucent dots and drooping chains of long tubular flowers that are white on the outside and purple on the inside of the flowers. It is a common plant in Florida. *Lonchocarpus* is a member of the LEGUME family.

Lonicera.   5
HONEYSUCKLE. Many species of evergreen and deciduous shrubs and vines, some hardy into zone 3. Because it is such a common landscape plant, and large numbers of people have long been exposed to the sweet, pervasive scent, allergy to the fragrance is not uncommon. Pollen from HONEY-SUCKLE has occasionally been implicated in allergy

but is fairly rare. In some southern states *L. japonica*, the JAPANESE HONEYSUCKLE, has naturalized and is rapidly taking over large areas of native woodland plants. This evergreen HONEYSUCKLE has a slightly higher potential for allergy than other species.

LOOSESTRIFE.
See *Lythrum.*

Lophophora.   ✣ 1
MESCAL BUTTON, PEYOTE. Small spineless cacti, native to Texas and northern Mexico. The crowns of these succulent plants yield the hallucinogenic alkaloid known as *peyote*, used by Native Americans of these areas.

LOQUAT.
See *Eriobotrya japonica.*

Loropetalum chinense.   5
Evergreen shrubs bearing small clusters of greenish-white flowers; hardy in zones 7–10.

Lotus.   3
PARROT BEAK, TREFOIL. Many species of evergreen shrubs and herbs. *L. berthelotii*, PARROT BEAK, is a spreading red-flowered frost-tender perennial. *L. corniculatus*, BIRD'S-FOOT TREFOIL, is a low-growing, very cold-hardy perennial with yellow flowers resembling PEA blossoms; it is used as a ground cover or as a pasture legume.

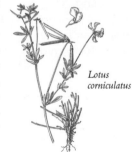

Lotus corniculatus

LOVAGE.
See *Levisticum officinale.*

LOVE APPLE.
See *Solanum.*

LOVE-IN-A-MIST.
See *Nigella damascena.*

LOVE-LIES-BLEEDING.
See *Amaranthus.*

LOVEJOY.
See *Episcia.*

LUCKY TREE.
See *Thevetia.*

LULO.
See *Solanum.*

Luma apiculata.   4
AMOMYRTUS. (Also known as *Myrtus luma.*) Large evergreen shrub or small tree for zones 9–10. Related to the MYRTLES, which it resembles.

Lunaria annua.   4
HONESTY, MONEY PLANT. Easy-to-grow biennial for sun or shade in all zones. HONESTY bears purple flowers on erect stalks which are followed by paper-thin, translucent pods that are often used for dried flower arrangements. On rare occasions people are allergic to these dried flowers, although almost no one is allergic to the flowers themselves.

LUNGWORT.
See *Pulmonaria.*

Lupinus.   3
LUPINE. Annuals, perennials, or sub shrubs of the LEGUME family. All parts of the plant are poisonous if eaten. All LUPINES need good drainage and full sun. When used as cut flowers, the pollen may pose an allergy problem.

Lupinus

Lycaste.
See ORCHIDS.

LYCHEE NUT.
See *Litchi chinensis.*

Lychnis (Viscaria).   3
CAMPION, CATCHFLY, MALTESE CROSS, MULLEIN PINK. Easy-to-grow annuals and perennials for sunny areas. Related to *Dianthus*, a few species are dioecious but are never sold sexed.

Lycium.   6
MATRIMONY VINE. Large group of deciduous or evergreen vines and shrubs of the POTATO family. Some species are separate-sexed but not sold sexed.

Lycopersicon lycopersicum.   3
TOMATO. TOMATO plants are not an important allergy problem for many, except that a few people are bothered by the smell of TOMATO leaves and, in rare cases, develop rashes upon contact with the leaves.

Lycopodium.   ✳10
CLUB MOSS, GROUND CEDAR, GROUND PINE, PRINCESS PINE, RUNNING MOSS, RUNNING PINE. Native species used as ground cover for moist, shady areas. Occasionally used in hanging baskets. These are not flowering plants but spore-bearing mosses that produce a vast number of spores. *Lycopodium* spores are gathered for many industrial uses; as a result, exposure to *Lycopodium* is quite common. The spores are still used in some cosmetics and, because of their high flammability, in fireworks. Swags of bright green *Lycopodium* are often brought indoors at Christmas time to use as decorations. Allergic response to *Lycopodium* spores is fairly common and often unusually severe, typical of which are hay fever and serious rash from contact. Those suffering an allergy to molds and spores should be careful around fireworks, and check all cosmetics to see if *Lycopodium* is listed as an ingredient. Poisonous if eaten.

LYCORIS.
See *Lilium*.

Lygodium japonicum.   4
Climbing ferns for shady areas of zones 8–10. They
need ample moisture to thrive.

Lyonia.   7
Shrubs grown in cool, moist soils of zones 6–10.
All parts of *Lyonia* are poisonous if eaten, making
the plants dangerous to livestock. Contact with the
leaves and sap may cause skin rash.

Lyonothamnus floribundus.   4
CATALINA IRONWOOD. Evergreen shrub or tree, to
60 feet. Needs good drainage and grows best near
the coast. The clusters of small white flowers do
not drop off cleanly after blooming.

Lysiloma thornberi.   5
FEATHER BUSH. An Arizona native fern-like shrub
or small tree for desert areas of zones 8–10; deciduous in the desert but may be semi-evergreen
elsewhere. It bears small white flowers.

Lythrum.   4
PURPLE LOOSESTRIFE. Hardy, invasive perennials for
bogs and wetlands.

M

Allergy Index Scale: *1* is Best, *10* is Worst.

❋ for *1* and *2*   ✳ for *9* and *10*

📷 See insert for photograph

Maackia.   *3*
Easy-to-grow Asian native deciduous shrubs or trees, hardy to zone 3. They bear clusters of pea-like white flowers.

Macadamia. 📷   *3*
MACADAMIA NUT TREE, QUEENSLAND NUT. Easy-to-grow tree wherever there is little frost, as in zone 10. Fast-growing from seed. Leaves are sharp-toothed and resemble HOLLY. It bears small white flowers in winter, followed by the edible nuts.

MACARTHUR PALM.
See *Ptychosperma*.

Macfadyena unguis-cati (Doxantha).   *3*
CAT'S CLAW, YELLOW TRUMPET VINE. Drought-tolerant perennial vine for zones 8–10 that grows best with good summer heat. Bears bright yellow, trumpet-shaped flowers and large, round, deep-green leaves. Claw-shaped tendrils make it able to cling to masonry. Can grow to 30 feet.

Maclura pomifera. 📷   *males* ✳ *9, females* ❋ *2*
BOWDOCK, BOWWOOD, HEDGE APPLE, OSAGE ORANGE. A thorny, deciduous separate-sexed tree, occasionally used for large hedges, common throughout the eastern United States. The wood is used to make strong, supple archery bows. Female OSAGE ORANGE bears large, round, inedible fruits called OSAGE APPLES or HEDGE APPLES, which are used to repel cockroaches. These female trees, which produce no pollen, make good choices for the allergy-free landscape.

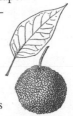

Maclura pomifera

The milky sap of *Maclura* is a contact allergen and the pollen is also allergenic. A member of the MULBERRY family, OSAGE ORANGE is very easy to grow and transplant. Male trees can be identified by the flowers, which are small, dull yellow balls on short stalks. Female trees bear larger, round, green ball-shaped flowers. There are a few selected, asexually grown clones, such as 'Fan d'Arc' and 'Altamont', but these are all pollen-producing males. Leaves are poisonous.

Macropiper.   *8*
KAWA-KAWA, PEPPER TREE. Shrubs or small trees from New Zealand. Rare in the United States.

Macrozamia.   *males* ✳ *9, females* ❋ *1*
A group of separate-sexed palms from Australia, grown in zone 10.

MADAGASCAR JASMINE.
See *Stephanotis*.

MADAGASCAR PERIWINKLE.
See *Catharanthus roseus*.

MADAGASCAR PLUM.
See *Flacourtia*.

MADEIRA NUT.
See *Juglans*.

MADEIRA VINE.
See *Anredera*.

MADRONE, MADRONO.
See *Arbutus*.

MAGIC FLOWER.
See *Cantua buxifolia*.

Magnolia.   *deciduous 6, evergreen 5*
Evergreen or deciduous trees and shrubs, for zones 3–10, depending on species.

M. *acuminata*, the CUCUMBER TREE or SWEET BAY, is a very large, tall, common deciduous shade tree hardy in zones 4–10.

M. *denudata*, the large CHINESE WHITE MAGNOLIA or LILY TREE, bears very large white flowers, and is hardy in zones 3–10. M. *grandiflora*, the COMMON BULL BAY or SOUTHERN MAGNOLIA TREE, is a common evergreen tree that gets quite tall and wide and bears large cup-shaped fragrant white flowers. It is hardy in zones 5–10.

M. *soulangiana*, the SAUCER MAGNOLIA or TULIP TREE, is a deciduous, often shrubby tree that puts on a big display of flowers early in spring before the leaves appear. It is good for areas where late frosts are a problem.

Allergy to *Magnolia* is only occasional and allergic response to the pollen is usually moderate, not severe. Those who live on a block lined with big *Magnolias*, or who have a large *Magnolia* in

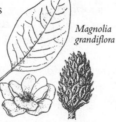

Magnolia grandiflora

their own yard, have a much greater chance of becoming hypersensitive than others.

Because deciduous *Magnolias* produce most of their flowers abundantly early in the year, their total bloom is much heavier than that of the evergreen varieties, which bloom off and on throughout much of the year.

The fragrance from some of the deciduous *Magnolias*, especially the CUCUMBER TREE, may cause negative odor challenges for some individuals.

MAGNOLIA VINE.
See *Schisandra*.

Mahernia.
See *Hermannia*.

Mahoberberis miethkeana.   ✳ 2
Hardy evergreen shrubs related to BARBERRY. Its dense growth habit, thick, round leaves, and sharp spines make it useful as a barrier shrub.

MAHOGANY.
See *Swietenia*.

MAHOGANY, MOUNTAIN.
See *Cercocarpus*.

Mahonia aquifolium. 📷   ✳ 2
OREGON GRAPE. Evergreen shrubs for zones 5–10, with thick, glossy leaves and edible (but tasteless) fruits.

MAIDENHAIR FERN.
See *Adiantum*.

MAIDENHAIR TREE.
See *Ginkgo biloba*.

MAIDEN'S WREATH.
See *Francoa ramosa*.

MALABAR PLUM.
See *Syzygium*.

MALAY APPLE.
See *Syzygium*.

Malcolmia maritima.   ✳ 1
VIRGINIAN STOCK. A fast-growing, unscented annual for full sun. (See also *Matthiola*.)

MALE LINDEN.
See *Tilia*.

MALLEE.
See *Eucalyptus*.

Mallotus japonica (Croton). 📷
males ✺ *10, females* ✳ *1*
A small, evergreen, separate-sexed tree from China and Japan, hardy only in zone 10. Large green leaves start out as red, resembling POINSETTIA bracts.

Male flowers are yellowish green; female flowers are reddish. Pollen from males is quite potent.

MALLOW.
See *Hibiscus; Lavatera.*

Malpighia glabra. 4
ACEROLA, BARBADOS CHERRY, WEST INDIAN CHERRY. An evergreen shrub occasionally raised commercially, especially in Southern Florida. Hardy in zones 9–10, the bushes grow to 15 feet and produce high yields of a small fruit that has the highest content of vitamin C of any fruit—3,300 milligrams per 100 grams of fruit, almost 100 times more vitamin C than in an orange. The fruits, or cherries, may be red, purple, yellow, or orange, depending on the strain of seed used. Highly productive cultivars can be bought occasionally; there is great variability among the seedling grown trees. Some trees bear leaves with tiny stinging hairs that can cause rash.

MALTESE CROSS.
See *Lychnis.*

Malus. 4
APPLE, CRABAPPLE. APPLES and CRABAPPLES are hardy in most zones and make handsome additions to the landscape.

APPLE trees are not known to cause much allergy, but those living in or next to orchards may well develop hypersensitivity to the pollen. People who are allergic to ROSES have a greater chance of developing allergy to APPLE blossom pollen because they are both in the ROSE or *Rosa* family.

APPLE pollen is heavy and does not travel far from the tree, so if planted away from the house, APPLES and CRABAPPLES present few allergy problems. Leaves and seeds are poisonous.

Mammea americana. 5
MAMEY. A tropical American fruit that looks, smells, and tastes much like an APRICOT. Large evergreen trees, they can occasionally be found in southern Florida. The leaves and sap of the MAMEY tree can cause rashes and serious swelling.

Mammillaria.
See CACTUS.

MANCHURIAN MAPLE.
See *Acer mandshuricum.*

MANDARIN ORANGE.
See *Citrus.*

Mandevilla (Dipladenia). 📷
deciduous 4, evergreen ✳ *2*
Evergreen and deciduous vines. The evergreen vines are beautiful but are difficult in most areas, even in milder parts of zone 10. The allergy potential from the evergreen *Mandevilla* is very low. The deciduous *M. laxa,* or CHILEAN JASMINE, is much hardier (zones 7–10), has very fragrant white flowers, and is easier to grow than the evergreen species. It has a higher allergy potential because of the possibility of negative odor reactions.

Mangifera indica. 📷 ✳10
MANGO. A tropical fruit tree for the mildest frost-free coastal areas of zone 10. It produces large, attractive, sweet fruit. MANGO is an especially interesting allergy plant; the trees bear three kinds of flowers—male only, female only, and complete flowers with both male and female parts in the same flower. As a result of this system, some highly allergenic pollen becomes airborne.

A relative of POISON IVY and POISON SUMAC, contact with the sap also may cause a rash. Typical of the allergic reactions to members of this group (*Anacardiaceae*), the onset of symptoms is delayed for several hours after exposure. Those who have been overexposed to POISON IVY or POISON OAK may develop a cross-allergic reaction to eating MANGO.

MANGOSTEEN.
See *Garcinia mangostana.*

MANGROVE PALM.
See *Nypa.*

MANILA GRASS.
See *Zoysia.*

MANILA PALM.
See *Veitchia.*

MANUKA.
See *Leptospermum.*

MANZANITA.
See *Arctostaphylos.*

MANZANOTE.
See *Olmediella betschlerana.*

MAPLE.
See *Acer.*

Maranta leuconeura.   ✳ 1
PRAYER PLANT. A houseplant, good in terrariums, that needs filtered light, warmth, and regular water.

MARGUERITE DAISY.
See *Anthemis; Chrysanthemum.*

MARIGOLD.
See *Tagetes.*

MARIPOSA LILY.
See *Calochortus.*

MARJORAM.
See *Origanum majorana.*

MARKING-NUT TREE.
See *Semecarpus.*

MARLOCK.
See *Eucalyptus.*

MARMALADE BUSH.
See *Streptosolen jamesonii.*

Marrubium vulgare.   ✳ 2
HOREHOUND. Hardy perennial herb of the MINT family.

MARSH GRASS.
See *Spartina.*

MARSH MARIGOLD.
See *Caltha palustris.*

MASCARENE GRASS.
See *Zoysia.*

MASTERWORT.
See *Astrantia.*

MATERNITY PLANT.
See *Kalanchoe.*

MATILIJA POPPY.
See *Romneya coulteri.*

Matricaria recutita.   7
CHAMOMILE. Annual herb used for chamomile tea. Plants have a smell of pineapple when crushed. See also *Chamaemelum nobile.*

MATRIMONY VINE.
See *Lycium.*

Matthiola.   6
STOCKS. Perennial usually grown as annual. Erect flower stalks with many fragrant individual flowers of purple, white, rose, blue, or yellow. Common cut flowers, STOCKS have a powerful fragrance, and those with hypersensitivity to perfumes may be allergic to them. The pollen is of little concern.

MATTRESS VINE.
See *Muehlenbeckia complexa.*

Mauritia flexuosa.   males 8, females ✳ 1
MORICHE PALM. Tall fan palm tree from Trinidad. An exception to most FAN PALMS, which are perfect-flowered and completely insect-pollinated, making them fine allergy-free landscaping choices. The MORICHE PALM, however, is separate-sexed, and the pollen-producing males can cause allergy. Male MORICHE PALMS are identified by their taller and thinner trunks; females are stockier and produce small fruits.

MAYBUSH, MAYDAY TREE.
See *Prunus padus.*

MAYFLOWER.
See *Claytonia.*

MAYPOP.
See *Passiflora.*

Maytenus boaria.   7
MAYTEN TREE. Small evergreen tree grown widely in zones 9–10. Resembling WILLOWS in appearance, they are related to *Euonymus.* These trees, when in full bloom, have numerous inconspicuous tiny, white-greenish flowers.

MAZARI PALM.
See *Nannorrhops.*

Mazus reptans.   ❋ 1
Hardy perennial ground cover with small clusters of flowers, blue with markings of yellow and white. A good rock garden plant that will not stand up to foot traffic.

MEADOW RUE.
See *Thalictrum.*

MEADOW SAFFRON.
See *Colchicum autumnale.*

MEADOWSWEET.
See *Filipendula.*

Meconopsis.   3
ASIATIC POPPY. Many species, all with large, brightly colored flowers. Some species are long-lived, quite hardy perennials, while others will grow for a year or two and then will die soon after flowering (monocarpic). Best grown in zones 3–7.

MEDITERRANEAN FAN PALM.
See *Chamaerops humilis.*

MEDLAR.
See *Mespilus.*

Melaleuca.   7
BOTTLEBRUSH, HONEY MYRTLE, CAJEPUT TREE. Popular landscape trees and shrubs from Australia, used often in zones 9–10. Brushy flower stalks may be red, yellow, white, purple, or cream colored and, like true BOTTLEBRUSH (*Callistemon*), the flowers have many exposed male stamens. *Melaleuca* occasionally has a strong smell and this may cause allergy in odor-sensitive people. *M. alternifolia* oil, claimed to cure almost anything, is widely marketed and may cause allergy. Cross-reactive responses between *Melaleuca* and *Callistemon* are common.

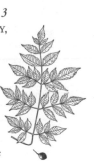

Melaleuca leucadendron

Melampodium.   7
Perennial, frost-hardy daisy, native to southwestern United States and Mexico.

Melia.   3
ARBOR SANCTA, BEAD TREE, CHINA BERRY, FALSE SYCAMORE, HOLY TREE, PATERNOSTER TREE, PERSIAN LILAC, PRIDE OF CHINA, PRIDE OF INDIA, SYRIAN BEAD TREE, TEXAS UMBRELLA TREE. A wide deciduous tree, hardy in zones 7–10, the *Melia* produces quantities of poisonous seeds that are used for making rosaries. People have been poisoned by chewing on these rosaries, and even a small number of seeds can be fatal to children.

Melia azedarach

Melianthus.   5
HONEYBUSH. Frost-tender ornamental and medicinal herbs for zone 10. Leaves give off foul odor when crushed.

Melicoccus.   *males 8, females* ❋ 1
HONEYBERRY, GENIPE, SPANISH LIME. Tall (to 60 feet) dioecious tree for zone 10, commonly used in Florida. Female *Melicoccus* produce an edible green fruit, yellow inside. Not sold sexed, the males produce allergenic pollen, but the females are fine choices for the allergy-free landscape.

Melilotus. 4

SWEET CLOVER. Tall, bushy varieties of clover that bear small stalks of white or yellow flowers. These cause more allergy than low-growing, creeping varieties of CLOVER.

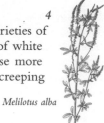

Melilotus alba

Meliosma. 4

Rare, hardy tree from China. Scented flowers are greenish yellow.

Menispermum. males 7, females ✳ 2

MOONSEED, YELLOW PARILLA. Native woody vines, grown for their foliage. MOONSEED is separate-sexed, and the males may cause allergy. Female vines can be recognized by their black fruits. *Menispermum* can be propagated by cuttings, and only the females, which are excellent choices for the allergy-free landscape, should be encouraged. All parts are highly poisonous.

Menispermum (female)

Mentha. 3

MINT. Hardy, sometimes invasive herbs for all zones, grown for their intensely scented, sometimes flavorful foliage. All MINTS require ample moisture to thrive.

Mentzelia. ✳ 2

BLAZING STAR, EVENING STAR. Hardy annuals and perennials for desert areas in full sun, with well-drained soil. *Mentzelia* grows to about 3 feet in some species and has large, bright yellow flowers with orange centers.

MERATIA.
See *Chimonanthus*.

MERCURY.
See *Chenopodium*.

Mertensia. ✳ 1

GIANT FORGET-ME-NOTS, MOUNTAIN BLUEBELLS, VIRGINIA BLUEBELLS. Tall, blue-flowered, very hardy, shade-loving plants that need acid soil and ample moisture.

Meryta sinclairii. males 8, females ✳ 1

PUKA. Houseplants grown for their attractive large leaves, *Meryta* is occasionally grown outside in mild parts of zone 10, where the plants may become small trees. Native to New Zealand, the females of this separate-sexed species are a good choice for allergy-free households.

MESCAL BEAN.
See *Sophora secundiflora*.

MESCAL BUTTON.
See *Lophophora*.

Mespilus. 3

HOSEDOUP, MEDLAR. A thorny tree that bears white or pink blossoms followed by small, pear-shaped fruit which is picked green and allowed to ripen off the tree, where it develops a flavor similar to spiced applesauce. Budded trees are often grafted onto QUINCE, PEAR, or HAWTHORN rootstocks.

MESQUITE.
See *Prosopis*.

MESSMATE.
See *Eucalyptus*.

Metasequoia glyptostroboides. 4

DAWN REDWOOD. A large, fast-growing deciduous conifer. A beautiful but messy tree that drops litter year round. Related to CYPRESS and with a flowering system seemingly designed to produce allergy, this tree is, nonetheless, rarely implicated in allergy. The DAWN REDWOOD was long considered by botanists to be extinct until a few living trees were found in a small, isolated valley in China in the 1950s. Seeds were brought to the United States, and they are now fairly common.

Metrosideros.   6
NEW ZEALAND CHRISTMAS TREE. Evergreen trees or big shrubs native to New Zealand and common in zone 10 of California. They do best near the coast, where they produce red flowers.

MEXICAN BLUE PALM.
See *Brahea armata.*

MEXICAN BUCKEYE.
See *Ungnadia.*

MEXICAN BUSH SAGE.
See *Salvia.*

MEXICAN FAN PALM.
See *Washingtonia robusta.*

MEXICAN FIRE PLANT.
See *Euphorbia.*

MEXICAN FLAME VINE.
See *Senecio.*

MEXICAN GRASS TREE.
See *Nolina longifolia.*

MEXICAN ORANGE.
See *Choisya ternata.*

MEXICAN PALO VERDE.
See *Parkinsonia aculeata.*

MEXICAN STAR.
See *Milla biflora.*

MEXICAN SUNFLOWER.
See *Tithonia rotundifolia.*

MEXICAN TEA.
See *Chenopodium.*

MEXICAN TULIP POPPY.
See *Hunnemannia.*

MICHAELMAS DAISY.
See *Aster.*

Michelia.   3
BANANA SHRUB. Evergreen shrubs or trees for zone 10; their large, white flowers, which resemble *Magnolia*, smell like ripe bananas. They need fertile soil, ample water, and partial shade to grow well.

Microcachrys.   7
An evergreen shrub, native to Tasmania, and grown in zone 10. It is related to *Podocarpus.*

Microcoelum.   8
WEDDEL PALM. Short palms from Brazil, grown in zones 9–10.

Microcycas.   males ✳ 9, females ✳ 1
PALMA CORCHO. Medium-sized palms from Cuba and used in zone 10.

Microlepia.   4
Shade-loving, dry-soil ferns for zone 10.

Micromeria.
See *Satureja.*

MIGNONETTE.
See *Reseda odorata.*

MILK BARREL.
See *Euphorbia.*

MILKBUSH.
See *Euphorbia.*

MILKWEED.
See *Asclepias.*

MILKWORT.
See *Polygala.*

Milla biflora.   ✳ 2
MEXICAN STAR. Bulbs for full sun in zones 9–10. The flat, star-shaped flowers are white with green stripes.

MILLET.
See *Panicum.*

MILO.
See *Sorghum.*

Miltonia.
See ORCHIDS.

MIMOSA.
See *Albizia julibrissin; Acacia.*

MIMOSA, PRAIRIE.
See *Desmanthus.*

Mimosa pudica.   3
SENSITIVE PLANT. Small, fast-growing houseplant or annual. A slight touch on the little leaves and the leaves quickly fold up, to reopen later. It needs a bright window when grown inside.

Mimulus.   ❋ 1
STICKY MONKEY FLOWER. (Also known as *Diplacus*.) Hardy native Californian sub shrub that bears yellow or orange flowers that resemble monkey faces. An easy-to-grow, loosely structured plant that requires good drainage.

Mina lobata (Quamoclit).   4
SPANISH FLAG. A perennial vine for zone 10; of the MORNING GLORY family, it has heart-shaped leaves and long red flowers that fade to yellow, then white. Quick from seed soaked overnight in warm water. Possible contact rash from the leaves.

MINER'S LETTUCE.
See *Montia.*

MING ARALIA.
See *Polyscias.*

MINIATURE FAN PALM.
See *Rhapis.*

MINT.
See *Mentha.*

Mirabilis jalapa.   4
FOUR O'CLOCKS. Drought-tolerant perennial in zones 7-10, but grown as annuals elsewhere. Tuberous roots can be dug and stored in cold winter areas. The 2-inch, trumpet-shaped red, yellow, or white flowers remain closed until afternoon. FOUR O'CLOCKS are pollinated by night-flying moths, drawn in by the fragrance of the flowers. This same fragrance may affect odor-sensitive individuals.

MIRACULOUS FRUIT.
See *Synsepalum dulcificum.*

MIRROR PLANT.
See *Coprosma repens.*

MIST FLOWER.
See *Eupatorium.*

MISTLETOE.
See *Phoradendron serotinum; Viscum cruciatum.*

MOCCASIN FLOWER.
See *Cypripedium.*

MOCK ORANGE.
See *Philadelphus; Murraya paniculata; Pittosporum.*

MOLDS.
Although not true plants, MOLDS are common in gardens and landscapes, where they are both infectious agents for some plants and beneficial catalysts in the process of natural decomposition and decay. Allergy to MOLD is very common and contact should be avoided. Fruit, especially if left in plastic bags, will mold quickly, and handling moldy fruit releases quantities of airborne spores.

Fresh air and sunlight are the natural enemies of most molds. In the garden, limit MOLD growth with judicious watering, pruning overhead trees to allow direct sunlight to penetrate the canopy, and by planting to encourage good air circulation. Compost heaps often harbor molds and sensitive individuals should let someone else turn the heap. Plants infested with molds or mildews should be discarded, not composted.

Natural fertilizers, especially cow manure, often harbor many MOLD spores. Often when new lawns are planted and allergies erupt, the lawn grass is blamed when actually it is MOLD spores in the fertilizer that trigger the reaction.

MOLE PLANT.
See *Euphorbia.*

Moluccella laevis. ✲ 2
BELLS OF IRELAND. Annuals grown for their unusual green flowers, borne on tall spikes.

Monadenium. ✱10
Group of about 50 species of succulent sub shrubs or herbs from eastern Africa, seldom seen in United States.

Monarda. 4
BEE BALM, HORSEMINT, OSWEGO TEA. Easy to grow in full sun or partial shade, these tall perennials are hardy in all zones. Large clusters of puffy rosy-red flowers are fragrant and attractive to butterflies and hummingbirds. The pungently scented leaves are used in tea. Pollen is not a problem, but the fragrance may affect some.

MONDO GRASS.
See *Liriope.*

MONEY PLANT.
See *Lunaria annua.*

MONGOLIAN LINDEN.
See *Tilia.*

MONKEY FLOWER.
See *Mimulus.*

MONKEY-HAND TREE.
See *Chiranthodendron pentadactylon.*

MONKEY PISTOL.
See *Hura.*

MONKEY-PUZZLE TREE.
See *Araucaria.*

MONKSHOOD.
See *Aconitum.*

MONK'S-PEPPER TREE.
See *Vitex.*

Monstera. 4
SPLIT-LEAF PHILODENDRON, SWISS CHEESE PLANT. (Also known as *Philodendron pertusum.*) Frost-tender evergreen tropical and subtropical vines for shady, protected areas of zones 9 and 10, and as houseplants elsewhere. Easy to grow, these large-leaved plants rarely flower indoors, but when they do, their pollen may trigger reactions. Outside these plants present little allergy potential. The sap of these big-leaved tropicals may also cause contact rash. All parts are poisonous.

Montanoa. 8
Large group of flowering shrubs or small trees, native to Mexico and the New World tropics. Hardy only in warmest parts of zone 10.

Montbretia.
See *Crocosmia; Tritonia.*

MONTEZUMA CYPRESS.
See *Taxodium.*

Montia. ✲ 1
MINER'S LETTUCE. Small herbs, many native, for moist, shady areas or full sun along the coast. Very common forest herb in the REDWOOD areas. The edible leaves have a spicy, peppery taste.

MOON CACTUS.
See *Selenicereus.*

MOON FLOWER.
See *Ipomoea.*

MOONSEED.
See *Cocculus laurifolius; Menispermum.*

MOOSEBERRY.
See *Viburnum*.

Moraea.
See *Dietes*.

MORAINE LOCUST.
See *Gleditsia*.

MORICHE PALM.
See *Mauritia flexuosa*.

MORNING COCKLE.
See *Silene*.

MORNING GLORY.
See *Ipomoea*.

MORTON BAY CHESTNUT.
See *Castanospermum australe*.

MORTON BAY FIG.
See *Ficus*.

Morus

MULBERRY. This large group of deciduous trees, shrubs, vines, and herbs is very important in the study of allergy. Different species of *Morus* have distinct flowering systems, producing varying degrees of allergy potential. Allergic reaction to *Morus* pollen is often severe, and in some western cities it is the primary cause of springtime asthma and hay fever.

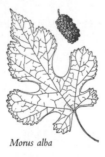
Morus alba

M. alba. 📷   *males* ✳ *10, females* ✽ *1*
WHITE MULBERRY, SILKWORM MULBERRY. Trees may be either male or female or in a few cases, both. There are some varieties sold for their fruit and these need further study before they can be rated. Over a dozen kinds of *M. alba* are sold as FRUITLESS MULBER-RIES; these all-male varieties are to be avoided.

M. australis.   *Not rated.*
AINO MULBERRY, JAPANESE MULBERRY, KOREAN MUL-BERRY. Heavy pollen producers; avoid use.

M. bombycis.   *Not rated.*
CHINESE MULBERRY. Avoid use.

M. 'Illinois Everbearing'.   *5*
A hybrid cross between WHITE and RED MULBERRY, developed for fruit production. This tree is hardy to 25° below zero.

M. nigra.   *5*
BLACK MULBERRY. A large tree hardy in zones 4–10. These are fruiting trees and although quite messy, not nearly as allergenic as some other species.

M. platanifolia.   ✳*10*
Most of these are all-male clones and are therefore to be avoided.

M. rubra.   *males 8, females* ✽ *1*
AMERICAN MULBERRY, PURPLE MULBER-RY, RED MULBERRY. A common large tree of the eastern United States, RED MULBERRY is almost always a fruiting tree.
Morus rubra

MOSES-IN-THE-CRADLE.
See *Rhoeo spathacea*.

MOSS CAMPION.
See *Silene*.

MOSS ROSE.
See *Portulaca grandiflora*.

MOTHER-IN-LAW'S TONGUE.
See *Sansevieria trifasciata*.

MOTH MULLEIN.
See *Verbascum*.

MOTH ORCHID.
See *Phalaenopsis*; ORCHIDS.

MOUNT ATLAS PISTACHE.
See *Pistache*.

MOUNTAIN ASH.
See *Sorbus*.

MOUNTAIN BLUEBELLS.
See *Mertensia*.

MOUNTAIN CAMELLIA.
See *Stewartia*.

MOUNTAIN HOLLY.
See *Nemopanthus*.

MOUNTAIN LAUREL.
See *Kalmia*.

MOUNTAIN MAHOGANY.
See *Cercocarpus*.

MOUNTAIN RIBBONWOOD.
See *Hoheria*.

MOUNTAIN SPRAY.
See *Holodiscus*.

MOURNING BRIDE.
See *Scabiosa*.

Muehlenbeckia.   7
MATTRESS VINE, WIRE VINE. Evergreen ground
cover or hanging basket vines, hardy in zones
6–10.

MUKU TREE.
See *Aphananthe*.

MULBERRY.
See *Broussonetia; Morus*.

MULGA.
See *Acacia*.

MULLEIN.
See *Verbascum*.

MULLEIN PINK.
See *Lychnis*.

Murraya paniculata.   4
MOCK ORANGE, ORANGE JESSAMINE. Evergreen
shrubs or small trees for zone 10 in frost-free areas
and partial shade. Fast-growing to 12 feet, the clustered white flowers have a JASMINE fragrance and
are very attractive to bees. Older shrubs bear small
red fruits. The plants are a good choice for big,
loose hedges. The heavy fragrance may adversely
affect odor-sensitive individuals.

Musa paradisiaca.   5
BANANA, PLANTAIN. Tall, frost-tender evergreen
trees that produce bananas. To grow best they need
ample water, fertile soil, warmth, and protection
from wind. In cooler areas, BANANAS are grown in
large pots and then moved inside when frost
threatens. The flowers are eaten in many areas, usually boiled. The fruit should be left on the trees until almost ripe, and then picked and brought inside
to ripen off the tree; BANANAS left to ripen on the
tree often cause indigestion.

Muscari.   ❈ 2
GRAPE HYACINTH. Bulbs hardy in all zones. The
spring-blooming blue flowers are held on stalks
rising above the grass-like foliage.

MUSHROOMS.
MUSHROOMS reproduce by spores, and spores, like
pollen, may cause allergies. Large globe-shaped
MUSHROOMS called PUFFBALLS are common in
many lawns and gardens. Stepping on these will
release millions of airborne spores.

MUSTARD.   6
See *Brassica*.

Myoporum.   ❈ 2
Evergreen shrubs or trees mostly from New Zealand
and Australia, for zones 9–10. Three species are com-

monly grown in Florida and California: *M. debile*, a low-growing ground cover; *M. laetum*, a fast-growing, drought- and salt-tolerant large shrub or small- to medium-sized tree that attains its maximum size near the coast; and *M. parvifolium*, a tall ground cover for banks. All *Myoporums* are easy and fast-growing, requiring initial watering until established, and then becoming quite drought resistant. A leaf held up to the sun reveals the pores (*myoporum*) clearly.

Myosotis. ✳ 2
FORGET-ME-NOTS.

Myrica. males ✷ 9, females ✳ 2
BAYBERRY, CALIFORNIA WAX MYRTLE, CANDLEBERRY, COMPTONIA, PACIFIC WAX MYRTLE, SWAMP CANDLE-BERRY, SWEET GALE, WAX MYRTLE. Evergreen or deciduous shrubs or trees, many native to United States. All *Myrica* berries yield a wax which is used to scent candles and perfumes. Many people are sensitive to the smell of *Myrica*, and even more are allergic to the abundant pollen. Some *Myricas* are separate-sexed, but female plants are hard to find. Allergy rating of all monoecious species is 8.

Myristica fragrans. males 8; females ✳ 1
NUTMEG. A large group of large tropical evergreen trees native to Indonesia, Grenada, and Australia, grown for their large brown seeds, which yield the spice nutmeg, and which are surrounded by a thin net or aril that is ground to yield the spice mace. NUTMEGS are separate-sexed trees and the males have potent pollen.

Myrrhis odorata. 4
SWEET CISELY. Hardy perennial, upright to 3 feet, SWEET CISELY roots are eaten fresh or cooked. The plants need fertile, moist soil, and partial shade to thrive.

Myrsine. 7
AFRICAN BOXWOOD, CAPE MYRTLE. A drought-tolerant shrub for zones 9–10, often used for foundation plantings and low hedges. The tiny flowers cause allergy if the plant is allowed to bloom. Most blooms are borne on older wood, so frequent

shearing reduces the allergy potential. A good substitute shrub for *Myrsine* is female *Podocarpus*.

MYRTLE.
See *Cyrilla racemiflora; Luma; Myrica; Myrsine; Myrtus; Umbellularia californica; Vinca*.

MYRTLE, HONEY.
See *Melaleuca*.

MYRTLE, JEWISH.
See *Ruscus*.

Myrtus communis. 3
TRUE MYRTLE. An easy-to-grow, drought-tolerant evergreen shrub or small tree (to about 16 feet), for zones 8–10. Very small, dark green leaves and small, white flowers makes this an attractive plant for full sun, but it may get leggy in the shade. Because it is easily shaped by shearing, it is often used for foundation plants, screens, tub plants, topiary, and hedges.

N

Allergy Index Scale: *1* **is Best,** *10* **is Worst.**

❄ for *1* and *2* ✹ for *9* and *10*

📷 See insert for photograph

NAKED LADY.
See *Amaryllis belladonna.*

NAMAQUALAND DAISY.
See *Venidium.*

Nandina domestica. ❄ *1*

HEAVENLY BAMBOO. Evergreen sub shrub. The plants are completely hardy in zones 7–10, and the roots are hardy to zone 6. There are many dwarf varieties available, and all *Nandina* make fine landscaping plants. Although it resembles BAMBOO, it is not related; *Nandina* plants have clusters of white flowers, followed by bright red, round, fleshy-coated little seeds, which persist on the plants for months. Easy to grow and fairly drought-tolerant in sun or partial shade, the color of the leaves is best in good light.

NANKING CHERRY.
See *Prunus tomentosa.*

Nannorrhops. ❄ *1*

MAZARI PALM. Four species of small- to medium-sized slow-growing palms from India, Afghanistan, and Iran, hardy in zones 8–10.

NANNYBERRY.
See *Viburnum.*

Narcissus. *4*

DAFFODIL. Trumpet-shaped yellow, white, or pale green flowers on these spring-blooming bulbs. Daffodils will persist and naturalize where conditions are perfect—fertile, fast-draining soil with ample moisture.

Allergic reactions are reported from handling DAFFODIL bulbs, but this is most common in bulb-packing sheds or with workers digging the bulbs. People working at cutting *Narcissus* for the commercial cut-flower trade also experience allergy to DAFFODIL pollen, sap, and foliage.

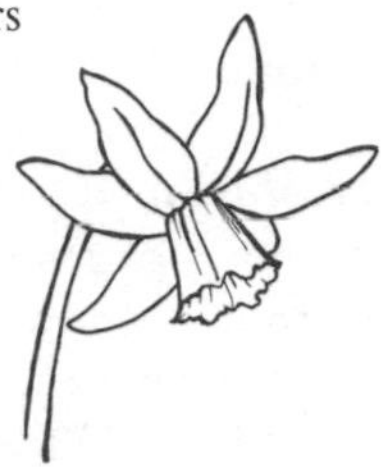
Narcissus

For the average gardener, or for those who buy an occasional bunch to bring indoors, the allergy potential is very small. However, allergy is well documented and some caution is advised. The bulbs and all parts of *Narcissus* contain toxic calcium oxylate crystals.

NASTURTIUM.
See *Tropaeolum.*

NATAL IVY.
See *Senecio.*

NATAL PLUM.
See *Carissa grandiflora.*

NAUPKA.
See *Scaevola.*

NECTARINE.
See *Prunus persica.*

NEEDLE PALM.
See *Rhapidophyllum hystrix; Yucca.*

Nelumbo. ❄ *1*

WATER LILY. Hardy flowering pond plants.

Nemesia strumosa. ❋ 2

Easy-to-grow annuals from seed; for full sun.

Nemopanthus. 7

CATBERRY, MOUNTAIN HOLLY. Native deciduous shrub of the eastern United States, hardy into zone 5. It resembles HOLLY (*Ilex*). CATBERRY needs moist soil and partial shade to grow well.

Nemophila. ❋ 1

BABY BLUE EYES. Fast-growing annuals from seed for full sun or part shade. *Nemophila* needs ample moisture.

Neolitsea. *males 8, females* ❋ 1

A group of about 80 evergreen trees native to Japan and Korea, all of which are separate-sexed; the males present a high potential for allergy. Trees grow 12 to 20 feet and females have small, usually black berries. *N. dealbata* is a tropical dioecious evergreen tree common in parts of Australia. Unlike most separate-sexed plants, *N. dealbata* is almost completely insect-pollinated and makes a good choice for the allergy-free landscape.

Neopanax (Nothopanax).

males 8, females ❋ 1

FIVE-FINGERS. Tall (to 25 feet) New Zealand native evergreen shrubs and trees, used in zone 10. *Neopanax* are characterized by their long, five-lobed, serrated leaves. The trees are separate-sexed and the males show high potential for allergy. Females are identifiable by their small dark purple fruits.

Neoregelia.

See *Bromelia*.

NEPAL CAMPHOR TREE.

See *Cinnamomum camphora*.

Nepenthes. *Not rated.*

A family of separate-sexed carnivorous herbs or vines from the Philippine Islands. Rarely seen in this country.

Nepeta. 5

CATMINT, CATNIP. Perennial hardy ground covers of the MINT family. They thrive in moist soil, in full sun to partial shade.

Nephelium lappaceum. *males 7, females* ❋ 1

HAIRY LYCHEE, RAMBUTAN. Large, tall, separate-sexed evergreen tropical fruit trees. Related to MANGOSTEENS, the female trees bear delicious fruit.

Nephrolepis. 4

SWORD FERN. A group of easy-to-grow, long-lived ferns. One species, *N. exaltata* 'Bostoniensis', the BOSTON FERN, and the more compact *N. exaltata* 'Bosteniensis Dallas', the DALLAS FERN, are popular houseplants. All ferns have spores, and spores can cause allergy, so with this in mind, do not hang houseplant or patio ferns directly over chairs or tables. In the garden, however, SWORD FERNS pose little allergy risk. They thrive in shady areas with good soil moisture.

Nephrosperma. 7

VAN HOUTTAN PALM. A tropical palm, to 30 feet, used in equatorial landscapes.

Nephthytis.

See *Syngonium podophyllum*.

Nerine. ❋ 2

A bulbous perennial bearing pink or red flowers, usually grown in pots but used outdoors in zones 7–10.

Nerium oleander. 📷 6

OLEANDER. Very common evergreen landscape shrubs and small trees in zones 8–10. All parts of the OLEANDER are very poisonous, as is the smoke from them when burned. In recent years a virus has been killing off many OLEANDER hedges in southern California, especially in some desert areas. There is no known cure for this virus and it is expected to spread. OLEANDERS are tough, drought-resistant, and flower well if pruned back occasionally. Pollen from OLEANDER is not a well-documented allergy factor, despite the fact that the plants bloom profusely and the pollen-bearing stamens are well exposed. The sap is known to cause rash, and the odd fragrance is allergenic for some individuals.

Nertera granadensis. ❋ 2
BEAD PLANT. Tender houseplants or ground cover for small areas in zone 10; best in partial shade with good moisture.

NERVE PLANT.
See *Fittonia*.

Nestegis. ❋ 9
Evergreen trees or shrubs, from New Zealand. Hardy only in zones 8–10. Related to OLIVES, these plants are dioecious but not yet sold sexed.

NET BUSH.
See *Calothamnus*.

NETTLES.
See *Urtica*.

NEW MEXICAN PRIVET.
See *Forestiera*.

NEW ZEALAND BRASS BUTTONS.
See *Cotula squalida*.

NEW ZEALAND BUR.
See *Acaena*.

NEW ZEALAND CHRISTMAS TREE.
See *Metrosideros*.

NEW ZEALAND FLAX.
See *Phormium tenax*.

NEW ZEALAND LACEBARK.
See *Hoheria populnea*.

NEW ZEALAND LAUREL.
See *Corynocarpus laevigata*.

NEW ZEALAND SPINACH.
See *Tetragonia*.

NEW ZEALAND TEA TREE.
See *Leptospermum scoparium*.

NICHOL'S WILLOW-LEAFED PEPPERMINT TREE.
See *Eucalyptus*.

Nicotiana. 3
FLOWERING TOBACCO. Frost-tender perennials for full sun, used as annuals in all zones.

Nidularium innocentii.
See *Bromelia*.

Nierembergia. ❋ 1
CUP FLOWER. White- or purple-flowered perennials, for full sun with ample water, in zones 7–10. The plants must be sheared yearly to maintain their shape. Most species are low-growing and mounded, but one is tall.

Nigella damascena. 3
LOVE-IN-A-MIST. Tall annuals with unusual blue flowers and large, light, 1-inch papery seed pods which are used in dried flower arrangements.

NIGHT-BLOOMING CACTUS.
See *Cereus; Selenicereus*.

NIGHT JASMINE.
See *Nyctanthes*.

NIGHT JESSAMINE.
See *Cestrum nocturnum*.

NIGHT PHLOX.
See *Zaluziyanskya capensis*.

NIGHTSHADE.
See *Solanum*.

NIKAU PALM.
See *Rhopalostylis sapida*.

NIKKO FIR.
See *Abies*.

NINEBARK.
See *Physocarpus.*

NIPA PALM.
See *Nypa.*

NOBLE FIR.
See *Abies.*

Nolana. ❊ 2
Annual vines that resemble MORNING GLORIES, with bright, large flowers. They are difficult to grow well, requiring full sun and very well-drained soil.

Nolina longifolia. 7
MEXICAN GRASS TREE. A desert relative of *Yucca* and *Agave*, these can cause allergies.

NORFOLK ISLAND PINE.
See *Araucaria.*

Normanbya. 8
BLACK PALM. A tall (to 60 feet) Australian native, used in zone 10.

NORSE FIRE PLANT.
See *Columnea.*

NORWAY MAPLE.
See *Acer platanoides.*

Nothofagus. 7
A group of deciduous and evergreen trees related to BEECH, hardy only in zones 8–10. Native to New Zealand and Australia.

Nothopanax.
See *Neopanax.*

NUT GRASS.
See *Cyperus.*

NUTGALL.
See *Rhus.*

NUTMEG.
See *Myristica fragrans; Torreya.*

Nyctanthes. 5
NIGHT JASMINE, TREE-OF-SADNESS. Small Asian trees or shrubs for zones 9–10, bearing fragrant white flowers that yield a perfume and an orange dye.

Nymphaea. ❊ 1
WATER LILY. Blooming aquatic plants hardy in all zones.

Nypa. 8
MANGROVE PALM, NIPA, NYPA PALM. Native to India and the Solomon Islands and occasionally planted in zone 10.

Nyssa. 📷 *males* ✹ *9, females* ❊ *1*
BEE GUM, PEPPERIDGE TREE, TUPELO, SOUR GUM, SWAMP GUM, WILD OLIVE. Native deciduous tree with attractive leaves and often exceptionally beautiful fall color. Thrives in continually moist soils. TUPELOS are separate-sexed trees; the males contribute to allergy, the females produce clusters of small, round blue berries, on 2-inch stems. The cultivar 'Miss Scarlet' is a pollenless female prized for its brilliant red fall color and ornamental blue fruit.

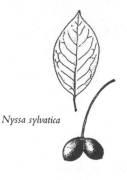

Nyssa sylvatica

O

Allergy Index Scale: *1* is Best, *10* is Worst.

✳ for *1* and *2*   ✸ for *9* and *10*

📷 See insert for photograph

OAK.
See *Quercus.*

OAK-LEAF HYDRANGEA.
See *Hydrangea quercifolia.*

OAK, TANBARK.
See *Lithocarpus densiflorus.*

OATS.
See *Avena.*

OAXACA PALMETTO.
See *Sabal.*

OBEDIENCE PLANT.
See *Physostegia virginiana.*

OCEAN SPRAY.
See *Holodiscus.*

Ochna serrulata.   ✳ *2*
BIRD'S-EYE BUSH. Evergreen shrub for zones 9–10. The large yellow flowers appear in early summer and are followed by red sepals, then black fruit which resemble a mouse's face and ears. Thrives in partial shade and moist, acidic soil; a good potted plant.

Ocimum.   ✳ *2*
BASIL. Annual culinary and decorative herbs, fast-growing from seed.

OCONEE BELLS.
See *Shortia galacifolia.*

OCOTILLO.
See *Fouquieria splendens.*

OCTOPUS TREE.
See *Schefflera.*

Odontoglossum.
See ORCHIDS.

Oemleria cerasiformis.   *males 6, females* ✳ *1*
INDIAN PLUM, OSO BERRY. A dioecious (separate-sexed) member of the ROSE family, this large decid-uous shrub is native from British Columbia to California and is used as an ornamental in zones 4–10. Only the female plants have small blue-black fruits.

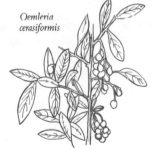

Oemleria cerasiformis

Oenothera. 📷   *3*
EVENING PRIMROSE. Hardy perennials and bienni-als for full sun, in all zones. *O. berlandieri* or *O. speciosa* is the MEXICAN EVENING PRIMROSE, with large pink flowers; it is fast-spreading and reseeds easily, sometimes becoming invasive. *O. biennis* is a tall wildflower. *O. missourensis*, the MISSOURI EVENING PRIMROSE, is a very hardy, low-growing, yellow-flowered perennial. Tall *O. tetragona*, or SUN DROPS, opens its yellow blooms in the daytime.

OIL PALM.
See *Corozo.*

OKRA.
See *Abelmoschus esculentus.*

OLD MAN.
See *Artemisia.*

OLD MAN CACTUS.
See *Cephalocereus senilis; Espostoa.*

OLD WOMAN.
See *Artemisia.*

Olea europaea. 📷   ✹10
OLIVE. Evergreen trees hardy in zones 8–10. OLIVES need good summer heat to make best fruit. Olive trees are easy to transplant and, as urban sprawl has taken over orchards, many have been moved into city landscapes. This is unfortunate because OLIVE blossoms are a primary cause of severe allergy. The bloom on OLIVES is heavy and the trees often are in bloom from April through June. The pollen is exceptionally light and buoyant and often becomes airborne. In many southern and western cities OLIVES produce the worst early summer pollen. If OLIVE trees are pruned hard each winter they will not bloom, but this is difficult if the trees are allowed to grow tall.

One variety, 'Swan Hill Olive' never flowers, making it an acceptable tree. Also worth noting is the fact that OLIVE trees will grow perfectly well in the tropics and subtropics but will almost never flower in these climates.

OLEANDER.
See *Nerium oleander.*

OLEANDER, YELLOW.
See *Thevetia.*

Olearia. 📷   8
ASTER TREE, DAISYBUSH. Many species of shrubs and small trees mostly from New Zealand and Australia. Several species of *Olearia* are used as landscape material in California and Florida, but these RAGWEED relatives produce a heavy bloom and have a relatively high allergy potential.

OLIVE.
See *Olea europaea.*

Olmediella betschlerana. 📷
males 7; females ✳1
COSTA RICAN HOLLY, GUATEMALAN HOLLY, MANZANOTE. Small- to medium-sized evergreen trees for zones 9–10. Separate-sexed, with male trees presenting some allergy potential. If pollinated, female trees produce hard, inedible green fruits the size and shape of a Japanese PERSIMMON. Young trees are frost-tender but acquire more hardiness as they age. Trees grow to about 30 feet tall and nearly as wide, are pest-free and have attractive large, glossy leaves that resemble those of HOLLY.

Olneya tesota.   4
DESERT IRONWOOD. Leguminous evergreen tree for desert areas of zones 8–10.

Oncidium.   group 1–3
DANCING-LADY ORCHIDS. A very large group of ORCHIDS from tropical South America. Greenhouse plants. Allergy ratings from 1 to 3, depending on species. See also ORCHIDS.

ONION.
See *Allium.*

Onoclea.   5
Tall, hardy ferns for moist, shady areas.

Onosma tauricum.   ✳2
GOLDEN DROPS. Perennials for sun or shade, hardy in zones 3–10. GOLDEN DROPS make excellent rock garden plants.

Ophiopogon.
See *Liriope.*

OPPOSSUMWOOD.
See *Halesia.*

Opuntia.
See CACTUS.

ORANGE.
See *Citrus.*

ORANGE BROWALLIA.
See *Streptosolen jamesonii.*

ORANGE CLOCK VINE.
See *Thunbergia.*

ORANGE JESSAMINE.
See *Murraya paniculata.*

Orbignya.   ✳9
BABASSU, COHUNE PALM. Twenty species of subtropical palm trees from Central and South America,
grown in zones 9–10. Some species reach 60 feet.

ORCHARD GRASS.
See *Dactylis.*

ORCHID CACTUS.
See *Epiphyllum.*

ORCHID PANSY.
See *Achimenes.*

ORCHID TREE.
See *Bauhinia.*

ORCHID VINE.
See *Stigmaphyllon.*

ORCHIDS.   ✳ 1
The largest group of plants in the world, ORCHIDS
come in many sizes, shapes, and colors. Some are
hardy into the coldest zones while others thrive
only in frost-free jungles. Many ORCHIDS, called
epiphytic, live in trees and need no soil. Other terrestrial ORCHIDS grow in the ground. All ORCHIDS
need good moisture and most potted ORCHIDS are
planted in containers of pure tree bark, or a mix of
bark and sand; these require regular fertilizing
every two weeks during the growing season. Most
ORCHIDS do best in partial shade, and a lath house
is a popular place in which to grow them. Because
ORCHIDS often have some of the world's fanciest
flowers, well designed to attract insect pollinators,
they rarely cause allergy.

OREGON BOXWOOD.
See *Paxistima.*

OREGON GRAPE.
See *Mahonia aquifolium.*

OREGON MYRTLE.
See *Umbellularia californica.*

ORGANPIPE CACTUS.
See CACTUS.

ORIENTAL ARBORVITAE.
See *Platycladus orientalis.*

Origanum majorana (Amaracus).   5
SWEET MARJORAM. Perennial culinary herb with
strongly scented leaves, for moist, shady areas. *Oil
of Marjoram* is known to cause skin rash.

ORNAMENTAL GRASS.
See *Festuca; Pennisetum.*

ORNAMENTAL PEAR.
See *Pyrus.*

Ornithogalum.   3
PREGNANT ONION, STAR OF BETHLEHEM. Bulbs for
sun or partial shade in zones 7–10. The bulbs are
poisonous.

Oryza.   7
RICE. A cultivated grain crop. Very few people
are allergic to eating rice, and a common diet
used to eliminate the possible causes of an unknown allergy is pears, lamb, and rice. The only
exception is found among those living close to
RICE paddies; although self-pollinated and the
pollen does not travel far, it is the cause of late fall
severe asthma in localities where it is grown.

OSAGE ORANGE.
See *Maclura pomifera*.

Oscularia. ✳ 1
Small, drought-resistant shrubby succulent plants for full sun in zone 10. They bear pink or purple flowers.

OSIER.
See *Cornus*.

Osmanthus. 📷 5
SWEET OLIVE. About 15 species of slow-growing, evergreen tall shrubs and small trees, some hardy to zone 6. *Osmanthus* grows best in partial shade with ample moisture. The tiny flowers have a powerful fragrance, suggestive of apricot, and this scent may trigger allergic reaction in odor-sensitive individuals. Some species are separate-sexed, but the male plants do not release much airborne pollen. *Osmanthus* is related to OLIVE and ASH, but unlike them, *Osmanthus* flowers have very few and very small male stamens.

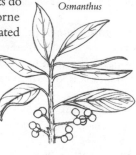
Osmanthus

Osmunda. 3
CINNAMON FERN, ROYAL FERN. Shade- and moisture-loving ferns, hardy into zone 3. The emerging fronds of *Osmunda* can be eaten, usually boiled like asparagus.

OSO BERRY.
See *Oemleria cerasiformis*.

Osteomeles. 4
Several species of deciduous and evergreen shrubs from China, New Zealand, and Hawaii, hardy to zone 7. The flowers of *Osteomeles* resemble those of HAWTHORN or *Cotoneaster*.

Osteospermum. 📷 6
AFRICAN DAISY. Several species of spreading, sun-loving, easy-to-grow ground covers, hardy in zones 9–10.

Ostrya. 📷 7
BEETLEWOOD, DEERWOOD, HARDTACK, HOP HORN-BEAM, STONEWOOD. Hardy deciduous trees of the BIRCH family, prized for their fine yellow autumn color. Although all may cause early spring allergy, they have a relatively short bloom period that lessens their overall impact. An occasional HOP HORNBEAM in the landscape is not much of a problem. The leaves of HOP HORNBEAM resemble those of ELM and they bear papery clusters of seeds that resemble ripe HOPS.

OSWEGO TEA.
See *Monarda*.

OURICURI PALM.
See *Syagrus*.

OX-EYE DAISY.
See *Heliopsis helianthoides scabra*; *Chrysanthemum*.

Oxalis. 📷 ✳ 1
SHAMROCK, SORREL, WOOD SORREL. Many species of small, low growing perennials and annuals characterized by their three- and four-lobed leaves, which resemble CLOVER. Some of this genus are difficult-to-eradicate weeds, but a few are shade-loving ground covers. The plants contain oxalic acid, which gives the stems a pleasantly tart flavor. The leaves are considered poisonous.

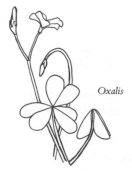
Oxalis

Oxydendrum. 📷 ❋ 2

LILY-OF-THE-VALLEY TREE, SORREL TREE, SOUR-WOOD, TITI. A slow-growing, tall (to 80 feet) native deciduous tree of the eastern United States, hardy in zones 5–10. *Oxydendrum* grows best in moist, acid soils. The large leaves turn a bright scarlet red or orange in autumn, and in the springtime the tree bears tiny tubular white flowers which attract bees.

Oxytropis. 6

CRAZYWEED, LOCOWEED. Perennial members of the LEGUME family, sometimes grown as ornamentals. Plants, seeds, and flowers are poisonous if eaten.

OZARK WHITE CEDAR.
See *Juniperus.*

P

Allergy Index Scale: *1* is Best, *10* is Worst.

✳ for *1* and *2*   ✸ for *9* and *10*

📷 See insert for photograph

Pachysandra. 6

JAPANESE SPURGE. Hardy in all zones, this common, spreading ground cover is widely used in zones 3–7, in moist areas of full sun to deep shade. Evergreen in the south and deciduous in the north, *Pachysandra* can cause allergies in any climate. A better choice for the allergy-free garden is *Vinca minor* in the north and *V. major* in the south.

Pachystachys lutea. ✳ *2*

GOLDEN CANDLE. A houseplant, or grown outside in the mildest parts of zone 10. Related to *Justicia* or SHRIMP PLANT, which it resembles. It grows best in partial shade, with good soil and ample water.

PACIFIC WAX MYRTLE.
See *Myrica*.

Paeonia. ✳ *2*

PEONY. Hardy, long-lived perennials that grow best in moist, sunny spots in zones 3–8. The plants bear large leaves and very large, showy red, pink, or white flowers. PEONIES refuse to grow in hot, dry areas and are impossible to grow in zones 9–10. TREE PEONIES are deciduous shrubs, some to 6 feet, that are hardy to zone 2; they produce exception-

ally large flowers, often fully double. Most PEONIES are hybrids and there is a wide selection from which to choose.

PAINTED DAISY.
See *Chrysanthemum; Pyrethrum*.

PAINTED FINGERNAIL PLANT.
See *Bromelia*.

PAINTED TONGUE.
See *Salpiglossis sinuata*.

PALM LILY.
See *Yucca*.

PALMA CHRISTI.
See *Ricinus communis*.

PALMA CORCHO.
See *Microcycas*.

PALMA PITA.
See *Yucca*.

PALMETTO.
See *Sabal*.

PALMETTO THATCH.
See *Thrinax*.

PALMYRA PALM.
See *Borassus*.

PALO VERDE.
See *Cercidium*.

PAMPAS GRASS.
See *Cortaderia selloana*.

PANAMIGA, PANAMIGO.
See *Pilea*.

Panax. ✳ *2*

GINSENG. Very winter-hardy perennial grown for its prized, medicinal roots. GINSENG is notoriously difficult to grow and requires moist, rather poor, acid soil, partial shade, and a deep mulch to thrive.

Pandanus. *males* ✸ *9, females* ✳ *1*
PANDUS PALM, SCREW PINE. Very large group of Old World tropical shrubs and trees, all separate-sexed. The males cause widespread allergy in Myanmar, Sri Lanka, and the Philippine Islands. Some species are used in tropical and subtropical landscapes in the United States.

Pandorea. ✳ *2*
BOWER VINE, WONGA-WONGA VINE. Large, vigorous evergreen vines for sun or shade in zones 9–10. They have large leaves and 2-inch, trumpet-shaped white, pink, or rose-colored flowers. Prune after blooming to encourage new growth.

PANDUS PALM.
See *Pandanus.*

Panicum. 5
PANIC GRASS, MILLET. A common grain crop.

PANSY.
See *Viola.*

PANSY ORCHID.
See *Miltonia*; ORCHIDS.

Papaver. 3
POPPY. Annuals and perennials for full sun. The RED FLANDERS POPPY or SHIRLEY POPPY is an annual variety that is fast from seed. *P. orientale*, the ORIENTAL POPPY is a perennial hardy to zone 2 and has very large, papery flowers in white, lilac, pink, red, or scarlet. *P. nudicale*, the ICELAND POPPY is grown as an annual, and flowers well during the winter months in zones 7–10. The bitter sap of all POPPIES is potentially poisonous.

PAPAYA.
See *Carica papaya.*

PAPERBARK MAPLE.
See *Acer griseum.*

PAPER MULBERRY.
See *Broussonetia papyrifera; Morus.*

Paphiopedilum.
See ORCHIDS.

PAPYRUS.
See *Cyperus.*

Parabenzoin. *males* ✸ *9, females* ✳ *1*
Two species of deciduous shrubs or small trees, native to Japan and China and used there in landscapes. Separate-sexed with males having high potential for allergy.

PARADISE PALM.
See *Howea.*

PARADISE TREE.
See *Simarouba.*

Parajubaea. 7
Two species of tall palms (to 20 feet) from sub-tropics, used in zones 9–10.

PARA NUT.
See *Bertholletia excelsa.*

PARA-PARA.
See *Pisonia.*

PARA RUBBER.
See *Hevea brasiliensis.*

Parkinsonia aculeata. 6
JERUSALEM THORN, MEXICAN PALO VERDE. Drought-tolerant, thorny deciduous desert tree, to 30 feet, that bears yellow flowers.

PARLOR IVY.
See *Senecio.*

PAROUOT PALM.
See *Acoelorrhaphe wrightii.*

PARROT BEAK.
See *Clianthus puniceus; Parrotia; Lotus.*

Parrotia. 📷   4
PARROT BEAK, PERSIAN IRONWOOD, PERSIAN WITCH HAZEL. Deciduous tree or large shrub for zones 8–9, prized for its autumn color.

PARSLEY PANAX.
See *Polyscias.*

Parthenium argentatum.   8
GUAYULE. Native to desert areas of the Southwest, GUAYULE is raised as a domestic rubber-producing plant and is one of only two plants used commercially in natural rubber production (see also *Hevea brasiliensis*). A 3-foot-tall shrub with small white or yellowish flowers, GUAYULE is drought-tolerant and needs fast-draining soil and high summer heat to grow well. GUAYULE is a RAGWEED relative, and it is possible that rubber produced from GUAYULE may be allergenic to those with sensitivity to RAGWEEDS.

P. hysterophorum, the POUND CAKE WEED, is a common weed in the southern United States that causes severe skin rash and inhalant allergy, and thus its allergy rating is 10. There are several other species of *Parthenium*, and all of them are, at best, suspect.

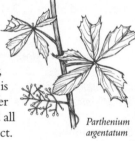

Parthenium argentatum

Parthenocissus.   4
BOSTON IVY, VIRGINIA CREEPER, WOODBINE. Several species of deciduous, long-lived clinging vines, some native to United States and others to Asia. Allergies to BOSTON IVY or VIRGINIA CREEPER are uncommon. Members of the GRAPE family, the grape-like fruits are mildly toxic if consumed.

Paspalum.   ✳9
BAHIA GRASS, DALLIS GRASS. Perennial, fast-growing, spreading grasses used for pastures and hay crops. There are many species worldwide: *P. dilatatum* or DALLIS GRASS, is a common forage grass in warmer parts of the United States, and it often escapes cultivation to become a large, crab-grass-like weed in lawns. In the lawn DALLIS GRASS flowers when still short and produces large amounts of allergenic pollen. BAHIA GRASS, another of this group, is used as a warm-climate lawn grass and also flowers when short.

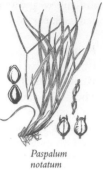

Paspalum notatum

Passiflora. 📷   3
MAYPOP, PASSION FLOWER, PASSION FRUIT. Mostly evergreen, some deciduous vines for zones 8–10. *P. edulis* produces a rich, sweet, flavorful fruit that is said to be an aphrodisiac. The vines are easy to grow, easily propagated from cuttings, and have very unusual large flowers, the parts of which are said to represent the Passion of Jesus Christ. The best fruit is produced when there are several plants for cross-pollination. Leaves and unripe fruit are poisonous.

PATERNOSTER TREE.
See *Melia.*

PATERSON PLUM.
See *Lagunaria patersonii.*

Paulownia tomentosa.   4
EMPRESS TREE. Large, fast-growing deciduous tree with very large heart-shaped leaves and many tubular lilac-blue colored flowers in spring. Hardy in zones 7–10, the EMPRESS TREE is a member of the TRUMPET VINE family and bears clusters of fragrant, trumpet-shaped flowers, which are edible and eaten fresh in salads. The tree needs good soil, full sun, and ample water to thrive. The wood is prized by carvers for its close grain and density. *Paulownia* is named for Anna Paulowna,

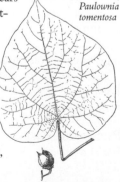

Paulownia tomentosa

princess of Holland and daughter of the Russian Czar Paul I.

PAUROTIS WRIGHTII.
See *Acoelorrhaphe*.

PAW PAW.
See *Asimina triloba*.

Paxistima.   ✳ 2
OREGON BOXWOOD. A low growing Pacific Northwest native evergreen shrub used for low hedges and ground covers. It needs good drainage but is otherwise not hard to grow.

PEACH.
See *Prunus persica*.

PEANUT.
See *Arachis hypogaea*.

PEAR, ORNAMENTAL, FLOWERING, EVERGREEN.
See *Pyrus*.

PEARLBUSH.
See *Exochorda*.

PEARLY EVERLASTING.
See *Anaphalis*.

PEAS, GARDEN.
See *Pisum sativum*.

PEAS, SWEET.
See *Lathyrus*.

PEASHRUB, SIBERIAN.
See *Caragana arborescens*.

PEASHRUB, SWAN RIVER.
See *Brachysema lanceolatum*.

PECAN.
See *Carya illinoensis*.

Pedilanthus tithymaloides.   ✴ 10
DEVIL'S BACKBONE, JAPANESE POINSETTIA, REDBIRD CACTUS, RIBBON CACTUS, SLIPPER PLANT. Houseplants or used outside in frost-free parts of zone 10. Not a type of cactus, but related instead to *Euphorbia*, the sap can cause severe skin rash.

Pediocactus.
See CACTUS.

PEE-GEE HYDRANGEA.
See *Hydrangea paniculata*.

Pelargonium.   5
GERANIUM. These are the tender showy-flowered houseplants and warm-climate perennials that most people know as GERANIUMS. They thrive in full sun and are remarkably drought-resistant. The large soft, slightly fuzzy leaves have a characteristic pungent odor and are occasionally zoned with dark green or purple or variegated. *Pelargoniums* release little pollen, but their fragrance and the smell of their leaves may affect odor-sensitive individuals.

IVY-LEAF GERANIUMS have waxy leaves without the characteristic odor. They tolerate some shade and, because of their lack of scent, are a better choice for the allergy-free garden.

Pellaea.   3
CLIFF-BRAKE, COFFEE FERN, BIRD'S-FOOT FERN. Shade- and moisture-loving ferns with attractive finely cut leaves, for zones 8–10.

PENCIL BUSH, PENCIL TREE.
See *Euphorbia*.

_____

Pennisetum.

P. clandestinum.   *Not rated.*
KIKUYUGRASS. A rapidly growing, sod-forming turf grass suitable for all southern areas. A South African male-sterile, female clone of this grass is a

very low pollen producer and may be a very useful low-allergy lawn grass.

P. setaceum. 📷 ✹*10*

FOUNTAIN GRASS. This is a large ornamental clump grass, hardy in all zones; it may naturalize in milder areas. It produces tall purplish seed heads that are held well above the plant. These and other ornamental grasses are gaining in landscape popularity because of the ease with which they are grown. FOUNTAIN GRASS causes frequent allergy, and its further use is discouraged.

PENNYROYAL.
See *Mentha.*

Penstemon. 📷 ❊ *2*

BEARD TONGUE. A large group of flowering perennials, one an Asian import but most native; various species are hardy throughout the United States. *Penstemon* is easy to grow, long-lived, and easy to propagate from cuttings. Plants grow in clumps from 1 to 6 feet tall depending on species. In California *P. heterophyllus* has become quite popular in recent years due to its good drought tolerance and wide range of flower colors.

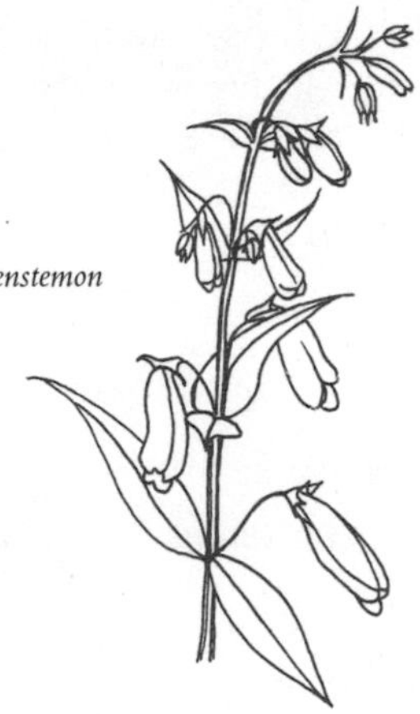
Penstemon

PEONY.
See *Paeonia.*

Peperomia. *4*

EMERALD LEAF, WATERMELON PEPEROMIA. Several species of attractive houseplants, usually low and spreading. All like semi-shade and ample moisture.

PEPPER.
See *Piper.*

PEPPER TREE.
See *Piper; Schinus; Vitex; Drimys; Macropiper.*

PEPPER VINE.
See *Piper.*

PEPPERIDGE TREE.
See *Nyssa sylvatica.*

PEPPERMINT.
See *Mentha; Eucalyptus.*

PEPPERMINT TREE.
See *Agonis flexuosa.*

PEPPERMINT WILLOW.
See *Eucalyptus.*

PEPPERWOOD.
See *Umbellularia californica; Zanthoxylum.*

PEREGRINA.
See *Jatropha.*

Perilla frutescens. *3*

SHISO. Tall, big-leafed annual that resembles *Coleus*, with its large edible leaves that taste like MINT. The long clusters of flower buds are also cooked in Japanese tempura batter. *Perilla* thrives in sun or partial shade with generous water.

PERIWINKLE.
See *Catharanthus; Vinca.*

Pernettya mucronata. ✣ 2

An evergreen shrub for zones 7–10. *Pernettya* produces tiny, pink, bell-shaped flowers followed by attractive bright purple, white, or black berries. It thrives in moist, acid soil, and needs partial shade in the hottest areas. A light yearly pruning keeps it compact.

Persea. 📷 3

AVOCADO. A large group of tender evergreen trees for zones 9–10. *P. americana*, the common edible AVOCADO, is not frost resistant and is most commonly grown as a houseplant outside of the warmest zones; 'Bacon' is among the hardiest cultivars. In fertile soil in areas with little frost, a mature AVOCADO, tree can grow to 70 feet. Because of its shallow roots, AVOCADO requires summer irrigation and year-round mulch. The pollen is rarely implicated in allergy.

P. borbonia, the RED BAY, SHORE BAY, or SWAMP BAY, is a large tree, native to the southeastern United States, which can reach 80 feet, although it is usually much smaller. It thrives in moist to wet soils in zones 8–10. *P. indica* is a smaller evergreen tree used mostly in California. *Persea* leaves are poisonous.

PERSIAN IRONWOOD.
See *Parrotia*.

PERSIAN IVY.
See *Hedera colchica*.

PERSIAN LILAC.
See *Melia*.

PERSIAN RANUNCULUS.
See *Ranunculus*.

PERSIAN VIOLET.
See *Exacum*.

PERSIAN WITCH HAZEL.
See *Parrotia*.

PERSIMMON.
See *Diospyros*.

PERUVIAN DAFFODIL.
See *Hymenocallis*.

PERUVIAN LILY.
See *Alstroemeria*.

PETTICOAT PALM.
See *Copernicia*.

Petunia. 📷 ✣ 2

Annuals and a few perennials that are very popular as container and bedding plants for full sun. Newer varieties, like the 'Carpet Series' (including 'Purple Wave'), grow low, spread, and have lots of flowers. *Petunias* need good soil, adequate moisture, and warm temperatures to grow well. Most require judicious dead-heading to encourage continuous bloom. *Petunias* were one of the first flowers I used in inhalant testing, and I never found anyone allergic to them.

PEYOTE.
See *Lophophora*.

Phacelia distans. 7

WILD HELIOTROPE. A small annual native to dry areas of the western United States, with fernlike leaves and coils of small, blue, bell-shaped flowers. It causes contact skin rash.

Phalaenopsis (MOTH ORCHID).
See ORCHIDS.

Phalaris. ✳ 9

CANARY GRASS, CANARY REED GRASS. An important, coarse, tall-growing forage grass for pastures.

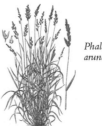

Phalaris arundinacea

Phaseolus. *4*

Beans. The flowers and fruit of beans are not of concern when it comes to allergies. However, contact with leaves can cause rash and old bean plants often have rust. Use care when pulling up old plants.

Phellodendron. *males 8, females ✻ 1*

Amur cork tree, cork tree. Ten species of large deciduous trees, all with thick, corky bark, for zones 4–10. Cork trees are separate-sexed and the tall (to 80 feet) males shed large quantities of airborne pollen with high allergy potential. Female trees produce small resin-scented black fruits. The compound leaves of *Phellodendron* resemble those of ash. 'His Majesty' and 'Macho' are male cultivars and should be avoided. No relation to *Philodendron*.

Phellodendron amurense

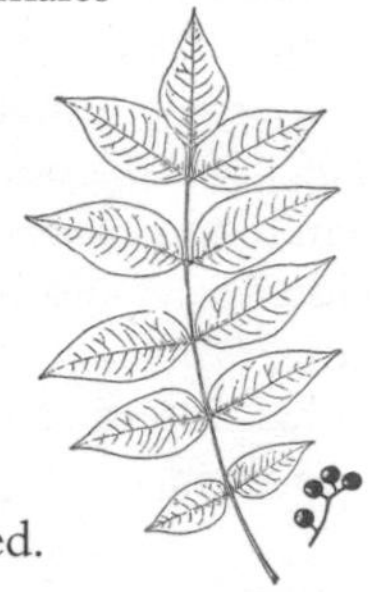

Philadelphus. *singles 4, doubles 3*

Mock orange. Many species of deciduous shrubs, most with fragrant white flowers, hardy in zones 3–10. Mock orange grows best in full sun or partial shade in hot areas. Not fussy about soil or watering, it should be pruned hard each year after blooming, thinning and removing the oldest wood to encourage new growth and continued bloom. *P. lewisii* is native to the northwestern United States and is the state flower of Idaho. *P. virginalis* is a hybrid with double flowers; the cultivar 'Minnesota Snowflake' is fully double and releases less pollen than single varieties. Certain kinds of *Philadelphus* are very fragrant, and these may affect some sensitive individuals.

Phillyrea decora. *males ✸ 9, females ✻ 1*

Jasmine box, privet, sharpberry tree. An evergreen shrub or small tree from the Mediterranean area, hardy in zones 6–10. These are separate-sexed plants, and because they are members of the olive family, the tiny white flowers of the males have high potential for allergy. Female shrubs produce small red fruits which turn purple in late fall.

Philodendron. *3*

Houseplants, used outside in frost-free parts of zones 9–10. Several hundred species of frost-tender evergreen perennials. Most of these plants seldom flower; the flowers of *Philodendron*, however, are designed to release airborne pollen, and in the tropics this group of plants contributes to allergy. As used in the United States, most *Philodendrons* are low-allergy-rated plants, with a caution for contact allergy from the sap. One species, *P. cordatum*, which is often confused with *P. oxycardium*, the oxheart philodendron, is implicated in causing skin rash in nursery workers. Poisonous if eaten.

Phleum. *✸ 10*

Timothy. A common pasture grass for northern areas. Timothy is among the worst of all grasses for causing allergy. If possible, farmers using it for hay should mow the first crop early to prevent flowering. Early cuts of hay provide less tonnage but higher food value.

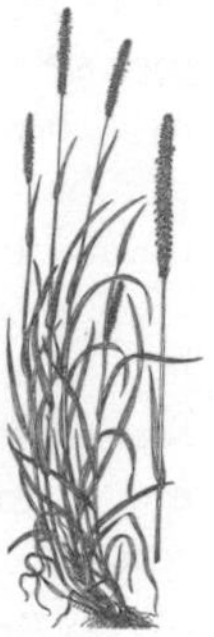

Phleum pratense

Phlomis fruticosa. *3*

Jerusalem sage. Tall, shrubby perennial with bright yellow flowers, hardy in all zones. Easy to grow and not fussy about soil. A member of the mint family.

Phlox. *4*

Annuals and perennials, a few hardy to zone 3. Several different colors are available. *Phlox* grows best in full sun with plenty of water; the perennial varieties are long-lived once established.

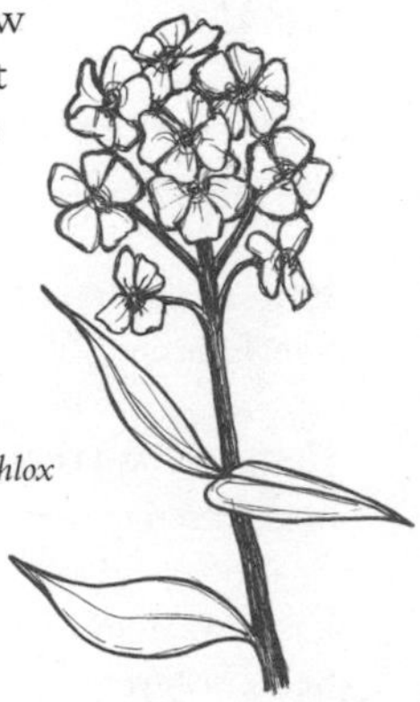

Phlox

Phoenix dactylifera. 📷 *males* ✻ *9, females* ✳ *1*
DATE PALM. The DATE PALM of commerce, is a tall, thin-trunked tree, cold-hardy to 10 degrees. Of the approximately 15 other species of DATE PALMS, none else is cold-hardy below 20 degrees. All members of this genus are separate-sexed, but no attempt has been made to sell them sexed, despite the fact that the trees are easy to propagate from root suckers, which produce young trees of the same sex as the parent. As with all separate-sexed trees, the males produce quantities of potent, air-borne pollen. CANARY ISLAND DATE PALMS are very common street trees in California, Florida, and all along the Gulf Coast, creating a corridor of allergy when they bloom. The pollen of male CANARY ISLAND PALMS is occasionally used to pollinate female *P. dactylifera* but results in smaller fruit.

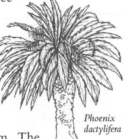
Phoenix dactylifera

PHOENIX TREE.
See *Firmiana simplex*.

Phoradendron serotinum. 6
AMERICAN MISTLETOE. A parasitic evergreen plant that grows on many species of trees. Most MISTLETOE is unisexual and can cause pollen allergies. MISTLETOE saps strength from the host trees and should be removed where possible. MISTLETOE berries that are brought inside as holiday decorations pose little allergy threat; they are poisonous, however.

Phormium tenax. ✳ *2*
NEW ZEALAND FLAX. Evergreen perennials for zones 7–10 that form tall clumps of broad grass-like bronze fronds marked with stripes. The red or yellow flowers, borne on tall, erect stalks, rise up out of the middle of these clumps; the entire plant may reach 12 feet. Although they look like a grass plant, *Phormium* is related to the *Agaves*.

Photinia. 📷 4
The deciduous *P. villosa* is hardy in zones 3–10. *P. × Fraseri* is a common evergreen shrub or small tree hardy in zones 9–10. *Photinia* flowers are usually white, occasionally pink, showy and, like the blossoms of the related PEAR, malodorous. When pruned hard, the new leaves grow back a bright red color, which slowly turn green as they mature. Despite its offensive smell, *Photinia* blossom is not a great contributor of allergenic pollen.

Phygelius capensis. ✳ *1*
CAPE FUCHSIA. An easy-to-grow perennial for zones 7–10, with pendulous, red tubular flowers.

Phyla nodiflora. ✳ *2*
LIPPIA. A drought-tolerant, low-growing perennial ground cover for zones 8–10, with small rose-colored flowers that attract bees. It does not compete well with weeds and becomes dormant in cold weather. It will tolerate desert conditions, but grows best with adequate water. *Phyla* is related to *Verbena*.

Phyllitis scolopendrium. 3
HART'S-TONGUE FERN. Long-lived hardy ferns for zones 5–10. They are popular potted plants, and will grow well in shady areas of their range.

Phyllostachys.
See BAMBOO.

Physalis. ✳ *2*
CHINESE LANTERN PLANT, GROUND CHERRY, STRAWBERRY TOMATO, TOMATILLO. Several species of annuals or frost-tender perennials, none of which cause allergy. The unripe fruits of some species, however, are poisonous.

PHYSIC NUT.
See *Jatropha*.

Physocarpus. 4
NINEBARK. Easy-to-grow deciduous shrubs for full sun or partial shade, hardy in zones 2–10. The white flowers resemble those of *Spiraea*.

Physostegia virginiana. 3
FALSE DRAGONHEAD, OBEDIENCE PLANT.   Hardy perennial for all zones. Tall, upright plants bear tubular, rose-colored flowers on long spikes that should be cut back after flowering.

Phytolacca. 5–8, depending on species
POKE, POKE BERRY, POKE SALAD, POKEWEED. A group of herbs, shrubs, or tree-like plants native to the tropics and to southeastern United States. Many have poisonous roots and leaves, and the fruits are especially toxic. *P. americana*, usually called POKE SALAD or PIGEON BERRY, has leaves that are boiled and eaten in spring when the plants are small. The water must be changed several times to leach out the poisonous properties. Once the toxins are removed, the leaves are highly nutritious and are used much as collard greens. Mature POKE plants have sap that is so dangerous that they should never be handled unless gloves are worn. Even small amounts of sap contacted through cuts or breaks in the skin can cause poisoning. The attractive red berries of POKE have also proven fatal to children on numerous occasions. In addition, the pollen from male POKE

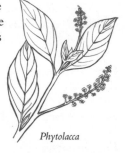
Phytolacca

plants is both allergenic and poisonous. In Brazil, Uruguay, and Argentina, *P. dioica*, a tall (to 60 feet) evergreen separate-sexed tree, is used in landscaping, where the males contribute to allergy. Several other species of *Phytolacca*, mostly herbs and flowers, are grown in China and Japan but these are perfect flowered and are not contributors to allergy.

Picea. 3
SPRUCE.   Large evergreen, coniferous trees, hardy to zone 1, native to wide areas of the Northern Hemisphere, including North America, China, Japan, Tibet, and Scandinavia. SPRUCE grow best in cool summer, cold winter areas (and do not thrive in hot, dry climates) where soil is deep, well-drained, moist, and acidic. They are related to

PINES, and like them, the pollen has a waxy coating which prevents it from irritating sensitive mucous membranes. As a result, SPRUCE, like PINE, is not an important tree in allergy even though it releases large amounts of pollen each year. Occasionally, some sensitive individuals may be allergic to the scent of SPRUCE.

There are many species of *Picea*, ranging from ground covers to tall, handsome pyramidal-shaped trees. The COLORADO BLUE SPRUCE (*P. pungens* 'Glauca') is a very popular slow-growing landscape tree. *P. abies*, the NORWAY SPRUCE is another common landscape plant that may reach 150 feet; it is also an important lumber tree.

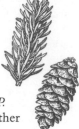
Picea pungens 'Glauca'

PICKEREL WEED.
See *Pontederia cordata*.

Pieris. 3
FETTERBUSH, LILY-OF-THE-VALLEY BUSH.   Eight species of evergreen flowering ground covers, shrubs, or small trees, hardy in all zones. Some *Pieris* are native to Asia and others to the United States, but all grow best in partial shade in cool summer areas with well-drained, moist, acidic, peaty or sandy soils. *Pieris* bears small, pink, drooping clusters of attractive buds, followed by white, pink, or occasionally red flowers. The leaves are glossy and handsome and the shrubs grow well alongside *Rhododendrons*, which share their cultural requirements. All parts of the plant are highly poisonous if eaten.

PIGEON BERRY.
See *Duranta; Phytolacca*.

PIGEON GRASS.
See *Setaria*.

PIGEON PLUM.
See *Coccoloba*.

PIGGY-BACK PLANT.
See *Tolmiea menziesii*.

Pilea.   *males 5, females* ❊ *1*

ALUMINUM PLANT, ARTILLERY PLANT, CREEPING CHARLIE, PANAMIGA, PANAMIGO. A large group of frost-tender herbs often used as houseplants. The male flowers have allergy potential, so it is best to remove any blooms as they appear.

PILI NUT.
See *Canarium ovatum.*

Pimelea prostrata, P. coarctata.   3
Small evergreen shrub with fragrant white flowers that grows best in full sun with moist, acid, well-drained soil.

PIMPERNEL.
See *Anagallis.*

Pimpinella anisum.   ❊ *2*
ANISE. Annual herb for all zones; easy to grow from seed in full sun with good moisture. The seeds and foliage are used to season foods.

Pinanga.   6
A group of more than 100 species of small- to medium-sized attractive palms used mostly in tropical landscapes.

PINCUSHION FLOWER.
See *Scabiosa.*

PINCUSHION TREE.
See *Hakea laurina.*

PINDO PALM.
See *Butia capitata; Cocos australis.*

PINE.
See *Pinus.*

PINE, WATER.
See *Glyptostrobus lineatus.*

PINEAPPLE *(Ananas comosus).*
See *Bromelia.*

PINEAPPLE FLOWER.
See *Eucomis.*

PINEAPPLE GUAVA.
See *Feijoa sellowiana.*

PINEAPPLE SAGE.
See *Salvia.*

PINK BALL DOMBEYA.
See *Dombeya.*

PINK CEDAR.
See *Acrocarpus fraxinifolius.*

PINK IRONBARK.
See *Eucalyptus.*

PINK POLKA-DOT PLANT.
See *Hypoestes phyllostachya.*

PINK POWDER-PUFF BUSH.
See *Calliandra.*

PINKS.
See *Dianthus.*

PIÑON, PINON NUT PINE.
See *Pinus.*

Pinus.   4
PINE, PINON, PINON NUT TREE. Evergreen coniferous trees and shrubs that are native to most temperate parts of the world, including Asia, Europe, and America. Some species are hardy into the coldest zones. In urban landscaping large PINE trees often overwhelm the area in which they are planted.

PINES shed enormous quantities of pollen, but because it is waxy and not highly irritative to mucous membranes, their potential for allergy is rather low and, when it occurs, not usually severe. Allergic reactions to the scent of cut PINE are reported but are also rare.

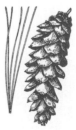

Pinus strobus

On the central coast of California most of the native MONTEREY PINES have died off recently. The small, low-growing varieties such as the MUGO PINE present even less allergy potential than larger types and are good choices for the allergy-free landscape. One *Pinus* species, *P. contorta,* the LODGEPOLE PINE from Colorado, is known to cause asthma. Use of LODGEPOLE PINE in landscaping should be discouraged.

Piper.
PEPPER. A group of more than 1,000 different species of evergreen vines, shrubs, and small trees, many of which have high allergy potential from their odor, contact with their leaves and sap, and their pollen. Some species are separate-sexed plants, but all are tropical or subtropical, only grown in the United States in a few frost-free areas and in greenhouses. All members of the *Piper* genus are high-allergy plants and should not be used in the allergy-free landscape.

P. betle.
BETEL. A large shrubby vine, common in Asia and India. The leaves are chewed along with slaked lime and nuts from *Areca catechu* (the BETEL NUT) as a stimulant.

P. kadsura.
A climbing shrub from Asia, used in landscapes in Japan and Korea.

P. methysticum.
KAVA-KAVA. A large shrub or small tree, the roots of which are used to produce a herbal remedy for stress relief. The extract is also used in teas and mouth sprays, as a calming agent.

P. nigrum.
BLACK PEPPER, PEPPER VINE, WHITE PEPPER. A large, woody vine that is the source of commercial pepper. Black pepper is made from the dried unripe fruits of the female vines. White pepper is made from ripe fruits.

Piqueria trinervia. ✳10
STEVIA. A small group of winter-blooming annuals and shrubs grown mostly in Mexico and Central America as florist crops for cut flowers. A high-allergy plant.

Pisonia. 7
BIRD-CATCHER TREE, PARA-PARA. Houseplants or evergreen shrubs or small trees in mildest parts of zone 10. From New Zealand and Australia, *Pisonia* bears tiny pink or white flowers.

Pistache. ⌨ *males 8, females* ✳ 1
A group of deciduous and evergreen trees and shrubs from the southwestern United States, Mexico, the Mediterranean region, and the Canary Islands. All species are separate-sexed, and the male plants have very high potential for causing allergy. *Pistache* is in the *Anacardiaceae* family of plants that includes POISON IVY, POISON OAK, and POISON SUMAC. Because of this close familial connection, it is probable that those with hypersensitivity to POISON IVY or POISON OAK may develop a severe allergy to either PISTACHIO nuts, their pollen, or both.

P. atlantica, the MOUNT ATLAS PISTACHE is a large, briefly deciduous separate-sexed tree for zones 8–10.

P. chinensis, the CHINESE PISTACHE TREE, is a deciduous tree to 60 feet, prized for its orange and red autumn color in zones 8–10, and for the ornamental, glossy, half-red, half-blue-green fruit of the female trees. A popular street tree in California, the cultivar 'Keith Davey' is a male and should never be used.

P. vera is a small- to medium-sized deciduous nut tree for hot summer areas of zones 8–10. Both sexes needed to produce the edible nuts.

Pisum sativum. ✳ 2
ENGLISH PEAS, GARDEN PEAS. Annual vines which produce edible peas and in some varieties, edible pods.

Pitanga.
See *Eugenia.*

PITCHER PLANT.
See *Sarracenia*.

Pithecellobium guadalupense. 8

BLACKBEAD TREE. A tropical tree used in zone 10, especially in Florida. There are a few other species of this genus that are also of interest in allergy. *P. unguis-cati*, the CAT'S CLAW is used in landscapes in south Florida, the West Indies, and Mexico. The flowers of this species resemble those of *Mimosa* and are capable of releasing airborne pollen.

Pittosporum. 📷 5

CAPE PITTOSPORUM, KARO, KOHUHU, MOCK ORANGE, QUEENSLAND PITTOSPORUM, VICTORIAN BOX. Easy to grow, glossy-leafed evergreen shrubs and trees native to Australia, New Zealand, Japan, China, and South Africa, used as common landscape plants in zones 9–10. They are fairly drought tolerant once established and not fussy about soil; they grow well in either sun or shade, but tend to legginess in deep shade. *Pittosporums* produce fragrant white flowers followed by rounded seed pods full of sticky seeds (their Latin name means "sticky seeds"), which may present a litter problem. The fragrance of some *Pittosporum*, especially *P. tobira*, can be very intense, particularly on warm, still summer evenings, and this fragrance may be allergenic for odor-sensitive individuals.

Pityrogramma. 3

GOLDBACK FERN. A native of the West Coast from California to Alaska and used in landscapes in shady, dry spots. It becomes summer dormant and looks best during the winter.

PLANE TREE.
See *Platanus*.

Planera aquatica. ✳10

PLANNER TREE, WATER ELM. A species of ELM-related deciduous trees, native to swampy areas of the southeastern United States and hardy into zone 7. This is one of the few members of the ELM family that produces separate male flowers, and as a result it is an especially heavy airborne pollinator.

PLANTAIN.
See *Musa*.

PLANTAIN LILY.
See *Hosta paradisiaca*.

Platanus. 📷 ✳9

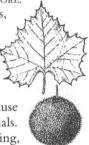

BUTTONBALL TREE, PLANE TREE, SYCAMORE. Big, fast-growing deciduous trees, some native, with attractive, peeling bark. Sycamore trees are used throughout the world and they cause allergy everywhere they're cultivated. Several species grown in zones 3–10. The fuzzy leaves may cause contact rash in sensitive individuals. When they bloom in early spring, SYCAMORES produce large amounts of airborne pollen, and allergy to SYCAMORE is common.

Platanus occidentalis

Platycarya. 8

A deciduous Chinese tree, hardy in zones 6–10. The bark of these relatives of the WALNUT is used to make a black dye.

Platycerium. 3

STAGHORN FERN. Dry, shade-loving epiphytic ferns which grow on trees or in hanging wire baskets in gardens in zones 9–10.

Platycladus orientalis. 8

ORIENTAL ARBORVITAE. Also known as *Thuja orientalis, Biota orientalis*. Evergreen coniferous shrubs, native to Korea and China, and hardy in zones 4–10. Extremely common landscape plants because of their tidy growth habits, these relatives of the CYPRESS cause allergy.

Platycodon grandiflorus. ✳2

BALLOON FLOWER. An easy-to-grow perennial for full sun or partial shade in all zones. Its balloon-like blue or white flowers appear in summer on the upright plants.

Plectranthus. ❋ *1*
SWEDISH IVY. Easy-to-grow houseplant related to *Coleus.*

Pleiogynium. males ❋ *9, females* ❋ *1*
BURDEKIN PLUM, HOG PLUM, QUEENSLAND HOG PLUM. Two species of separate-sexed trees from the Philippine Islands, New Guinea, and Australia. Grown in California, Hawaii, and Florida, the HOG PLUM is a large (to 60 feet) evergreen tree, the females of which produce small fruits popularly used in jellies and jams.

Pleione.
See ORCHIDS.

Pleroma.
See *Tibouchina.*

PLOVER EGGS.
See *Adromischus.*

PLUM, FLOWERING.
See *Prunus.*

PLUM, PATERSON.
See *Lagunaria patersonii.*

PLUM YEW.
See *Cephalotaxus.*

PLUMBAGO.
See *Ceratostigma; Plumbago auriculata.*

Plumbago auriculata. 3
CAPE PLUMBAGO. *Plumbago* is a large group of over 300 species, none of which is important in allergy. The CAPE PLUMBAGO is a large, sprawling shrub with sky-blue flowers, native to Ethiopia, which thrives on neglect in sunny areas of zone 10. Good bank cover plants. (See also *Ceratostigma.*)

PLUME CEDAR.
See *Cryptomeria.*

Plumeria. 4
FRANGIPANI. Frost-tender evergreen and deciduous shrubs and small trees for sheltered locations of zone 10, or as greenhouse plants. *Plumeria* are easy to propagate from cuttings and make good container plants. Their extremely fragrant flowers may affect those with odor sensitivity. Flowers and leaves are poisonous.

PLUMS, PRUNES.
See *Prunus.*

Poa. ❋10
BLUEGRASS. *P. pratensis,* KENTUCKY BLUEGRASS, is a popular lawn grass for northern areas, where it must be mowed often to keep it low and nonflowering. The common annual weed grass, *P. annua,* blooms at any height and also produces allergenic pollen.

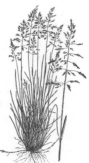

Poa pratensis

Podocarpus. 📷 *males* ❋ *9, females* ❋ *1*
FERN PINE, YEW PINE. A small group of separate-sexed coniferous evergreen shrubs or trees with leaves rather than needles. The female trees produce small, round, fleshy covered seeds. *P. macrophyllus,* the YEW PINE, is a very common shrub in California and is hardy in zones 9–10. Several dwarf forms are sold for use as a ground cover or low hedges. 'Select Spreader' is a low-growing male cultivar that should be avoided for its allergy potential.

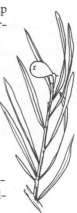

Podocarpus

P. gracilior, the FERN PINE, is a medium- to large-sized tree, occasionally used to make a dense, large hedge. *P. henkelii* is a handsome long-leafed shrub or small tree for zones 8–10, occasionally sold as LONG-LEAFED YELLOWWOOD.

Podocarpus are not related to PINE but rather to YEWS (*Taxus*).

POHUTUKAWA.
See *Metrosideros.*

POINCIANA.
See *Caesalpinia.*

POINSETTIA.
See *Euphorbia.*

POINTED-LEAF MAPLE.
See *Acer argutum.*

POISON BERRY.
See *Solanum.*

POISON ELDER.
See *Rhus.*

POISON IVY.
See *Rhus.*

POISON OAK.
See *Rhus diversiloba; Rhus toxicodendron.*

POKE, POKE BERRY, POKE SALAD, POKEWEED.
See *Phytolacca.*

POKER PLANT.
See *Kniphofia.*

POLECAT BUSH.
See *Rhus.*

Polemonium.   ❋ 2
JACOB'S LADDER. Hardy perennials best in cool summer areas in moist soil with good drainage. They bear stalks of blue or lavender flowers held erect above ferny foliage.

Polianthes tuberosa.   4
TUBEROSE. Tender tuberous perennial for the mildest areas of zone 10, *Polianthes* is used mostly as a potted plant. The powerfully fragrant, tubular white flowers are borne on tall spikes and may affect perfume-sensitive individuals.

POLKA-DOT PLANT.
See *Hypoestes phyllostachya.*

Polyandrococos.   7
A palm tree from Brazil, with small, edible fruit, used in zones 9–10, especially in Florida.

POLYANTHUS.
See *Primula polyantha.*

Polygala.   3
BIRD-ON-THE-WING, CANDYWEED, MILKWORT, SENECA SNAKEROOT, SWEET PEA SHRUB, VIOLET TREE, YELLOW BACHELOR'S BUTTON. Large group of evergreen perennials, shrubs, and small trees for light soils and partial shade of zones 7–10. Many species are frost-tender. The common name MILKWORT is derived from the belief that the plants could increase the flow of milk in cows.

Polygonatum.   ❋ 2
SOLOMON'S SEAL. Tall perennials of the LILY family, hardy in all zones. They grow in shady, moist areas, where they bear white or green-white bell-shaped flowers. Plants are poisonous.

Polygonum.   7
KNOTWEED, FLEECEFLOWER, SILVER LACE VINE, SMARTWEED. Many species of worldwide distribution: herbs, ground covers, vines, annuals, or perennials, of varying hardiness. The Latin name means "many joints," and refers to the many joints or nodes found along the stems of these plants. SMARTWEED is a common weed which thrives in almost any moist area and gets its name from the fact that the juice or sap can "smart" or burn the skin. All *Polygonum* members may cause skin rash from their caustic sap, and some species may also cause airborne allergy. All parts of plant are poisonous.

Polygonum

Polypodium.   *Individually rated.*
The largest group of ferns, with over 7,000 species.

Polypogon.   5
BEARDGRASS, RABBIT'S FOOT GRASS. Small annual, ornamental grass with large, fluffy heads. It often naturalizes.

Polyscias.   ✳ 1
PARSLEY PANAX, MING ARALIA. Tall, shrubby houseplants or small trees in tropical zone 10. *Polyscias* grows best in partial shade.

Polystichum.   5
SHIELD FERN, HOLLY FERN, HEDGE FERN, WESTERN SWORD FERN. Large group of easy-to-grow landscape ferns, some hardy to zones 4–5. All grow best in shady spots in the garden.

POMEGRANATE.
See *Punica granatum.*

POMPOM TREE.
See *Dais cotinifolia.*

POND CYPRESS.
See *Taxodium.*

PONDWEED, CAPE.
See *Aponogeton distachyus.*

Pontederia cordata.   ✳ 2
PICKEREL WEED. Pond plant for all zones; it bears tall stalks of blue flowers.

PONYTAIL.
See *Beaucarnea recurvata.*

POOR-MAN'S ORCHID.
See *Schizanthus.*

POPLAR.
See *Lirodendron; Populus.*

POPLAR, TULIP.
See *Liriondendron.*

POPLAR, YELLOW.
See *Liriodendron.*

POPOLO, YELLOW.
See *Solanum.*

POPPY.
See *Papaver.*

Populus. 📷
males ✱ *9, females* ✳ *1*

ASPEN, COTTONWOOD, POPLAR. More than 30 species of large, fast-growing, deciduous trees, members of the WILLOW family, hardy in all zones and under conditions ranging from arid deserts to wetlands, depending on species. Almost all species of *Populus* are separate-sexed; male trees often cause widespread and severe allergy, and in many areas, POPLAR pollen is the primary cause of springtime allergy. Female trees cause no allergy but are often maligned for the "cotton," seeds, and fruit that they shed. Because they shed their seeds, each with its parachute of highly visible "cotton" at the same time that RAGWEEDS, COYOTE BUSH, CHINESE ELM, and other highly allergenic plants are shedding their pollen, female POPLARS are unfairly blamed for the resulting allergy. (Female trees often mature to larger, longer-lived, rounder specimens than do male trees.) Trees sold as COTTONLESS COTTONWOODS or COTTONLESS POPLARS are males, and highly suspect in the allergy-free landscape.

Populus deltoides (female flowers)

The following named cultivars are all males and should be avoided: 'Androscoggin', 'Cordeniensis', 'Majestic', 'Mojave Hybrid', 'N. E. 17', 'N. E. 308', 'Wheeler', as should *P. songarica* (*P. manchurica*).

P. 'Volunteer' is a highly rated female RUSSIAN POPLAR, and *P. wilsoni* is a large female tree with reddish twigs and leaves that are bluish above and white below. *P.* 'Noreaster' is one of the best, a sterile female. All three are excellent choices for the allergy-free landscape.

P. alba.

WHITE POPLAR. The cultivar 'Nivea' is female; 'Pyramidalis' is a male.

P. canadensis.

BLACK POPLAR. The cultivars 'Incrassata', 'Marilandica', and 'Regenerata' are females and good choices for the allergy-free landscape. 'Eugenei', 'Gelrica' or DUTCH POPLAR, 'Prairie Sky', and 'Robusta' are male and should be avoided.

P. × canadensis (P. deltoides × P. nigra).

CAROLINA POPLAR. These are male hybrids.

P. candicans.

BALM-OF-GILEAD. Also known as P. × Jackii, P. balsamifera, and P. ontariensis. These are female trees, and fine choices for the allergy-free landscape. 'Candicans Aurora' is a named female cultivar. 'Candicans Variegata' is a beautiful female tree that is often used as a big shrub. Cut to the ground each fall, it resprouts with huge, variegated leaves, splashed with pink and white. The cultivar 'Macrophylla' is a male and should not be used. The hybrid P. × candicans 'White' is a male.

P. × canescens.

The cultivar 'Tower' is a male tree; avoid use.

P. deltoides.

Among named cultivars, 'Carolin' and 'Siouxland' are males; 'Cordata' is a female.

P. fremontii.

'Zappetini' is a male.

P. × Jackii.

The named cultivar 'Generosa' can be either male or female; female trees are identified by their catkins, which are twice as long as the male in this cultivar. Both 'Northwest' and 'Saskatchewan' are male.

P. lasiocarpa.

CHINESE NECKLACE POPLAR. A native of China, this is a rare example of a POPLAR that has bisexual flowers. It has very large leaves, and the pollen does not present much allergy potential.

P. nigra.

BLACK POPLAR. There are many named cultivars of BLACK POPLAR, but unless the trees are sexed, it is best to avoid use. The THEVES POPLAR 'Afghanica' is also named P. thevestina, P. usbekistanica, and P. nigra 'Ozbekistanica'. The THEVES POPLAR is a tall, narrow tree, similar in appearance to LOMBARDY POPLAR (P. n. 'Italica'), except that it is fuller and longer-lived. THEVES POPLAR is female, as is the variety P. n. 'Charkowiensis', which is a larger tree. 'Elegans' and 'Italica' are male.

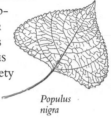

Populus nigra

P. nigra 'Italica'.

This is the tall, skinny LOMBARDY POPLAR that grows so tall and fast but then dies off almost as quickly. Although this is the most widely planted POPLAR in the world, 'Italica' (or 'Lombardi') is a male and should be avoided.

P. × petrowskiana.

'Waller' is a female.

P. × 'Pseudograndidentata'.

This is a WEEPING POPLAR, occasionally sold as P. pendula. It is a male.

P. simonii.

SIMON POPLAR. 'Fastigiata' and 'Pendula' are males.

P. tomentosa.

CHINESE WHITE POPLAR. Both sexes are sold; use only the female.

P. tremula.

EUROPEAN ASPEN. The varieties 'Erecta' and 'Pendula' are male.

P. tremuloides.

QUAKING ASPEN. 'Pendula' is a female.

PORCUPINE PALM.
See *Rhapidophyllum hystrix.*

PORK-AND-BEANS.
See *Sedum.*

PORT ORFORD CEDAR.
See *Chamaecyparis.*

Portulaca grandiflora. ❋ 2
MOSS ROSE. An annual for hot, sunny spots. Bright rose-like, little flowers in many colors cover these succulent bedding plants.

Portulacaria. ❋ 2
ELEPHANT'S FOOD, PURSLANE TREE. Tall succulent with many tiny, fleshy leaves borne on thick fleshy stalks. Easy to grow in sun or shade in protected areas of zones 9–10. Houseplant elsewhere, in good light.

POT MARIGOLD.
See *Calendula.*

POTATO VINE, POTATO BUSH.
See *Solanum.*

Potentilla. 3
CINQUEFOIL. Hardy evergreen and deciduous perennials and shrubs for all zones. Most *Potentilla* have bright yellow flowers but some are red, orange, or white. Several species are low-growing ground covers for partial shade with ample water.

POTHOS.
See *Epipremnum aureum.*

POUND CAKE WEED.
See *Parthenium hysterophorum.*

POVERTY GRASS.
See *Corema; Hudsonia.*

PRAIRIE MIMOSA.
See *Desmanthus.*

PRAIRIE TEA.
See *Croton monanthogynus.*

Pratia angulata. ❋ 1
New Zealand perennial native used in desert areas of zones 7–10 as a ground cover, although it needs ample water. *Pratia* bears small white or blue flowers.

PRAYER PLANT.
See *Maranta leuconeura.*

PREGNANT ONION.
See *Ornithogalum.*

PRICKLEWEED.
See *Desmanthus.*

PRICKLY ASH.
See *Zanthoxylum.*

PRICKLY PEAR.
See OPTUNIA.

PRICKLY POPPY.
See *Argemone.*

PRIDE-OF-BOLIVIA.
See *Tipuana tipu.*

PRIDE OF CHINA.
See *Melia.*

PRIDE OF INDIA.
See *Melia.*

PRIDE OF MADEIRA.
See *Echium fastuosum.*

PRIMROSE TREE.
See *Lagunaria patersonii.*

Primula. 📷 4
PRIMROSE, AURICULA. Hardy perennials often used as annuals. In hot areas PRIMROSES are best used as potted flowers, or in the garden for winter color or as early spring annuals. PRIMROSES do not produce

allergenic pollen, but some species, especially *P. malacoides* and *P. obconica*, frequently are the cause of severe skin rashes and lesions from simple contact with the plants.

PRINCESS FLOWER.
See *Tibouchina urvilleana*.

PRINCESS PALM.
See *Dictyosperma*.

PRINCESS PINE.
See *Lycopodium*.

PRIVET.
See *Ligustrum; Phillyrea*.

PRIVET, SWAMP.
See *Forestiera*.

Prosopis. ✸9

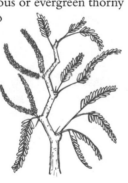

Prosopis

MESQUITE, SCREW BEAN, TORNILLO. Twenty or more species of summer-deciduous or evergreen thorny shrubs or trees, native to desert areas of southwestern United States and Mexico. With its fernlike foliage and numerous pollen-shedding small yellow flowers, MESQUITE is a major allergy plant in some areas.

Protea. 5
South African shrubs and trees, many with large, unusual flowers, which are favored as centerpieces for large flower arrangements. They are hardy only in zones 9–10.

Prunella. ✳ 2
HEAL-ALL, SELF-HEAL. Creeping perennial ground cover with medicinal properties, for shade with ample moisture.

Prunus. 📷
ALMOND, APRICOT, CHERRY, PEACH, PLUM, NECTARINE. *Prunus* is a large group of over 400 species of deciduous shrubs and trees, mostly native to the Northern Hemisphere.

Many species of *Prunus* are popular and useful landscape shrubs and trees. Following are some of the most common.

P. caroliniana 7
CAROLINA LAUREL CHERRY. A native evergreen small tree for zones 7–10.

P. ilicifolia. 7
HOLLYLEAF CHERRY. An evergreen ornamental shrub or small tree for zones 8–10.

P. laurocerasus. 6
ENGLISH LAUREL, ZABEL LAUREL. An ornamental evergreen shrub, commonly used as a hedge in zones 7–9.

P. lusitanica. 5
PORTUGAL LAUREL. An evergreen ornamental shrub with thick leathery leaves and white flowers. Hardy only in warm winter areas.

P. lyonii. 📷 7
CATALINA CHERRY. An ornamental flowering shrub for zones 8–10.

P. maackii. 5
AMUR CHOKECHERRY. A cold-hardy, highly ornamental cherry tree with incredibly beautiful bark, best in zones 4–7.

P. padus. 7
BIRD CHERRY. Tall ornamental cherry hardy to zone 4.

P. sargentii. 7
SARGENT CHERRY. A large tree, with small fruit that is very attractive to birds.

P. serrula. [📷]   5

BIRCH BARK CHERRY. A large flowering tree with handsome leaves and bark, hardy to zone 4.

P. serrulata.   7

JAPANESE FLOWERING CHERRY. A popular and common flowering cherry, hardy to zone 4. Double-flowered varieties are far less potent allergy trees.

P. virginiana.   6

CHOKECHERRY. Shrub or small tree, hardy even in zone 2. CHOKECHERRY produces many dark red bitter fruits. The leaves, stems, and unripe fruit of this species are extremely poisonous, by far the most toxic of all *Prunus* species.

The fruiting members of the *Prunus* genus (following) rarely present severe allergy problems, except for ALMONDS, which are known to produce copious amounts of highly irritant pollen.

P. armeniaca. [📷]   ✳ 2

APRICOTS are hardy in most zones, but do not fruit regularly in any but the mildest winter areas. Good trees often can be grown from seed, although they may take 3 or more years to fruit. They are especially beautiful when in bloom, and many have excellent fall color. Allergy to apricots is usually confined to those living in or near orchards; as the occasional yard tree, APRICOTS are a very good choice for the allergy-free landscape. *P. glandulosa* is the FLOWERING APRICOT.

P. avium, P. cerasus.   5

CHERRIES. CHERRIES are hardy, deciduous flowering trees that need a certain amount of winter cold to thrive. They will not grow well in zones 9 and 10. SOUR CHERRY (*P. avium*) is hardier than SWEET CHERRY (*P. cerasus*) and will grow as far north as zone 3. All varieties need good drainage to thrive. Pollen allergy is not common. Those living in or near orchards are most at risk. FLOWERING CHERRIES (*P. lannesiana or siebold,* see also *P. serrulata*) are commonly used as landscape and street trees and are a major source of pollen; double-flowered varieties release less pollen than single-flowered.

P. communis.   ✳10

ALMONDS. In allergy studies ALMONDS stand out as the cause of severe allergy. People living in or close to ALMOND orchards are most likely to develop allergy, and although there is occasionally a cross-over allergic reaction to eating ALMONDS, this is less common.

P. domestica, P. insititia. [📷]   3

PLUMS. *P. cerasifera*, the PURPLE-LEAF PLUM, is a common landscape tree with several cultivars, notably 'Newport' and 'Krauter Vesuvius', that produce little pollen. *P. blireana*, another hardy red-leafed plum, is also a low pollen producer. The smaller, shrubby *P. cistena*, the DWARF RED-LEAF PLUM, is also not a high-risk tree but has a slightly higher potential for allergy.

P. persica.   3, 4

PEACH, NECTARINE. Certain varieties of *P. persica* are hardy into zones 4 and 5, but most are not hardy past zone 6. The blossoms are pink and quite attractive; flowering varieties bloom very early and put on great shows. These flowering types have a greater allergy potential than do fruiting varieties. Nonetheless, allergy to PEACH OR NECTARINE is uncommon, although the fuzz on peaches is sometimes the cause of rash or inhalant allergy.

In areas with foggy nights, PEACH and NECTARINE are often afflicted with peach leaf curl, a fungal disease. They are best grown where spring and summer nights are warm and dry. Allergy rating for fruiting peach and nectarine is 3; for flowering peach and nectarine, 4; and for double-flowered peach and nectarine, 3.

P. tomentosa.   4

NANKING CHERRY. Fruiting bush cherry with edible fruit; the most hardy of any semisweet-fruited cherries. Zones 3–7.

Pseudolarix kaempferi (Chrysolarix).   3

GOLDEN LARCH. A deciduous conifer with attractive foliage and good, bright yellow fall color. A native of China, it grows best in moist, acid soil in zones 6–8. Not an important allergy tree, despite its abundant pollen.

Pseudopanax. *males 8, females* ✣ *1*

LANCEWOOD. Separate-sexed evergreen shrubs or small trees from New Zealand and Chile, grown in protected areas of zones 9–10. Female plants produce very small, one-seeded fruits.

Pseudophoenix. 5

CHERRY PALM. Four species of palm trees from the subtropics, used in zone 10.

Pseudotsuga. 3

BIG-CONE SPRUCE, DOUGLAS FIR. Five species of evergreen conifers, all large, tall trees, one native to Japan, the rest to the Pacific Northwest and hardy in zones 5–10. Although *Pseudotsuga* releases abundant pollen, none of the genus are important allergy offenders because the pollen has a waxy coating that keeps it from being easily absorbed. DOUGLAS FIR, a giant tree, occasionally reaching a height of 300 feet, is perhaps the most important lumber tree in the world. Small DOUGLAS FIRS are often used as Christmas trees and have the same aromatic smell as their close relatives, the PINES. DOUGLAS FIR was named after David Douglas, a famous Scotch plant explorer who first discovered and named many species of the Pacific coast. Douglas made three cross-continental trips searching for new plants before his untimely death in 1834, at the age of 35, at the hands of natives in the Sandwich Islands (Hawaii).

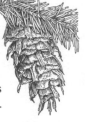

Pseudotsuga taxifolia

Pseudowintera. 6

Evergreen shrub or small tree, native of New Zealand and occasionally used in California.

Psidium. 📷 3

GUAVA. Many species of mostly evergreen shrubs or small trees, often cultivated for the sweet yellow fruits with pink flesh. The hardiest of the true GUAVAS is *P. littorale* 'Lucidum', the small, reddish, STRAWBERRY GUAVA, which grows in most areas of zone 9. *P. guajava*, the COMMON GUAVA, is a zone 10 shrub which needs heat to produce sweet fruit. Although the pollen-bearing stamens are well-exposed in *Psidium* flowers, and may present allergy problems if directly contacted, as a whole the genus does not pose allergy potential.

Psylliostachys suworowii. 4

Annuals grown for their large leaves and spikes of pinkish lavender flowers, resembling STATICE, which are often used in dried flower arrangements.

Ptelea. *males 7, females* ✣ *1*

HOP TREE, WAFER ASH. A deciduous shrub or small tree, related to and having flowers that smell like *Citrus*. HOP TREE is hardy to zone 3 if grown in a moist, shady spot. Separate-sexed; only the females produce the flat, hop-like seed pods.

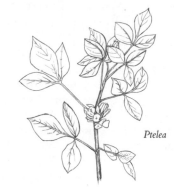

Ptelea

Pteridium aquilinum. 5

BRACKEN FERN. A native fern, hardy in all zones, which may become invasive. The emerging fronds, called *fiddleheads*, are edible, although recent research indicates that they may contain a carcinogen. The spores may cause allergy.

Pteris. 5

BRAKE. Subtropical ferns, often grown as houseplants.

Pterocarpus. 3

ROSEWOOD, SANDALWOOD. Large group of tropical trees, with aromatic wood much prized for fine furniture.

Pterocarya. 📷   7
WINGNUT TREE. A small group of deciduous trees related to WALNUT, which are grown for their attractive leaves and flowers. Various *Pterocarya* are hardy in zones 6–10, depending on species.

Pterostyrax. 📷   4
EPAULETTE TREE, WISTERIA TREE. Deciduous trees from Asia, grown in zones 7–10. The long clusters of white flowers are followed by small hairy seeds, which may be irritating to the skin. The flowers, however, present few pollen problems.

Ptychococcus.   7
A group of palm trees native from New Guinea to the Solomon Islands.

Ptychosperma.   7
ALEXANDER PALM, MACARTHUR PALM. A group of about 30 palm trees, many from Australia and occasionally used in zone 10. All can cause allergy.

Pueraria lobata.   3
KUDSU. The vine that took over the South. An Asian native, KUDSU has been planted in many southern areas as a pasture or hay crop because the feed value of the leaves is as good as alfalfa. It has escaped cultivation, however, and has become a rampant, invasive weed throughout much of the South, often smothering native flora and buildings with its fast-growing vines.

PUERTO RICAN HAT PALM.
See *Sabal.*

PUKA.
See *Meryta sinclairii.*

Pulmonaria.   ❋ 2
JERUSALEM SAGE, LUNGWORT. Perennials hardy in all zones, these shade-loving plants require ample moisture to bear their blue, purple, or red flowers.

Punica granatum. 📷   ❋ 2
POMEGRANATE. Deciduous shrubs or small trees, hardy to zone 7, but growing best in full sun, in hot summer areas of zones 8–9. Good heat is required to ripen sweet fruit. The large, orange flowers are followed by round fruits that require heat and adequate moisture to ripen fully. Although occasionally grown as an ornamental, POMEGRANATES are good fruit trees, with the variety 'Wonderful' producing the largest fruit. *Punica* is easy to propagate from dormant cuttings.

PURPLE CONEFLOWER.
See *Echinacea purpurea.*

PURPLE HEART.
See *Setcreasea pallida.*

PURPLE-LEAF PLUM.
See *Prunus.*

PURPLE LOOSESTRIFE.
See *Lythrum.*

PURPLE MULLEIN.
See *Verbascum.*

PURPLE OSIER.
See *Salix.*

PURPLE RAGWORT.
See *Senecio.*

PURPLE SAGE.
See *Salvia.*

PURPLE VELVET PLANT.
See *Gynura aurantiaca.*

PURPLELEAF ELDER.
See *Sambucus.*

PURSLANE.
See *Portulaca.*

PURSLANE TREE.
See *Portulacaria oleracea.*

PUSSY EARS.
See *Calochortus; Cyanotis.*

PUSSY TOES.
See *Antennaria.*

PUSSY WILLOW.
See *Salix.*

Putranjiva.   ✳ *10*
Small group of large trees native to India, Sri
Lanka, and the former Borneo, all with great po-
tential for allergy.

PUYA.
See *Bromelia.*

Pyracantha. 📷   *5*
FIRETHORN.   Several species of evergreen, thorny
shrubs or small trees with small white flowers followed by round, reddish-orange berries. The
berries are poisonous but are eaten by some birds.
Hardy in zones 7–10, *Pyracantha* is a common landscape shrub despite its long thorns and the fact that
the malodorous flowers tend to attract flies. The
odor may cause allergy in sensitive individuals.
Pyracantha is closely related to HAWTHORN and
Cotoneaster, and may serve as a host for the bacterial disease, fireblight.

Pyrethrum.   *7*
PAINTED DAISY.   A daisy-flowered plant from which
the botanical insecticide *pyrethrum* is derived. Those
working in *pyrethrum* processing plants often
become very allergic to the flowers and dust from
the flowers. *Pyrethrum* is a common insecticide
used in pet flea powders, and pet owners may
exhibit allergy to this flower-based powder. See
also *Chrysanthemum.*

Pyrostegia venusta.   *3*
FLAME VINE. Big, fast-growing evergreen vine with
long tubular orange flowers, for zone 10. FLAME
VINE needs heat to grow well.

Pyrrosia lingua (Cyclophorus).   *4*
JAPANESE FELT FERN.   Slow-growing, shade-loving
small ferns for zones 9–10.

Pyrus.   *ornamentals 4, fruiting varieties 3*
BRADFORD PEAR, PEAR. Deciduous fruit trees hardy
to zone 4 but growing best in zones 7–9. PEAR
blossoms are attractive but malodorous, athough
the strong smell does not carry far in the air. The
pollen is not usually an allergen. Among the many
ornamental, flowering, nonfruiting PEARS grown,
the most common and popular is the pyramidal
BRADFORD PEAR. ASIAN PEARS, which have large
sweet fruit, rounder than the common pear, are
also prized for their good autumn color.

PEARS often suffer from fireblight, a bacterial disease which can kill entire branches or even whole
trees. Fireblight is spread through airborne spores
and direct contact, so diseased branches should be
burned, not composted. It is worst during cool,
damp weather. Excessive growth encourages fireblight, so use of nitrogen fertilizers is not advised.

Q

Allergy Index Scale: *1* **is Best,** *10* **is Worst.**

❇ for *1* and *2* ✸ for *9* and *10*

📷 See insert for photograph

QUACKGRASS.
See *Agropyron*.

QUAILBUSH.
See *Atriplex*.

Quamoclit lobata.
See *Mina lobata*.

Quamoclit pennata.
See *Ipomoea*.

QUEEN ANNE'S LACE.
See *Daucus*.

QUEEN PALM.
See *Arecastrum romanzoffianum*.

QUEEN'S TEARS.
See *Billbergia*.

QUEEN'S WREATH.
See *Antigonon*.

QUEENSLAND HOG PLUM.
See *Pleiogynium*.

QUEENSLAND KAURI.
See *Agathis robusta*.

QUEENSLAND LACEBARK.
See *Brachychiton discolor*.

QUEENSLAND NUT.
See *Macadamia*.

QUEENSLAND PITTOSPORUM.
See *Pittosporum*.

QUEENSLAND POPLAR.
See *Homalanthus populifolius*.

QUEENSLAND UMBRELLA TREE.
See *Brassaia actinophylla*.

Quercus. 📷 *deciduous 8, evergreen* ✸ *9*
OAK. With over 400 species of deciduous or evergreen hardy shrubs or trees worldwide, OAKS are important timber and landscape plants in much of the temperate world. All OAKS make acorns, the usually large, capped oak seeds. Acorns are eaten by many wild animals and in the past were sometimes used as food by native peoples.

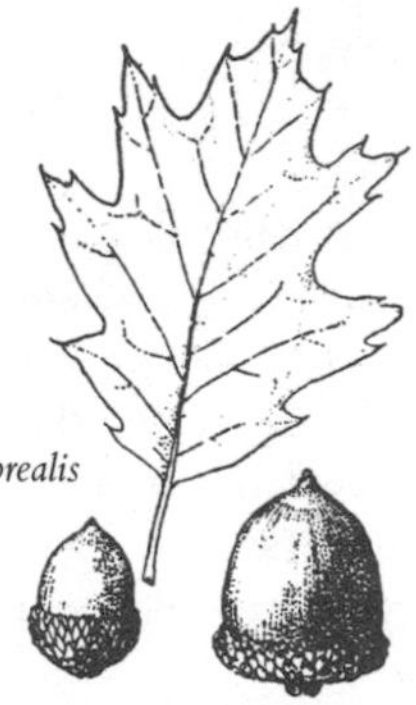

Quercus borealis

OAKS are pollinated by the wind, and they produce abundant pollen that provokes a great deal of allergy in areas with many OAKS. In some cities, planted landscape OAKS are the most common street trees and these in turn contribute to frequent allergic attacks. The large deciduous trees usually flower while the branches are still bare of leaves or as the new leaves are budding out. The evergreen OAKS often bloom later; in California they are often at their peak round the first of June. (In California there are so many kinds of OAKS, both native and planted, all of them blooming at different times, that parts of the state have a perennial OAK pollen allergy season.)

Some OAKS produce much more pollen than others, and an occasional OAK tree does not ever bloom. It is hoped that in the future, nurserymen will seek out non-blooming OAKS and graft them onto OAK seedlings.

The literature on OAK allergy suggests that there are distinct differences in degree of severity between the allergy potentials of the different species of OAKS, but as yet, we are forced to group them into two, oversimplified groups, evergreen and deciduous. Some bright graduate student could do us all a wonderful service by sorting out the actual allergy potential of each kind of OAK, how much pollen each releases, and exactly how allergenic each kind of pollen is.

Allergy to OAK pollen is such that if someone is allergic to the pollen of RED OAK, for example, they will usually also be allergic to pollen of WHITE OAK or any other OAK. The actual degree of allergy from each species varies greatly and as yet is something of a mystery. Most OAKS produce heavy pollen loads, but the evergreen or LIVE OAKS often produce the most pollen and produce it for a longer time. In California, *Q. agrifolia*, the COASTAL LIVE OAK, is a major allergy tree.

A large, spreading OAK tree may be the centerpiece of a landscape, and most people would be reluctant to remove it. If someone with allergies had a big OAK, he or she would be wise to get skin tested for OAK pollen, and if positive, to undergo desensitizing shots for OAK. For OAKS that are not too large in height, it is hoped that the future will bring us some sort of non-toxic spray that could be used to knock down the huge amount of male flowers before they can release their pollen. Pollen from all types of OAK is also known to sometimes cause skin rashes from contact.

Quillaja saponaria. 4
SOAP BARK TREE. A tall evergreen tree from Chile, hardy in zones 8–10. Soap is made from the bark of some species.

QUINCE.
See *Chaenomeles.*

QUINOA.
See *Chenopodium.*

R

Allergy Index Scale: *1* **is Best**, *10* **is Worst**.

✳ for *1* and *2*   ✺ for *9* and *10*

📷 See insert for photograph

RABBIT'S FOOT GRASS.
See *Polypogon*.

RABBIT'S PEA.
See *Tephrosia*.

RAGWEED.
See *Ambrosia*.

RAGWORT.
See *Senecio*.

RAIN LILY.
See *Zephyranthes*.

RAISIN TREE.
See *Hovenia dulcis*.

RAMBUTAN.
See *Nephelium lappaceum*.

RAMONA.
See *Salvia*.

RAMONTCHI.
See *Flacourtia*.

Ranunculus. 📷   5
BUTTERCUPS, CROWFOOT, PERSIAN RANUNCULUS.
Colorful tuberous perennials usually grown as annuals, *Ranunculus* flowers (sometimes fully double)
are held aloft on tall, wiry stems. They begin
blooming in early spring and grow best in cool
weather. *R. repens* is a true perennial, hardy in all
zones, and useful as a ground cover for moist soils.
As cut flowers, they pose some allergy potential.
All parts of *Ranunculus* are poisonous if eaten.

RAPE.   6
See *Brassica*.

Raqulia australis.   4
Low-growing, spreading perennial for zones 8–10.
It requires full sun and good drainage to thrive.

RASPBERRY.
See *Rubus*.

RATTAN PALM.
See *Rhapis humilis*.

RATTLEBOX.
See *Crotalaria*.

RATTLESNAKE GRASS.
See *Briza maxima*.

RED-APPLE ICEPLANT.
See *Aptenia cordifolia*.

RED BAY.
See *Persea borbonia*.

RED-BERRIED GREENBRIER.
See *Smilax*.

RED CEDAR.
See *Juniperus; Thuja*.

RED CHOKEBERRY.
See *Aronia arbutifolia*.

RED ELDER.
See *Sambucus*.

RED ESCALLONIA.
See *Escallonia*.

RED FIR.
See *Abies*.

RED GUM.
See *Eucalyptus*.

RED-HOT POKER.
See *Kniphofia uvaria*.

RED MAPLE.
See *Acer rubrum*.

RED OSIER.
See *Cornus*.

REDBIRD CACTUS.
See *Pedilanthus tithymaloides*.

REDBUD.
See *Cercis*.

REDONDO CREEPER.
See *Lampranthus*.

REDTOP.
See *Agrostis*.

REDWOOD.
See *Sequoia sempervirens*.

REDWOOD, DAWN.
See *Metasequoia glyptostroboides*.

REDWOOD, FORMOSAN.
See *Taiwania cryptomerioides*.

REED, GIANT.
See *Arundo donax*.

Rehmannia elata. ✳ 2
Tall, erect perennial for sun or shade in zones 9–10. The tubular multicolored flowers of *Rehmannia* persist over a long blooming period.

Reinwardtia indica. 4
YELLOW FLAX. Large shrublike perennial for zones 9–10. The bright yellow flowers bloom in late fall and early winter.

Reseda odorata. 4
MIGNONETTE. Fragrant, fast-growing warm-season annuals. The strongly fragrant blooms may present a challenge to the odor-sensitive.

Retinispora.
See *Chamaecyparis*.

Rheum. 4
RHUBARB. RHUBARB flowers cause limited allergy, but usually only in those living next to fields of *Rheum*. Nevertheless, these flowers are highly suspect given some of their allergenic cousins.

Rhamnus (Cascara). 📷 ✻ 9
BEARBERRY, BUCKTHORN, CAROLINA BUCK-THORN, CASCARA SAGRADA, COFFEEBERRY, HOLLYLEAF REDBERRY, INDIAN CHERRY. A large group of mostly deciduous shrubs or small trees, native to the United States and Asia, especially China and Japan; some are hardy to zone 3. In California *R. californica*, the COFFEE-BERRY, is a commonly used native shrub, recently popular in the past wave of drought-tolerant native-based landscaping. All the *Rhamnus* species cause allergy and this is well known and long documented. *Rhamnus* flowers are small, numerous, and usually an off-white or greenish color; the pollen that they release triggers widespread and severe allergy. The inner bark of some species is boiled and used as a laxative. The fresh leaves and the seeds of some species are poisonous if eaten.

Rhamnus purshiana

Rhaphiolepis indica.   4

INDIA HAWTHORN. Several species of evergreen shrubs, some to 12 feet, common in zones 9–10. *Rhaphiolepis* grows in full sun or part shade, but flowers more profusely and holds its compact shape better in full sun. Although the attractive *Rhaphiolepis* is very common in urban landscapes, its overuse may eventually contribute to further allergy problems as urban biodiversity continues to decrease.

Rhapidophora aurea.

See *Epipremnum*.

Rhapidophyllum hystrix.   5

BLUE PALMETTO, NEEDLE PALM, PORCUPINE PALM. Clumpy, short, native palms; the hardiest of all the palm species, they will grow in zone 7.

Rhapis.   *males 6, females* ❋ 1

BAMBOO PALM, LADY PALM, MINIATURE FAN PALM, SLENDER LADY PALM. Small palms often used as houseplants, or outside in zones 9–10. Native to China, *Rhapis* are separate-sexed, but are not sold sexed. The female plants produce small one-seeded fleshy fruits.

RHINO'S HORN.

See *Agave attenuata*.

RHODES GRASS.

See *Chloris*.

Rhododendron. 📷   *azalea 3, rhododendron 4*

AZALEA, RHODODENDRON. A very large group of about 800 species of deciduous and evergreen shrubs or small trees. In general AZALEAS are lower-growing than RHODODENDRONS, but all have colorful, extremely showy flowers, often in large, impressive clusters. They thrive in the partial shade of large deciduous trees, in deep, peaty, well-drained acid soil with a steady supply of moisture. Because they are completely unforgiving as far as drought is concerned, it is advisable to keep these plants deeply mulched at all times.

Rhododendron pollen is relatively heavy and not usually airborne; the male stamens are exposed, however, and direct contact with the pollen is possible. Tall plants should be used at the back of the garden, where the danger from dropping pollen is lessened. All parts of AZALEA and RHODODENDRON are poisonous.

Rhodosphaera rhodanthema.   ❋10

YELLOWWOOD. A separate-sexed Australian timber tree, to 40 feet. Female trees produce large one-seeded, non-edible fruits.

Rhoeo spathacea.   ❋ 2

MOSES-IN-THE-CRADLE. A large-leaved plant with large white flowers that resemble small boats; for sheltered spots in zones 9–10.

Rhoicissus capensis.   ❋ 2

EVERGREEN GRAPE. *Rhoicissus* is used as an attractive vine or ground cover in zones 9–10; as houseplant in cooler zones.

Rhopaloblaste.   8

A group of tropical palms.

Rhopalostylis.   8

FEATHER-DUSTER PALM, NIKAU PALM. A group of subtropical palms used in zones 9–10.

RHUBARB.

See *Rheum*.

Rhus. 📷   *males* ❋ 10, *females* 7

AFRICAN SUMACH, CHINESE VARNISH TREE, FRAGRANT SUMAC, LAUREL SUMAC, LEMONADE BERRY, NUTGALL TREE, POISON ELDER, POISON IVY, POISON OAK, POLECAT BUSH, SMOOTH SUMAC, SUGAR BUSH, SUMAC, VINEGAR TREE, WILLOW SUMACH. About 150 species of evergreen or deciduous shrubs and trees, from many regions. Most are separate-sexed, and the light, buoyant pollen produced by males of the species presents a distinctly serious allergy potential.

The most well-known of the allergenic *Rhus* are poison sumac (*R. vernix*), poison ivy (*R. radicans*), and poison oak (*R. toxicodendron*), and cross-allergic reactions to the pollen of other *Rhus* species are a distinct possibility for those already hypersensitive to these three noxious weeds.

Although several of the *Rhus* species are prized as landscape shrubs because of their ease of growth and their good fall color, no members of this genus are recommended for allergy-free landscapes because even the female plants present a host of allergy problems from contact rashes to odor allergies.

In southern Italy, *R. coriaria*, the TANNER'S SUMAC, is grown as a source of tannin for leather making. In Japan, *R. orientalis*, is a vine with similar properties to our native POISON IVY. In east Asia, Japan, and India, *R. succedanea*, the WAX TREE, is used to make both a commercial wax and a lacquer. Both the wax and the lacquer may cause allergy.

In Japan the native *R. verniciflua* or VARNISH TREE, which is often described as "poisonous to touch," is used to make varnish or lacquer. It is occasionally grown in the United States in zones 9–10, even though varnish or lacquer produced from the sap of this tree has been implicated as causing severe contact rash in individuals who handle furniture coated with this lacquer.

R. integrifolia, a California native, has berries that are occasionally used as a substitute for lemons in lemonade; those who suffer allergy to any *Rhus* species should not drink this beverage. *R. ovata*, or SUGARBUSH, is a large, drought-tolerant evergreen shrub native to the southwestern United States. Female plants (with red berries) are rated at 4, while males are rated at 9. Since *Rhus* species are separate-sexed, only the female plants have fruit. Because *Rhus* males produce allergenic pollen, in addition to all the other potential problems, the males should never be used. Cross-reactive responses between all different species of *Rhus* are well known, and since allergy to poison ivy and poison oak is so common, none of these plants can be recommended. Even the VOCs released into the air when the plants are pruned are capable of causing allergy.

Lastly, it is important to realize that allergic response to *Rhus* species is almost always a delayed reaction. The actual allergy may not occur until hours, or even days, after the initial exposure.

RHYNCHOSPERMUM.
See *Trachelospermum*.

RIBBON BUSH.
See *Homalocladium platycladum*.

RIBBON CACTUS.
See *Pedilanthus tithymaloides*.

RIBBONWOOD.
See *Hoheria*.

Ribes.   *males 7, females* ✳ *1*
CURRANT, GOOSEBERRY. Very cold-hardy evergreen or deciduous shrubs grown in all zones, some for their fruit and others as landscape plants. There is a *Ribes* for almost any landscape situation ranging from shade to full sun, and from dry to moist soils. CURRANTS do not usually have thorns and GOOSEBERRIES are usually prickly.

R. alpinum, the ALPINE CURRANT; *R. diacanthum; R. fasciculatum; R. orientale*; and *R. tenue* are all separate-sexed plants, although rarely sold sexed.

R. bracteosum, glandulosum, and *viburnifolium* all have malodorous flowers, leaves, or both, and should be avoided.

Both *R. nigrum*, the BLACK CURRANT, and *R. sativum*, the RED CURRANT, are grown for their fruit and do not pose an allergy problem. *R. uva-crispa*, the common, large-fruited GOOSEBERRY, is a prickly plant that also is fine for the allergy-free garden. *R. odoratum*, which has fragrant, yellow, complete flowers, also presents no allergy problem.

RICE.
See *Oryza*.

RICE PAPER PLANT.
See *Tetrapanax papyriferus*.

Ricinus communis.   ✳10
CASTOR BEAN, CASTOR-OIL PLANT, PALMA CHRISTI, WONDER TREE. The CASTOR BEAN is native to tropical Africa but has naturalized in the tropics, subtropics, and other warm regions around the world. A common large weedy shrub or small tree in

zones 9–10, and used as an annual landscape foliage plant in all other zones, CASTOR BEAN poses a severe allergy threat. Many acres of it were planted in the midwestern United States during World War II, and by the second season of this crop large numbers of allergies to CASTOR BEAN appeared in people living close to these fields.

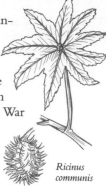

Ricinus communis

Seed from these plantings escaped cultivation, and CASTOR BEAN is a common and pernicious weed in many areas. Allergy to *Ricinus* is common and severe, including asthma.

A member of the *Euphorbia* or SPURGE family, CASTOR BEAN plants produce large amounts of light, airborne pollen, and the watery sap causes skin rash, as can simple contact with the leaves, flowers, or seeds.

The odd-looking, mottled seeds, or "beans" of *Ricinus* contain a deadly poison called *ricin*. *Ricoleic acid*, which is used in textile finishing and in the manufacture of some soaps, is also made from *Ricinus*, and cross-allergic reactions to these products are possible.

Those who are already allergic to CASTOR BEAN may have cross-allergic reactions to rubber from *Hevea brasiliensis*, which is a related plant.

RIVER WATTLE.
See *Acacia*.

Robinia. 5

BLACK LOCUST, FALSE ACACIA, GUMMY ACACIA, LOCUST, SILVER CHAIN TREE, SMOOTH ROSE ACACIA, WHYA TREE. *Robinia* is a group of several species of large, fast-growing deciduous, often thorny, flowering trees of the LEGUME family. All have

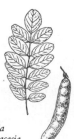

Robinia pseudoacacia

very hard, durable wood and are well adapted to growing in hot, dry summer areas; some species are cold-hardy to zone 3. Because they cast a light, filtered shade, they are prized lawn trees. Some named cultivars are spineless. All *Robinias* have seeds, flowers, and leaves that are poisonous if eaten. (See also *Gleditsia; Laburnum.*)

Rochea coccinea. ✳ 2

A tall, fleshy-leafed plant with bright red flowers that is grown as a greenhouse succulent or used outside in zone 10. It needs peaty, well-drained soil to thrive.

ROCK JASMINE.
See *Androsace*.

ROCK MAPLE.
See *Acer glabrum*.

ROCK PALM.
See *Brahea edulis*.

ROCKBERRY.
See *Empetrum*.

ROCKCRESS.
See *Arabis*.

ROCKROSE.
See *Cistus*.

ROCKY MOUNTAIN RED CEDAR.
See *Juniperus scopulorum*.

ROHDEA JAPONICA.
See *Lilium*.

ROMAN CANDLE.
See *Yucca*.

ROMAN LAUREL.
See *Laurus nobilis*.

ROMAN WORMWOOD.
See *Artemisia*.

Romneya coulteri.   *4*

MATILIJA POPPY. Very large perennial POPPY for zones 9–10. Its gray-green leaves and huge white flowers can reach 8 feet. The MATILIJA POPPY needs perfect drainage and is best grown on hillsides in sunny spots. All parts are poisonous.

Rondeletia.   *3*

Evergreen shrubs to 12 feet, for zone 10. *Rondeletia* bears long, tubular pink or yellow flowers in dense clusters.

Rosa. 📷   *Varies by variety.*

ROSES. A large group of over 100 species, hardy in all zones, according to species. Allergy to the fragrance of ROSES is more common than is allergy to the pollen, and any allergic response is usually low to moderate. Fully double roses release far less pollen than single-flowered varieties.

ROSES grow best in full sun to partial shade and require fertile, well-drained soil and ample moisture to thrive. Many roses are easy to grow from dormant cuttings, which can often be rooted simply by using long cuttings, direct-stuck in a partially shaded spot. Roses are best purchased bare root in spring. Because they are susceptible to many diseases including mildew, rust, and black spot, many garden ROSES are heavily sprayed. Both the spores of ROSE diseases and the chemicals used to control them may trigger allergic responses. Remove and replace disease-prone varieties with disease-resistant ones (a process rosarians refer to as "shovel-pruning").

When insects or diseases are a problem a soap-water spray is usually enough to afford control. The botanical product *Neem* is nontoxic and also controls both insects and disease.

The very best roses for an allergy-free garden are highly disease resistant, have either light or absent fragrance, and are fully double.

Good choices for the allergy-free garden include 'Sally Holmes', a disease-resistant single that is a very low pollen producer; 'Iceberg', a semi-double white that releases almost no pollen (I've found that 'Iceberg' is also the best all-around white garden rose); 'New Day', a yellow; 'Olympiad', a red; 'Gene Boerner' a pink; 'Singing in the Rain', a salmon-colored rose; 'Honor', another good white; and 'Touch of Class,' a rosy-coral hybrid tea that produces minimal amounts of pollen and has won many a blue ribbon. Miniature roses are also a good choice, because they release small amounts of pollen.

There is little point in trying to rate ROSES as a group, because of their incredible diversity. Very lightly scented or unscented ROSES with fully double blooms and many petals, combined with disease resistence, would rate at 2. MULTIFLORA ROSES with many highly fragrant, small flowers would rate as high as 5. Double ROSES with very high fragrance, such as 'Double Delight' or 'Fragrant Cloud' rate 4, unless they are cut and brought into the house. In that case, depending on the season, they could rate as high as 6, as ROSES are more fragrant in warm weather.

(To reduce the amount of pollen released by your ROSES, do not destroy EARWIGS, a common albeit minor pest of ROSES. Earwigs usually eat only the pollen-producing stamens and don't bother with the petals. Cucumber beetles also happily dine on rose pollen.)

ROSARY PEA, ROSARY VINE.
See *Abrus; Ceropegia.*

ROSE ACACIA.
See *Robinia.*

ROSE APPLE.
See *Syzygium.*

ROSE MALLOW.
See *Hibiscus.*

ROSE-OF-SHARON.
See *Hibiscus syriacus.*

ROSEMARY.
See *Rosmarinus officinalis; Ceratola.*

ROSEWOOD.
See *Pterocarpus; Tipuana tipu; Vauquelina californica.*

Rosmarinus officinalis. 6

ROSEMARY. Evergreen erect or prostrate shrubby herbs for zones 8–10, with small, highly aromatic leaves and numerous small, sky-blue flowers. ROSEMARY is very drought-resistant and grows best in well-drained soil, in full sun. The fragrance is objectionable to many and allergenic to some.

ROTENONE.
See *Tephrosia*.

ROYAL BAY.
See *Laurus nobilis*.

ROYAL FERN.
See *Osmunda*.

ROYAL PALM.
See *Roystonea regia*.

Roystonea regia. 7

CUBAN ROYAL PALM. A common allergy tree in Cuba.

RUBBER PLANT.
See *Ficus elastica decora*.

RUBBER TREE.
See *Ficus; Hevea brasiliensis; Parthenium; Sapium*.

Rubus.

BLACKBERRY, BOYSENBERRY, LOGANBERRY, RASPBERRY. Large group of prickly fruiting vines; one species is separate-sexed but most are perfect flowered. Group not rated.

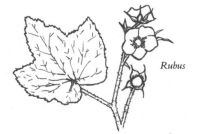

Rubus

Rudbeckia. 6

BLACK-EYED SUSAN, GLORIOSA DAISY. Annuals, biennials, and perennials, hardy in all zones.

RUE.
See *Ruta*.

Rumex. 8

DOCK, DOCK SORREL, SORREL, SPINACH. Large group of perennial herbs, some common weeds, others cultivated for their edible leaves and stalks, and others grown for their flowers, which are often used in dried flower arrangements. Numerous species of *Rumex* are important allergy plants and many of them cause some degree of allergy. Their use as dried flowers should be avoided.

R. hydrolapathum, R. hymenosepalus, R. patientia, and R. venosus present less allergy potential and are rated at 4.

Rumohra adiantiformis (Aspidium). 4

LEATHERLEAF FERN. A moisture-loving fern for either part shade or full sun in zone 10.

RUNNING MOSS, RUNNING PINE.
See *Lycopodium*.

Ruprechtia. males 8, females ❋ 1

BISCOCHITO. A group of separate-sexed tropical and subtropical shrubs and trees, native from Mexico to South America, and occasionally used in landscapes in Florida.

RUPTURE WORT.
See *Herniaria*.

Ruscus. 7

BOX HOLLY, BUTCHER'S BROOM, JEWISH MYRTLE. Evergreen shrub-like plants for shady areas, native to the Mediterranean region and hardy in zones 8–10. These separate-sexed plants are used as ground cover and as cut flowers.

RUSSIAN OLIVE.
See *Elaeagnus angustifolia*.

Ruta.   4
RUE. Numerous species of strongly scented herbs, the odor of which may bother sensitive individuals. Contact skin rash is common.

RUTABAGA.
See *Brassica.*

RYE.
See *Secale cereale.*

RYEGRASS.
See *Lolium.*

S

Allergy Index Scale: *1* is **Best**, *10* is **Worst**.

✳ for *1* and *2*   ✸ for *9* and *10*

📷 See insert for photograph

Sabal. 📷   5

BERMUDA PALM, BUSH PALM, CABBAGE PALMETTO, DWARF PALM, OAXACA palmetto, palmetto, PUERTO RICAN HAT PALM, SCRUB PALMETTO, SONORAN PALM, TEXAS PALM. A group of about 20 species of closely related small, FAN-LEAVED palms, some to over 60 feet. This group of PALMS has complete flowers that are insect-pollinated, but still produce some airborne pollen. Common in zones 8–10 and hardier than most PALMS, the SABAL PALMETTO causes allergy only in those areas where it is extremely common. A few of these in a garden should pose little threat.

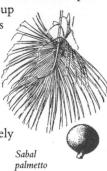

Sabal palmetto

Saccharum.   4

SUGAR CANE. Tall GRASSES used in the production of cane sugar. Unlike many GRASSES, these are bisexual and do not cause as much allergy as might be supposed; also, SUGAR CANE is almost always harvested before it flowers.

SAFFLOWER.
See *Carthamus tinctorius.*

SAFFRON.
See *Crocus.*

SAFFRON, FALSE.
See *Carthamus tinctorius.*

SAGE.
See *Salvia.*

SAGEBRUSH.
See *Artemisia.*

Sageretia thea.   5

An occasionally thorny, evergreen, flowering shrub, native to China and hardy in zones 7–10. The small white flowers are followed by one-seeded purplish black fruits. A relative of *Rhamnus* or BUCKTHORNS, *Sageretia* causes less allergy.

Sagina subulata.   ✳ 1

IRISH MOSS, SCOTCH MOSS. A low-growing, moss-like, spreading perennial hardy in all zones. Although difficult to establish, *Sagina* is useful as ground cover in partially shaded, moist areas.

SAGISI PALM.
See *Heterospathe.*

SAGO CYCAS.
See *Zamia.*

SAGO PALM.
See *Cycas revoluta.*

SAGUARO CACTUS.
See *Carnegiea gigantea.*

ST. AUGUSTINE GRASS.
See *Stenotaphrum secundatum.*

ST. JOHN'S BREAD.
See *Ceratonia siliqua.*

ST. JOHN'S WORT.
See *Hypericum*.

ST. MARY'S THISTLE.
See *Silybum*.

Saintpaulia ionantha.   ✼ 1
AFRICAN VIOLET. Houseplants for filtered light. The handsome blue, lavender, white, or pink flowers are held above a rosette of fuzzy leaves. AFRICAN VIOLETS are easy to propagate from leaf cuttings, rooted in water. The plants need acid-based potting soil and regular light feedings of complete fertilizer to thrive.

SALAL.
See *Gaultheria*.

Salix.

OSIER, PUSSY WILLOW, SALLOW, WEEPING WILLOW, WILLOW. A large genus of mostly deciduous shrubs and trees, with over 500 species worldwide. Various species are adapted to grow anywhere from desert washes to frozen tundras, and are native to every continent except Australia. The common WILLOWS and WEEPING WILLOW are useful in damp spots where most trees fail to flourish. They grow quickly and may be used to form a quick-growing tall hedge. Low-growing WILLOW SHRUBS are used as ground covers.

Because most WILLOWS are easily propagated from cuttings, a number of clones exist. WILLOWS are often mentioned as potent allergen-producing plants, but because they are separate-sexed, the females of the species are excellent choices in the allergy-free landscape.

S. acutifolia.   ❋ 10
The cultivars 'Blue Streak' and 'Lady Aldenham' (despite her name!) are male trees.

S. aegyptiaca.   ❋ 9
This species bears flowers of both sexes on the same tree; do not use.

S. alba.   *males* ❋ *10, females* ✼ *1*
WHITE WILLOW. A group of common European trees. The cultivar 'Cardinalis' is a small, narrow, female tree. 'Chrysostela', 'Liempde', and 'Tristis' are male cultivars.

S. 'Americana'.   ❋ 10
A male clone.

S. arbutifolia.   ❋ 10
This is one of the worst WILLOWS for allergy; avoid its use.

S. 'Austree Hybrid'.   ❋ 10.
A new, fast-growing male clone marketed in Australia and California.

S. babylonica.   *males* ❋ *10, females* ✼ *1*
CHINESE WEEPING WILLOW. In Asia, Europe, and the United States, female clones are available; in India, however, a male clone exists. 'Annularis', the RINGLEAF WILLOW, is female.

Salix babylonica

S. calcodendron.   ✼ 1
To 40 feet; a female.

S. cantabrica.   ✼ 1
A large shrub; a female.

S. caprea.   *males 6, females* ✼ *1*
GOAT WILLOW, SALLOW. 'Kilmarnock' is a male with scented flowers that cause less allergy than most male WILLOWS. 'Weeping Sally' is a female weeping PUSSY WILLOW.

S. cinerea.   *males 6, females* ✼ *1*
'Variegata' is male; however, the flowers of this species are scented and it will cause less allergy than other *Salix* males.

S. daphnoides.   *males* ❋ *10, females* ✼ *1*
The cultivars 'Aglaia' and 'Continental Purple' are male.

S. fragilis.   *males* ✳ *10, females* ✳ *1*
BRITTLE WILLOW, CRACK WILLOW. 'Decipiens' is a male cultivar; 'Bedford Willow' is a female tree.

S. kinuiyanagi.   *males* ✳ *10, females* ✳ *1*
The cultivar 'Kishu' is a small male tree; 'Kioryu' is a small female tree.

S. 'Maerd Brno'.   ✳ *1*
A small female tree.

S. matsudana.   ✳ *1*
The variety known as *S. babylonica* 'Pekinensis', is female. 'Navajo' is a large female WILLOW that grows well under desert conditions. *S. matsudana* 'Tortuosa', the CORKSCREW WILLOW, is a female.

S. × pendulina.   *males 5, females* ✳ *1*
This is a rare bisexual WILLOW. The cultivars 'Blanda' and 'Elegantissima' are female. 'Elegantissima' is similar in appearance to *S. babylonica*, the WEEPING WILLOW, but is more cold hardy. It is one of the best big WEEPING WILLOWS.

S. purpurea.   *males* ✳ *10, females* ✳ *1*
PURPLE OSIER. The cultivar 'Eugene' is a male.

S. repens.   *males 6, females* ✳ *1*
The cultivar 'Boyd's Pendulous' is a male.

S. reticulata.   *males 6, females* ✳ *1*
This low-growing ground cover WILLOW is a male.

S. × rubens.   *males* ✳ *10, females* ✳ *1*
The cultivar 'Basfordiana' is male; 'Sanguinea' is a small female tree.

S. sachalinensis.   *males* ✳ *10, females* ✳ *1*
The cultivar 'Sea' is a male tree.

S. × sepulcralis.   *males* ✳ *10, females* ✳ *1*
Also known as *S. × salamonii*; this is a female tree. A named variety, 'Chrysocoma', goes by many names: *S. alba* 'Aurea Pendula', 'Niobe', or 'Vitellina Pendula Nova'; *S. babylonica* 'Aurea'; the Niobe weeping willow or the golden weeping

willow. All are essentially the same tree and all are male.

S. × sericans.   ✳ *10*
A male hybrid.

S. triandra.   *males* ✳ *10, females* ✳ *1*
'Black Maul' is a male cultivar.

S. × tsugaluensis.   ✳ *1*
WILLOW SHRUB. The cultivar 'Ginme' is a female with attractive reddish branchlets.

S. uva-ursi.   *males 5, females* ✳ *1*
BEARBERRY. A very hardy (to zone 1), low-growing, spreading species used as a ground cover or bank cover. Not sold sexed; it would be a very useful plant if a female clone could be identified.

SALLOW.
See *Salix*.

SALLY.
See *Eucalyptus*.

Salpiglossis sinuata.   ✳ *2*
PAINTED TONGUE. An annual for warm sunny spots, it bears colorful flowers that resemble *Petunias*. *Salpiglossis* make good cut flowers.

SALT CEDAR.
See *Tamarix*.

SALTBUSH.
See *Atriplex*.

SALTGRASS.
See *Distichlis*.

Salvia.   ✳ *2*
CREEPING SAGE, GREASEWOOD, MEXICAN BUSH SAGE, PINEAPPLE SAGE, PURPLE SAGE, RAMONA, SAGE, SCARLET SAGE, VERVAIN. A large group of over 700 species of mostly evergreen perennials, herbs, sub shrubs, and

shrubs, bearing small flowers of white, blue, lavender, purple, or bright red. Many *Salvias* thrive in
hot, dry areas, while others do best in cool, moist
situations. Some, like *Salvia azurea*, or BLUE SAGE,
are hardy in zones 3–10, while many others, such
as *S. leucantha* or MEXICAN BUSH SAGE, do not grow
outside of zones 8–10. *Salvias* are identifiable by
their square stems. Many plants are called SAGE, and
most of them are types of either *Salvia* or
Artemisia. *S. officinalis* is true culinary SAGE. The
Artemisias contribute greatly to allergy but *Salvias*
do not. Most *Salvias* thrive in full sun; in warm
winter areas cut the plants back hard at least once
a year, after a heavy bloom.

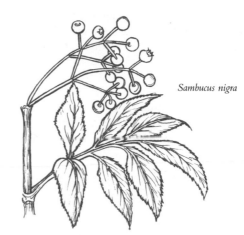

Sambucus nigra

Sambucus. 📷

BLACK ELDER, DANEWORT, DEVIL'S WOOD, ELDER-
BERRY, PURPLELEAF ELDER, RED ELDER, STINKING
ELDER, WALLWORT. Where it is common, ELDER-
BERRY causes allergy, although certain species are
worse than others. The plants are prized for their
(usually) edible fruits, although all fruit must be
thoroughly cooked before eating. Eaten raw, the
fruit is mildly toxic. ELDER tea is made from the
leaves, but should be used with caution because
too much can cause illness. The sap of ELDERBERRY
stems causes irritation to the skin, eyes, and nose in
some. ELDERS thrive in moist soil and partial shade.
Stems, leaves, and unripe fruit are very poisonous.

S. caerula. 6
BLUE ELDER, STINKING ELDER. A tree, to 50 feet, this
species gets one of its common names from its
malodorous leaves.

S. canadensis. 4
AMERICAN ELDER. A large shrub bearing black edible fruit, much loved by birds.

S. nigra. 5
BLACK ELDERBERRY. A European ELDERBERRY
grown for its sweet black fruit, which is used in jellies and wines.

S. pubens. 6
RED ELDER. RED ELDER is often found growing
wild throughout the United States; the fruit is attractive but poisonous.

The BOX ELDER, a variety of MAPLE, is not related to
Sambucus, nor is the SWAMP ELDER (*Iva*). Both BOX
ELDER and SWAMP ELDER are potent allergy plants.

SAN JOSE HESPER PALM.
See *Brahea*.

SAND VERBENA.
See *Abronia*.

SANDALWOOD.
See *Pterocarpus*.

SANDBOX TREE.
See *Hura*.

SANDHILL SAGE.
See *Artemisia*.

SANDWORT.
See *Arenaria*.

Sanguinaria canadensis. 3
BLOODROOT. A hardy perennial with large leaves and white-pink flowers, for moist, shady areas of zones 2–7. The thick, fleshy roots exude a blood-red sap when cut.

Sansevieria trifasciata. ❈ 1
BOWSTRING HEMP, MOTHER-IN-LAW'S TONGUE, SNAKE PLANT. A common houseplant with stiffly erect, long, narrow leaves with light margins. *Sansevieria* thrives on neglect, needing little in the way of fertilizer, light, or water.

SANTA LUCIA FIR.
See *Abies.*

Santalum. 7
SANDALWOOD. Several species of evergreen shrubs and trees from India to Australia to Hawaii with aromatic wood. *Santalum* is the sandalwood oil source.

Santolina. 7
GREEN SANTOLINA, GRAY SANTOLINA, LAVENDER COTTON. A shrubby perennial for full sun in zones 7–10. *Santolina* bears small, daisy-like yellow flowers; the bruised leaves release a pungent odor.

Sanvitalia procumbens. 4
CREEPING ZINNIA. A native annual of Mexico for sunny areas.

SAPPHIRE BERRY.
See *Symplocos.*

Sapindus. males 8, females 3
CHINESE SOAPBERRY, SOAPBERRY, WILD CHINA TREE. A dozen species of shrubs and trees, some native, some Asian, for zones 8–10 and commonly used in Florida and California. Some species of *Sapindus* are separate-sexed, but all cause allergy. All parts of the *Sapindus* tree are poisonous if eaten, and contact with leaves or, especially, sap, can cause contact dermatitis. The female trees bear small yellow-orange fruits that are occasionally used to make soap. Do not use soap made from *Sapindus* berries.

Sapium. 📷 males ❈ 10, females 5
CHINESE TALLOW TREE. The Japanese native *S. japonica* is hardy only in zones 8–10; *S. sebiferum*, the CHINESE TALLOW TREE, is hardy in zones 4–10. As members of the *Euphorbia* family, *Sapiums* share in its diverse allergenic properties. Some of the genera are separate-sexed, but all have a distinctly high allergy potential. The sap of all *Sapium* is poisonous and may cause skin rash; the pollen is also toxic and the cause of allergy. Contact with the leaves of some species may cause rash.

Sapium sebiferum

Sapodilla. 3
A large group of tropical and subtropical trees and shrubs with milky latex sap that is used to make, among other things, chewing gum.

Saponaria. 3
SOAPWORT. A group of low-growing, mat-forming perennials and annuals, hardy in any zone. The small flowers are usually pink.

SAPOTE, WHITE.
See *Casimiroa edulis.*

Sarcobatus. ❈9
GREASEWOOD. A spiny shrub native to the western United States. The hard yellow wood is much used as quick-kindling firewood.

Sarcococca. 📷 7
SWEET BOX, SWEET SARCOCOCCA. Evergreen shrubs of the BOXWOOD family, native to China and commonly used as shrubs for shady areas in zones 8–10. The scent of its flowers may cause allergy in perfume-sensitive individuals, and the pollen has allergenic potential.

Sarracenia. 3
PITCHER PLANT. Odd insect-catching perennials native to the United States. One species, *S. purpurea*, is a bog plant and is hardy into zone 3.

SARSAPARILLA, WILD.
See *Schisandra; Smilax.*

Sassafras. *males 7, females* ✻ *1*

Three species of large deciduous trees, one native to the southeastern United States and two native to China. The bark is used to make an aromatic oil and a tea. *Sassafras* is separate-sexed; the females are identifiable by their small dark fruits.

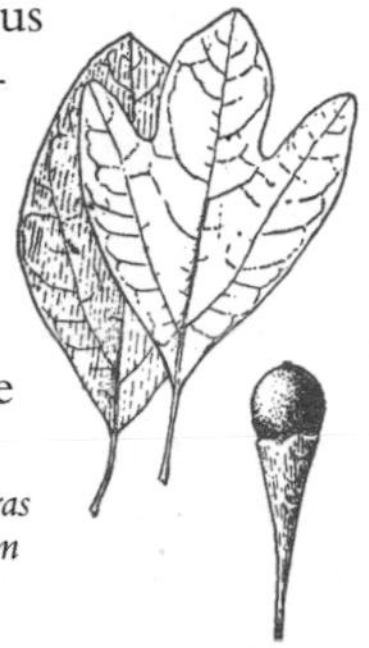

Sassafras albidum

SATINWOOD.
See *Zanthoxylum.*

Satureja (Micromeria). 3

CALAMINT, SUMMER SAVORY, YERBA BUENA, WINTER SAVORY. Annual and perennial herbs of the MINT family, *Satureja* are hardy in all zones. The fragrant leaves are used for tea.

SAUROMATUM.
See *Lilium.*

SAVIN.
See *Juniperus.*

SAVORY.
See *Satureja.*

SAWLEAF ZELKOVA.
See *Zelkova.*

Saxifraga. 3

BERGENIA, SAXIFRAGE. A group of over 300 species of small perennials, often grown for their attractive foliage. Some species are used as houseplants and others as garden plants, thriving in partial shade with average moisture.

Scabiosa. 3

PINCUSHION FLOWER. Annuals and perennials with many small, pom-pom-shaped, pastel flowers; most interesting for the tall stamens, held well above the petals, and resembling pins stuck into a pincushion. Thriving in full sun, *Scabiosa* are slightly fragrant and highly attractive to butterflies. They make a long-lasting cut flower if placed in water immediately after cutting. Because of the highly exposed, pollen-producing stamens, avoid directly inhaling the fragrance of *Scabiosa* flowers.

Scaevola. 3

BEACH NAUPKA. Spreading, drought-resistant, shrubby perennials covered with mauve flowers, for zone 10.

SCARLET GILIA.
See *Ipomopsis.*

SCARLET MAPLE.
See *Acer rubrum.*

SCARLET SAGE.
See *Salvia.*

SCARLET WISTERIA TREE.
See *Sesbania tripetii.*

Scheelea. 7

A group of about 40 species of large, slow-growing, thick-trunked tropical palm trees, used as landscape trees in zones 9–10.

SCHEFFLERA.
See *Brassaia actinophylla.*

Schinus. *males* ✸ *10, females 7*

PEPPER TREE. Twenty-eight species of separate-sexed South American evergreen trees. All members of *Schinus* are heavy flowering and the males produce abundant pollen, much of which becomes airborne. *Schinus* is a member of the *Anacardiaceae* family, with many noxious close relatives like POISON IVY, POISON SUMAC, and POISON OAK; people with sensitivity to these plants are at increased risk of allergy from *Schinus* pollen.

Although these trees are called PEPPER TREES and have a peppery odor, they are not true PEPPER plants; true black and white PEPPERS come from *Piper nigrum*, which is not related to *Schinus*. The red *Schinus* berries, called "peppercorns" by many, are sometimes combined with the black and white seeds of true PEPPER to produce a colorful mixture. *Schinus* seeds, however, are not edible and may cause allergy in those using this combination.

Because the plants are separate-sexed, the female trees do not produce pollen, automatically making them superior to the males. Nonetheless, all *Schinus* trees may cause skin rashes, eye inflammations, facial swellings, and odor allergies. The pollen, in addition to causing respiratory allergy, can also cause skin irritation. Allergies caused by *Schinus* are usually delayed, and identifying the cause of the reaction may be difficult.

S. molle, called the CALIFORNIA PEPPER TREE, AUSTRALIAN PEPPER, PERUVIAN PEPPER TREE, or PIRUL is a common street tree in zones 9–10, and especially so in California, where many mistakenly believe it to be a native species. *S. terebinthifolius*, the BRAZILIAN PEPPER TREE, or CHRISTMAS BERRY TREE, is another widely used species, especially in Hawaii, Florida, and California. *Terebinthifolius* means "turpentine scented" in Latin, and the crushed leaves emit a powerful, pungent odor when crushed. Of all the members of the genus, this is the most highly allergenic. The leaves are poisonous if eaten, the pollen is allergenic, mere contact with the leaves will cause rash for some, and when the plants are pruned or clipped, the volatile organic compounds (VOCs) released cause irritation to the eyes and/or respiratory tract.

The trees are not normally sold sexed; a named cultivar of *S. molle*, 'Shamel,' is a male.

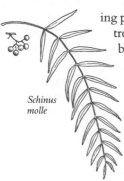

Schinus molle

S. latifolius, a popular landscaping plant in its native Chile, is a small tree with white flowers followed by small lavender fruits. *S. polygamous*, a spiny, narrow tree, also from Chile, is commonly used in California. *S. lentiscifolius* is a Brazilian native, commonly used as a landscape shrub because of its white flowers and pink fruits. *S. longifolius* is a small tree used in Argentina.

Schippia. ✳ 1
A tall (to 30 feet) slim-trunked palm tree from Belize.

Schisandra. males 7, females ✳ 1
BAY STAR VINE, MAGNOLIA VINE, WILD SARSAPARILLA. Separate-sexed vining shrubs, some hardy in zones 5–10. One species is native to the United States and the others are from China. The female vines bear red berries when fertilized.

Schizanthus. ✳ 2
BUTTERFLY FLOWER, POOR-MAN'S ORCHID. Easy-to-grow annuals for partial shade. They bear small colorful flowers, resembling ORCHIDS, on tall, drooping stems.

Schizocentron.
See *Heterocentron*.

Schizostylis.
See *Lilium*.

Schlumbergera. 📷 ✳ 2
CHRISTMAS CACTUS, CRAB CACTUS. Houseplants or outside in zone 10 in partial shade. *Schlumbergera* need regular watering and frequent feeding to thrive.

Sciadopitys. 7
UMBRELLA PINE. A slow-growing Japanese native evergreen tree, to 100 feet. The UMBRELLA PINE grows best in shaded, moist soil. It is unrelated to PINES.

Scilla. 3
SQUILL, BLUEBELLS. Easy-to-grow, blue-flowered perennials from bulbs; some species of *Scilla* are hardy in all zones. *Scilla* is quite poisonous, and some gardeners claim that if gophers eat it, they die. See also *Endymion*.

Scindapsus pictus. 3
Vining houseplants that resemble *Pothos*, but need a sunny window to thrive. The sap may cause rash.

Scirpus.   5
LOW BULRUSH. A tall reedy plant for wetlands or to edge ponds.

SCOTCH BROOM.
See *Cytisus*.

SCOTCH HEATHER.
See *Calluna*.

SCOTCH MOSS.
See *Sagina*.

SCREW BEAN.
See *Prosopis*.

SCREW PINE.
See *Pandanus*.

SCRUB PALMETTO.
See *Sabal*.

SEA ASH.
See *Zanthoxyllum*.

SEA BUCKTHORN.
See *Hippophae*.

SEA FIG.
See *Carpobrotus*.

SEA GRAPE.
See *Coccoloba*.

SEA HOLLY.
See *Eryngium*.

SEA LAVENDER.
See *Limonium*.

SEA PINK.
See *Armeria*.

SEA POPPY.
See *Glaucium*.

SEA URCHIN.
See *Hakea*.

SEASIDE DAISY.
See *Erigeron*.

Secale cereale.   *Not rated.*
RYE. A cool-season grain crop, unrelated to RYE-GRASS (*Lolium*), which is a common, allergenic lawn grass. There are five species of *Secale*, both annuals and perennials. RYE is not a major allergy plant because the pollen is heavy and does not travel far.

SEDGE.
See *Carex; Cyperus*.

Sedum.   ✱ 2
DONKEY TAIL, PORK-AND-BEANS, STONECROP. A large group of about 600 species of succulent perennials, hardy in zones 3–10, depending on species. *Sedum* flowers may be yellow, red, orange, or lavender. They are easy plants to grow, doing best in full sun but tolerant of light shade. They are easily propagated from cuttings.

Selenicereus.   ✱ 1
MOON CACTUS, NIGHT-BLOOMING CEREUS. Tall, night-blooming CACTUS.

SELF-HEAL.
See *Prunella*.

Semecarpus.   ✸10
MARKING-NUT TREE, VARNISH TREE. About 40 species of tropical and subtropical trees, the sap of which is used to make a black dye, used for ink. Both the dye and ink have allergenic properties, and the leaves of *Semecarpus* can cause very severe contact skin rash.

Semele androgyna.   7
CLIMBING BUTCHER'S VINE. A separate-sexed native of the Canary Islands, *Semele* is used as a greenhouse plant and is occasionally mistaken as a relative of *Asparagus*, to which it is unrelated.

SEMINOLE BREAD.
See *Zamia*.

Sempervivum.   ❋ 1
HENS-AND-CHICKS, HOUSELEEK. Easy-to-grow, drought-tolerant creeping succulents for sunny spots in zones 7–10, and as houseplants in sunny rooms elsewhere.

SENECA SNAKEROOT.
See *Polygala*.

Senecio (Jacobaea, Kleinea). 📷
7 to ❋*10, depending on species.*
CALIFORNIA GERANIUM, CANDLE PLANT, CINERARIA, DUSTY MILLER, FLAME VINE, GERMAN IVY, GOLDEN RAGWORT, HOT-DOG CACTUS, INCHWORM, KENYA IVY, LEOPARD'S BANE, NATAL IVY, PARLOR IVY, PURPLE RAGWORT, SPEARHEAD, STRING OF BEADS, TANSY RAGWORT, TAPE WORM, VELVET GROUNDSEL, WATER IVY, WAX VINE. Also known as *Kleinia repens*. A very large genus of nearly 3,000 species of annuals, biennials, perennials, vines, and shrubs, with worldwide distribution. Forming a group of plants whose uses range from flower garden herbs to landscape plants to weeds, all are implicated in causing some degree of allergy.

Because of the close relationship between *Senecio* and ragweed, *Senecio* pollen is a cause of airborne allergy and, in areas where they are numerous, may be the primary cause of summer and fall allergies. Most *Senecio* species bear small yellow flowers but a few, like the CINERARIA, bear larger, more colorful flowers that do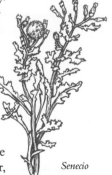

Senecio

not release as much pollen as the small-flowered species. With many members of the genus, there is a distinct chance of contact skin rash from the leaves and flowers. The flowers and leaves of most *Senecio* are poisonous if eaten.

SENNA.
See *Cassia*.

SENSITIVE PLANT.
See *Mimosa pudica*.

SENTRY PALM.
See *Howea*.

Sequoia sempervirens.   6
COAST REDWOOD. One of the tallest trees in the world, hardy in zones 8–10. There are many cultivars of REDWOOD, including a few dwarf or weeping varieties. *Sequoia* pollen causes allergy, although it is neither common nor severe. The large forms of REDWOOD should not be used as landscape plants, because they soon outgrow their surroundings.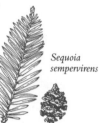

Sequoia sempervirens

Sequoiadendron giganteum.   6
BIG TREE, GIANT SEQUOIA. A giant REDWOOD that grows inland on the western slopes of the Sierra Nevada. Hardier than the COAST REDWOOD, it thrives in zones 4–10. It has the largest trunk diameter of any tree in the world. *Sequoiadendron* is unsuitable as a landscape tree, because of its immense mature size.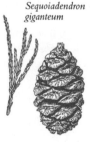

Sequoiadendron giganteum

SERVICE BERRY.
See *Amelanchier*.

Sesbania tripetii.   3
SCARLET WISTERIA TREE. Fast-growing deciduous shrub or small tree for sunny areas of zones 8–10. *Sesbania* is occasionally grown in large pots.

Setaria.   8
BRISTLEGRASS, PIGEON GRASS, FOXTAIL MILLET. European grasses used in warm zones of the United States.

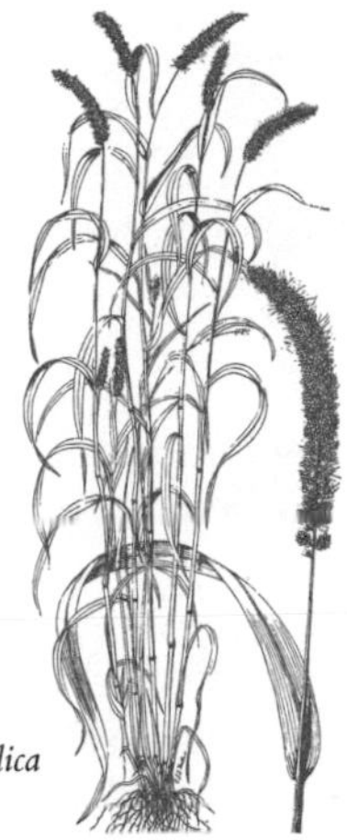
Setaria italica

Setcreasea pallida. ❊ *2*
PURPLE HEART. An easy-to-grow perennial for shady areas of zone 10, or as a houseplant elsewhere. The leaves, stems, and flowers are purple.

SHADBLOW, SHADBUSH.
See *Amelanchier.*

SHAGBARK HICKORY.
See *Carya ovata.*

SHAMROCK.
See *Oxalis.*

SHARPBERRY TREE.
See *Phillyrea decora.*

SHASTA DAISY.
See *Chrysanthemum.*

SHE-OAK.
See *Casuarina.*

SHEEP BUR.
See *Acaena.*

Shepherdia. *males 6, females* ❊ *1*
BUFFALO BERRY, SOAPBERRY. Three species of separate-sexed deciduous shrubs or small trees, hardy to zone 2. Adapted to dry, cold, rocky soils, female BUFFALO BERRY plants produce small edible fruits that are used for jelly.

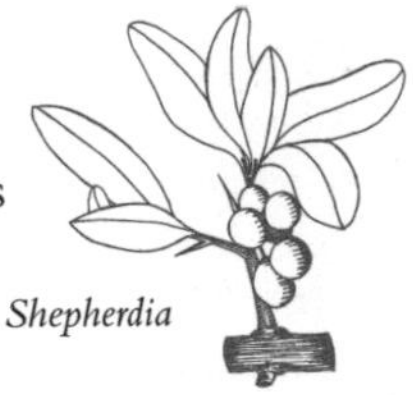
Shepherdia

Shibataea.
See BAMBOO.

SHIMPAKU.
See *Juniperus chinensis.*

SHISO.
See *Perilla frutescens.*

SHOOTING STARS.
See *Dodecatheon.*

SHORE BAY.
See *Persea borbonia.*

Shortia. ❊ *2*
FRINGE BELLS, FRINGED GALAX, OCONEE BELLS. Attractive small evergreen plants for shady areas in zones 3–8.

SHRIMP PLANT.
See *Justicia.*

SIBERIAN PEASHRUB.
See *Caragana arborescens.*

Sibiraea. 7
Several species of deciduous shrubs from Asia, used in zones 5–8.

SIERRA LAUREL.
See *Leucothoe.*

SIERRA MAPLE.
See *Acer glabrum.*

Silene. *3*
CAMPION, CATCHFLY, COCKLE, CUSHION PINKS, EVENING LYCHNIS, INDIAN PINK. MORNING COCKLE, MOSS CAMPION. Tall, easy-to-grow annuals and perennials, for all zones; some species are adapted

to dry areas and others to wet locations. Some *Silenes* are separate-sexed, but even the males of the *Silene* genus are not important allergy plants.

SILK TASSEL.
See *Garrya.*

SILK TREE.
See *Grevillea; Albizia julibrissin.*

SILKY CAMELLIA.
See *Stewartia.*

Silphium. 5
COMPASS PLANT. A small group of tall, hardy, flowering perennials, excellent for sunny spots in the back of flower borders.

SILVER CHAIN TREE.
See *Robinia.*

SILVER FIR.
See *Abies.*

SILVER LACE VINE.
See *Polygonum.*

SILVER LINDEN.
See *Tilia.*

SILVER MAPLE.
See *Acer saccharinum.*

SILVER PALM.
See *Coccothrinax.*

SILVER TREE.
See *Leucodendron.*

SILVER WATTLE.
See *Acacia.*

SILVERBELL TREE.
See *Halesia.*

SILVERBERRY.
See *Eleagnus commutata.*

Silybum. 5
ST. MARY'S THISTLE. Tall perennials often naturalized as weeds.

Simarouba. 8
ACEITUNO, BITTERWOOD, PARADISE TREE. Large tropical evergreen trees, often separate-sexed, for zone 10.

Simmondsia. *males 8, females* ✳ 1
GOATNUT, JOJOBA. Two dozen species of separate-sexed, evergreen shrubs, adapted to desert conditions. *Simmondsia* is often raised for its seeds, from which JOJOBA oil, a high-quality oil used as a substitute for whale oil, is pressed.

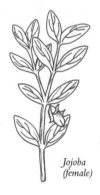

Jojoba (female)

Sinningia. ✳ 2
Many species from Mexico to Brazil. Perennials or shrubs, none are hardy outside of zones 9–10. *S. speciosa* is the florist's GLOXINIA, a plant beautiful when purchased, but one that never seems to thrive in the garden.

Sinofranchetia chinensis. *males 7, females* ✳ 1
A tall, separate-sexed vining shrub native to China.

Sinowilsonia henryi. 8
A small deciduous flowering tree from China.

Siphokentia.   7
Several species of palms from Molucca Islands, used in zone 10.

Sisyrinchium.   ❋ *1*
BLUE-EYED GRASS. Easy-to-grow, spreading perennials with grassy foliage and small blue flowers, spreading. Related to the IRIS.

Skimmia japonica.   6
A red-flowered evergreen shrub from Japan, hardy to zone 8.

SKUNK CABBAGE.
See *Veratrum.*

SKUNKBUSH.
See *Rhus.*

SKY FLOWER.
See *Duranta; Thunbergia.*

SLENDER LADY PALM.
See *Rhapis.*

SLIPPER PLANT.
See *Pedilanthus tithymaloides.*

SMARTWEED.
See *Polygonum.*

Smilacina.   3
FALSE SOLOMON'S SEAL. A shade-loving woodland perennial for zones 3–9.

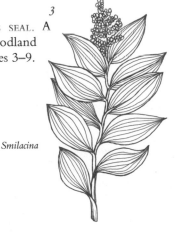
Smilacina

Smilax.   7
CARRION FLOWER, JACOB'S LADDER, RED-BERRIED GREENBRIER, WILD SARSAPARILLA. Separate-sexed vines, many species native to the southern United States. Some species may form small shrubs under the right conditions.

SMOKE BUSH.
See *Cotinus.*

SMOKE TREE.
See *Cotinus; Dalea.*

SMOOTH ROSE ACACIA.
See *Robinia.*

SMOOTH SUMAC.
See *Rhus.*

SNAIL VINE.
See *Vigna.*

SNAIL'S TRAIL.
See *Acanthus mollis.*

SNAILSEED.
See *Coccoloba; Cocculus laurifolius.*

SNAKE LILY.
See *Dichelostemma.*

SNAKE PLANT.
See *Sansevieria.*

SNAKEROOT.
See *Cimicifuga; Eupatorium.*

SNAPDRAGON.
See *Antirrhinum majus.*

SNAPDRAGON, FALSE.
See *Chaenorrhinum.*

SNEEZEWEED.
See *Helenium.*

SNOW-IN-SUMMER.
See *Cerastium tomentosum.*

SNOW-ON-THE-MOUNTAIN.
See *Euphorbia.*

SNOWBALL BUSH.
See *Viburnum.*

SNOWBELL TREE.
See *Styrax.*

SNOWBERRY.
See *Symphoricarpos.*

SNOWDROP TREE.
See *Halesia; Styrax.*

SNOWDROPS.
See *Galanthus.*

SNOWFLAKE.
See *Leucojum.*

SNOWFLAKE TREE.
See *Trevesia.*

SOAP BARK TREE.
See *Quillaja saponaria.*

SOAP TREE.
See *Yucca.*

SOAPBERRY.
See *Sapindus; Shepherdia.*

SOAPWELL.
See *Yucca*

SOAPWORT.
See *Saponaria.*

SOCIETY GARLIC.
See *Tulbaghia violacea.*

SODA APPLE.
See *Solanum.*

Solandra maxima. 3
CUP-OF-GOLD VINE. Large-flowered, night-fragrant evergreen vine for warmest parts of zone 10. *Solandra* thrives in the humidity of coastal areas; its heavy vines, lacking tendrils, need support. Poisonous.

Solanum. 📷
APPLE OF SODOM, DEADLY NIGHTSHADE, JERUSALEM CHERRY, LOVE APPLE, LULO, NIGHTSHADE, EGGPLANT, POISON BERRY, POTATO TREE, POTATO VINE, SODA APPLE, WHITE POTATO, YELLOW POPOLO. *Solanum* is a very large genus of over 1,500 species, including potatoes; eggplants; pepino; many domesticated flowers, shrubs, and vines; a few trees; and numerous weeds and wildflowers. In most species, the leaves, flowers, and berries are poisonous.

In medieval times young women put drops of juice of NIGHTSHADE in their eyes, to enlarge the pupils and make them brilliant (a beauty practice that often resulted in blindness). The Latin name for NIGHTSHADE, *Belladonna,* reflects this practice.

Allergy to POTATOES and EGGPLANTS is rare, as is allergy to *Solanum.* More likely, however, are poisonings caused by ingesting the attractive orange or yellow fruits of various *Solanum* species, especially those of JERUSALEM CHERRY, *S. pseudocapsicum.* A few species of *Solanum* produce edible fruits, notably the GARDEN HUCKLEBERRY and EGGPLANT. One species, WONDERBERRY, is used as a sugar substitute.

Solanum

Soleirolia soleirolii. 3
ANGEL'S TEARS, BABY'S TEARS. A small-leafed evergreen ground cover in zones 9–10; it becomes winter dormant in zones 6–8. BABY'S TEARS grows best in shade and requires ample water to thrive. In sunnier areas, it is more compact.

Solidago. 📷   8

GOLDENROD. A tall, bright-yellow, flowering perennial, hardy in all zones but most common in the East and Midwest. Much has been written about GOLDENROD and allergy, with many claiming that because it blooms at the same time as most RAGWEEDS, it is unfairly blamed for allergy. GOLDENROD, however, is related to RAGWEED and can cause allergy, albeit far less than its more potent cousin. *Solidago* pollen is heavier and less likely to become airborne than RAGWEED pollen. Thirty percent of those who suffer from RAGWEED allergy are also allergic to GOLDENROD pollen. Limit plantings to far from the house. GOLDENROD may cause contact skin rash.

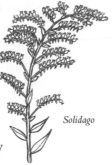

Solidago

Solidaster.   7

A hybrid of *Aster* and *Solidago* (GOLDENROD). Not the best combination for the allergy-free garden.

Sollya heterophylla.   3

AUSTRALIAN BLUEBELL CREEPER. Evergreen vine or shrub for zones 9–10. The BLUEBELL CREEPER needs excellent drainage to thrive; when in bloom, it is covered with small, bell-shaped bright blue flowers. A *Pittosporum* relative.

SOLOMON'S SEAL.
See *Polygonatum.*

SONORAN PALM.
See *Sabal.*

Sophora.   5

A large group of deciduous, leguminous trees. The largest is *S. japonica,* the CHINESE SCHOLAR or JAPANESE PAGODA TREE, which bears small yellow-white flowers followed by small bean-like pods. The seeds are poisonous if eaten in quantity; in very small doses, the seeds cause hallucinations and a deep, coma-like sleep, lasting for up to three days.

S. secundiflora, the MEXICAN or TEXAS MOUNTAIN LAUREL or MESCAL BEAN TREE, is well adapted to hot, dry areas, where it can grow to 50 feet. It bears long lavender flowers and its seeds are extremely poisonous—to a small child, a single seed may be fatal.

Sophora
japonica

Sorbaria sorbifolia.   5

FALSE SPIRAEA. A large, deciduous shrub for zones 3–9 that bears clusters of small white flowers. The FALSE SPIRAEA blooms on new wood only.

Sorbus.   4

MOUNTAIN ASH. A group of about 80 species of deciduous trees and large shrubs, producing small, edible fruits, hardy to zone 3. MOUNTAIN ASH has leaves resembling true ash, but it is a member of the rose family. They are beautiful trees when in full bloom and are also attractive when heavy with small red or orange fruit, which is used to make the sweetener Sorbital. The pollen of *Sorbus* may cause limited allergy.

Sorghum.   6– ✹10

GRAIN SORGHUM, GYP CORN, JOHNSON GRASS, MILO, SUDANGRASS. GRAIN SORGHUM causes limited allergy but the weed *S. halepense,* or JOHNSON GRASS, is a major allergy plant.

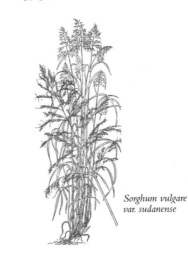

Sorghum vulgare
var. sudanense

SORREL.
See *Oxalis; Rumex.*

SORREL TREE.
See *Oxydendrum.*

SOUR GUM.
See *Nyssa.*

SOUR WEED.
See *Oxalis.*

SOURWOOD.
See *Oxydendrum.*

SOUTH AMERICAN LILY.
See *Alstroemeria.*

SOUTHERNWOOD.
See *Artemisia.*

SPANISH BAYONET.
See *Yucca.*

SPANISH BROOM.
See *Genista; Spartium junceum.*

SPANISH CEDAR.
See *Cedrela.*

SPANISH FIR.
See *Abies.*

SPANISH FLAG.
See *Mina lobata.*

SPANISH LIME.
See *Melicoccus.*

SPANISH SHAWL.
See *Heterocentron elegans.*

SPANISH TEA.
See *Chenopodium.*

Sparaxis.   ❋ 2
Perennial corms for zones 9–10.

Sparmannia africana.   6
AFRICAN LINDEN. An evergreen tree for zones 9–10, or grown as a houseplant elsewhere.

Spartina.   7
CORDGRASS, MARSH GRASS. Native grass that grows in southern coastal tidewater regions.

Spartium junceum.   7
SPANISH BROOM. A large evergreen shrub for dry, sunny areas of zones 8–10. Under optimum conditions, it may become invasive. All parts of these plants, including the seeds, are poisonous.

Spathiphyllum.   ❋ 2
Houseplants prized for their large dark green leaves and unusual, large, long-lasting white flowers.

SPEAR LILY.
See *Doryanthes palmeri.*

SPEARHEAD.
See *Senecio.*

SPEEDWELL.
See *Veronica.*

Sphaeropteris.   5
TREE FERNS. Over 100 species of very large, tall, tree-like FERNS, some hardy in zone 10 in shady locations. Although strikingly beautiful, TREE FERNS drop spores that trigger allergic reactions, so placement is important. Also, the stems have many tiny, sharp hairs that can cause rash.

SPICEBERRY.
See *Ardisia.*

SPICEBUSH.
See *Calycanthus; Lindera.*

SPIDER FLOWER.
See *Cleome spinosa.*

SPIDER LILY.
See *Hymenocallis; Crinum.*

SPIDER PLANT.
See *Chlorophytum comosum.*

SPIDERWORT.
See *Tradescantia.*

SPIKED CABBAGE TREE.
See *Cussonia.*

SPINACH.
See *Rumex; Spinacia.*

SPINACH, WILD.
See *Chenopodium.*

Spinacia.   5
SPINACH. A popular cool-weather garden veg-
etable plant, SPINACH is separate-sexed and related
to other species that cause a great deal of allergy. In
recent years, SPINACH has had its reputation tar-
nished as highly nutritious leafy green because of
the allergenic properties of the leaves.

SPINDLE TREE.
See *Euonymus.*

SPINY-CLUB PALM.
See *Bactris.*

Spiraea.   6
BRIDAL WREATH. Many species of mostly decidu-
ous shrubs of the Northern Hemisphere, most
bearing heavy panicles of small, bright white flowers. Allergy to *Spiraea* is not common, but may be
severe when it does occur. It is best planted far
from doors and windows.

SPLIT-LEAF PHILODENDRON.
See *Monstera.*

SPOON FLOWER.
See *Dasylirion.*

SPREKELIA.
See *Lilium.*

SPRING BEAUTY.
See *Claytonia.*

SPRING STAR FLOWER.
See *Ipheion uniflorum.*

SPRUCE.
See *Picea.*

SPURGE.
See *Euphorbia.*

SPURGE LAUREL.
See *Daphne.*

SPURGE NETTLE.
See *Cnidoscolus.*

SQUAWBERRY.
See *Viburnum.*

SQUAWBUSH.
See *Rhus.*

SQUIRREL CORN.
See *Dicentra.*

Stachys byzantina.   3
LAMB'S EAR. Small perennials grown for their soft,
fuzzy gray leaves; for sun or shade in zones 3–10.
They bear inconspicuous purple flowers on erect
stalks.

Stachyurus.   ✳ 2
A group of shade-loving deciduous shrubs from
China, hardy in zones 7–10, but growing best in
zones 7–8. *Stachyurus* is prized for its bright green
leaves, drooping clusters of little yellow flowers,
and good fall color.

STAGHORN FERN.
See *Platycerium.*

Stapelia. ✻ 2
CARRION FLOWER, STARFISH FLOWER. Unusual succulents with large, malodorous star-shaped flowers. They are popular in zones 9–10, and are occasionally used as potted plants.

Staphylea. 3
BLADDERNUT. Attractive shrubs or small trees, native to North America, for zones 5–9.

STAR APPLE.
See *Chrysophyllum cainito.*

STAR BUSH.
See *Turraea obtusifolia.*

STAR JASMINE.
See *Trachelospermum.*

STAR LILY.
See *Zigadenus.*

STAR OF BETHLEHEM.
See *Campanula; Ornithogalum.*

STARFISH FLOWER.
See *Stapelia.*

STARFLOWER, SPRING.
See *Ipheion uniflorum.*

STATICE.
See *Limonium.*

Stauntonia. 7
Several species of evergreen, woody climbing vines from Japan and China, and hardy to zone 8. *Stauntonia* bears fragrant white flowers and thrives in moist, shady spots with rich soil.

STEER'S HEAD.
See *Dicentra.*

Stenocarpus sinuatus. 3
FIREWHEEL TREE. An evergreen tree for zone 10, adopted by the Rotary Club as its mascot plant.

Slow growing and slow to come into bloom, the bright red, round flower clusters cover the plant. Young plants have beautiful foliage and are occasionally used as houseplants.

Stenolobium.
See *Tecoma.*

Stenotaphrum secundatum. 4
ST. AUGUSTINE GRASS. A broad-leafed, coarse, perennial lawn grass for zones 9–10. If it escapes cultivation to unmowed areas, it will grow tall, flower, and cause allergy. In the well-tended lawn, however, ST. AUGUSTINE GRASS rarely grows tall enough to bloom and produce pollen.

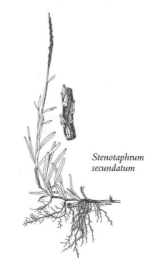

Stenotaphrum secundatum

Stephanotis. 7
MADAGASCAR JASMINE, WAX FLOWER VINE. An evergreen flowering vine for the very mildest coastal areas of zone 10, or grown as a houseplant or greenhouse plant elsewhere. The waxy white flowers are very fragrant, and may affect those with odor sensitivities. *Stephanotis* grow best with roots in shade and tops in sun. Recent reports from Holland documented asthma outbreaks among nursery workers exposed to the sap of the WAX FLOWER VINE.

Sterculia.
See *Brachychiton.*

Sternbergia lutea. ❋ 2

Small flowering plants from bulbs, hardy in all zones. Similar to *Crocus.*

Stevia. ✳ 9

A large group of perennial herbs and shrubs native to the tropics of North and South America. *S. serrata* is common in zones 8–10 and in Mexico. *S. rebaudiana* is used to make a strong natural sweetener. Another plant called STEVIA is *Piqueria trinervia,* another highly allergenic perennial flower.

Stewartia. 📷 3

MOUNTAIN CAMELLIA, SILKY CAMELLIA, STUARTIA. Attractive deciduous shrubs or small trees bearing large, showy flowers and with good fall color. They are hardy to zones 4 or 5, but grow best in zones 5–8. *Stewartia* thrives only in cool, moist, well-drained, acid soil, in partial shade. Several of the larger, less hardy species are Asian natives; *S. ovata* is native to the mountains of North Carolina and Tennessee.

STICKY MONKEY FLOWER.
See *Mimulus.*

Stigmaphyllon. ❋ 2

AMAZON VINE, BRAZILIAN GOLDEN VINE, BUTTERFLY VINE, GOLDEN CREEPER, ORCHID VINE. Vigorous evergreen vines, native to tropical America and bearing bright yellow, orchid-like flowers, for zone 10.

STINK TREE.
See *Ailanthus.*

STINKING CEDAR, STINKING YEW.
See *Torreya.*

STINKING ELDER.
See *Sambucus.*

STOCK.
See *Matthiola.*

Stokesia laevis. 6

STOKES ASTER. Perennials bearing blue, purple, or white flowers, hardy in all zones.

STONE COTTON TREE.
See *Eucommia ulmoides.*

STONECRESS.
See *Aethionema.*

STONECROP.
See *Sedum.*

STONEFACE.
See *Lithops.*

STONEWOOD.
See *Ostrya.*

STORAX.
See *Styrax.*

Stranvaesia. 4

Evergreen shrubs or small trees, native to Asia, and hardy in zones 8–10. The small white flowers appear in June and are followed by clusters of bright red berry-like fruits, occasionally used for Christmas decorations.

STRAWBERRY.
See *Fragaria.*

STRAWBERRY GERANIUM.
See *Saxifraga.*

STRAWBERRY GROUND COVER.
See *Waldsteinia fragarioides.*

STRAWBERRY TOMATO.
See *Physalis.*

STRAWBERRY TREE.
See *Arbutus.*

STRAWFLOWER.
See *Helichrysum.*

STREAM ORCHID.
See *Epipactis gigantea.*

Strelitzia. 📷   ✳ 1

BIRD-OF-PARADISE. *S. regina*, the BIRD-OF-PARADISE, is the official flower of the city of Los Angeles, despite the fact that it is native to South Africa and the tropics. The long-stemmed orange and blue flowers are popular in floral arrangements.

S. nicolai, the GIANT BIRD-OF-PARADISE, grows much larger and taller, resembling a BANANA tree. The flowers are very large and more unusual than beautiful. These tree-like plants are often used with good effect in indoor shopping mall landscaping.

The BIRDS-OF-PARADISE are not known to cause allergy, and the design of their flowers keeps pollen inside. Because it produces no airborne pollen and lacks the insect needed to pollinate it, BIRD-OF-PARADISE rarely sets seed in the United States. The flowers can be hand-pollinated and the resulting seeds are large and black, with a small fuzzy orange tuft.

Streptocarpus.   ✳ 2

CAPE PRIMROSE. Perennials for the mildest parts of zone 10 and houseplants elsewhere. *Streptocarpus* grows best in cool, moist, partial shade outdoors, and inside requires cultural conditions similar to those for AFRICAN VIOLETS, to which they are related.

Streptosolen jamesonii.   ✳ 2

FIREBUSH, MARMALADE BUSH, ORANGE BROWALLIA. An evergreen vining shrub for zones 9–10, or popular as a greenhouse plant in other zones. *Streptosolen* bears bright, orange-red flowers in large clusters. It needs full sun and good drainage with ample water to thrive.

STRING OF BEADS.
See *Senecio*.

STRIPED MAPLE.
See *Acer pensylvanicum*.

STUARTIA.
See *Stewartia*.

Styrax. 📷   4

JAPANESE SNOWBELL, SNOWBELL TREE, SNOWDROP TREE, STORAX. A group of about 100 species of deciduous and evergreen shrubs and trees, some Asian and others native to the United States. Some species of *Styrax* are hardy to zone 3. The small attractive flowers are usually white, lightly scented, and appear in early summer. Although the pollen is innocuous, the sap of some *Styrax* species may cause rash.

SUCCULENTS.
Listed individually; in general most succulents pose little allergy potential.

SUDANGRASS.
See *Sorghum*.

SUGAR BUSH.
See *Rhus ovata*.

SUGAR CANE.
See *Saccharum*.

SUGAR MAPLE.
See *Acer saccharum*.

SUGARBERRY.
See *Celtis*.

SUMAC.
See *Rhus*.

SUMMER CYPRESS.
See *Kochia*.

SUMMER HOLLY.
See *Comarostaphylis diversifolia*.

SUMMER HYACINTH.
See *Galtonia candicans*.

SUMMER SAVORY.
See *Satureja*.

SUMMERBERRY.
See *Viburnum*.

SUNFLOWER.
See *Helianthus*.

SUNROSE.
See *Halimium; Helianthemum nummularium*.

SURINAM CHERRY.
See *Eugenia*.

SWAMP BAY.
See *Persea borbonia*.

SWAMP CANDLEBERRY.
See *Myrica*.

SWAMP CYPRESS.
See *Cyrilla racemiflora; Glyptostrobus lineatus*.

SWAMP GUM.
See *Nyssa sylvatica*.

SWAMP HAW.
See *Viburnum*.

SWAMP PRIVET.
See *Forestiera*.

SWAN RIVER DAISY.
See *Brachycome iberidifolia*.

SWAN RIVER PEASHRUB.
See *Brachysema lanceolatum*.

SWEDISH IVY.
See *Plectranthus*.

SWEET ALYSSUM.
See *Lobularia*.

SWEET BAY.
See *Laurus nobilis; Magnolia*.

SWEET BOX.
See *Sarcococca*.

SWEET BRUSH.
See *Cercocarpus*.

SWEET CISELY.
See *Myrrhis odorata*.

SWEET CLOVER.
See *Melilotus*.

SWEET FERN.
See *Comptonia peregrina*.

SWEET GALE.
See *Myrica*.

SWEET GUM.
See *Liquidambar*.

SWEET HAKEA.
See *Hakea*.

SWEET LAUREL.
See *Laurus nobilis*.

SWEET MARJORAM.
See *Origanum*.

SWEET OLIVE.
See *Osmanthus*.

SWEET PEA.
See *Lathyrus*.

SWEET PEA SHRUB.
See *Polygala*.

SWEET PEPPERBUSH.
See *Clethra*.

SWEET POTATO.
See *Dioscorea*.

SWEET ROCKET.
See *Hesperis matronalis*.

SWEET SULTAN.
See *Centaurea*.

SWEET VERNAL GRASS.
See *Anthoxanthum*.

SWEET WILLIAM.
See *Dianthus*.

SWEET WOODRUFF.
See *Galium odoratum*.

SWEETBERRY.
See *Viburnum*.

SWEETLEAF.
See *Symplocos*.

SWEETSHADE.
See *Hymenosporum flavum*.

SWEETSPIRE.
See *Itea ilicifolia*.

Swietenia.   3
MAHOGANY. Six species of large evergreen tropical or zone 10 trees, occasionally used as street trees.

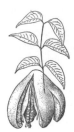

*Swietenia
mahagoni*

SWISS CHARD.
See *Beta vulgaris*.

SWISS CHEESE PLANT.
See *Monstera*.

SWORD FERN.
See *Nephrolepis;* FERNS.

Syagrus.   6
COCOS PALM, LICURI PALM, OURICURI PALM. A group of palms from South America, occasionally used in the United States in zones 9–10. Some species of *Syagrus* are used for palm oil.

SYCAMORE.
See *Platanus*.

SYCAMORE MAPLE.
See *Acer pseudoplatanus*.

Sycopsis.   7
Six species of monoecious evergreen shrubs or trees from China, the Himalayas, and the Philippine Islands, with showy male flowers.

Symphoricarpos.   3
CORALBERRY, INDIAN CURRANT, SNOWBERRY, WAXBERRY, WOLFBERRY. Deciduous shrubs native to the United States and China, used for their ornamental red fruits and attractive foliage. Easy to grow, some of the hardier species will grow into zone 3. SNOWBERRY thrives in sun or shade, in almost any kind of soil.

Symphytum officinale.   3
COMFREY. Hardy perennial herb for all zones. Traditionally, COMFREY was grown as a medicinal herb and a nutritious pot green or forage crop, but modern research indicates that the leaves contain a low-level poison.

Symplocos.   4
SAPPHIRE BERRY, SWEETLEAF. A large group of trees and shrubs from Eurasia, the Americas, and Australia. *S. paniculata*, the SAPPHIRE BERRY, grows to 40 feet and is hardy to zone 5.

Syngonium podophyllum.   ❋ 2
AFRICAN EVERGREEN, ARROWHEAD VINE. Occasionally sold as *Nephthytis afzelii*. A common and popular, easy-to-grow houseplant that resembles *Philodendron*. Because they produce separate male flowers, *Syngonium* may cause allergy, but as houseplants they rarely flower.

Synsepalum dulcificum. ❋ 2

MIRACULOUS FRUIT, WONDERBERRY. A tall shrub (to 12 feet), native to West Africa. Grows in zone 10 only. It bears white flowers, followed by small, succulent, oblong red fruits. After chewing the fruit, sour foods taste sweet. At one time showing promise as an artificial sweetener, MIRACULOUS FRUIT has been abandoned as a commercial venture. A member of the *Sapote* family.

SYRIAN BEAD TREE.
See *Melia*.

Syringa. 6

LILAC. Deciduous shrubs or small trees, hardy to zone 3. *S. vulgaris*, the common LILAC, is a tall shrub bearing clusters of highly fragrant flowers in early spring. The intensely sweet fragrance may produce allergic reactions in those with odor sensitivities. As a member of the OLIVE family, LILAC has allergenic pollen, but because it is rarely airborne, it does not present much allergy potential. LILACS should be planted away from doors and windows.

Syzygium. 6

AUSTRALIAN BUSH CHERRY, EUGENIA, JAMBU, JAVA APPLE, JAVA PLUM, LILLY-PILLY TREE, MALABAR PLUM, MALAY APPLE, ROSE APPLE, WAX APPLE. Over 400 species worldwide of evergreen shrubs and trees, some quite large, for zones 9–10.

Some species are raised for their edible plumlike fruits and one, *S. aromaticum*, is the source of CLOVES. *Syzygium* belong to the MYRTLE family, and those who are allergic to *Eucalyptus* should avoid them. Although the genus has not been well studied for allergy potential, the flowers are numerous, produced over a very long period, and have exposed, pollen-producing stamens, all of which suggest a good potential for allergy.

The most commonly used species in the United States (zones 9–10) is *S. paniculatum*, the AUSTRALIAN BUSH CHERRY, often sold as *Eugenia myrtlifolia*. This is usually seen as a landscape shrub or hedge plant, although when left unsheared it quickly grows into a large tree. Easy to grow in any soil and somewhat drought-tolerant when estab-

lished, BUSH CHERRY must be kept closely sheared to prevent flowering. Its small purple fruits, thought by many to be poisonous, are edible but certainly not delicious.

T

Allergy Index Scale: *1* is **Best**, *10* is **Worst**.

✳ for *1* and *2*   ✻ for *9* and *10*

📷 See insert for photograph

Tabebuia.   5

TRUMPET VINE TREE. Large evergreen flowering trees from the tropics and subtropics, occasionally used in zone 10. Two species, *T. avellanedae*, and *T. chrysotricha* (the GOLDEN TRUMPET TREE), are hardier than others of this genus. In the United States, these trees rarely get taller than 25 feet, but in the tropics they may grow to 100 feet. They are closely related to the hardy CATALPA TREE, which is known to cause allergy. Because these three trees have many similarities, use *Tabebuia* as a landscape tree with discretion. *Tabebuia* pollen is heavy and does not fall far from the tree; plant these trees away from the house.

Tagetes. 📷   6

MARIGOLD. Very common annual flowers, usually yellow, gold, or orange. They are frost tender, easy and fast from seed, and grow best in full sun. MARIGOLDS are classified as either FRENCH or DWARF MARIGOLDS (*T. patula*), or AFRICAN or TALL MARIGOLDS (*T. erecta*), despite the fact that MARIGOLDS are native to neither Africa or France, but to Mexico and Central America. One species, *T. signata* (MEXICAN MARIGOLD), is known to cause severe skin rash.

The fragrance of MARIGOLD is offensive to some and may cause allergy in perfume-sensitive individuals. Although allergy to MARIGOLDS is not common, the plants are related to RAGWEEDS and share some similarities. Fully double varieties hide their pollen deep within the flower and generally present less of an allergy potential than single-flowered varieties. The pollen is long-spined, light and may become airborne, yet most allergy from MARIGOLDS is from direct contact with the open flowers.

Taiwania cryptomerioides.   8

FORMOSAN REDWOOD, TAIWAN CEDAR. An evergreen coniferous tree discovered in 1904 in the mountains of Taiwan. A rare tree in the United States, *Taiwania* closely resembles the JAPANESE CEDAR (*Cryptomeria japonica*), but is more closely related to BALD CYPRESS. Because both of these species are well-documented allergy producers, it can be assumed *Taiwania* is also a potential allergen.

TALA PALM.
See *Borassus*.

TALL FESCUE.
See *Fescue elatior*.

TALL OATGRASS.
See *Arrhenatherum elatius*.

TALLHEDGE BUCKTHORN.
See *Rhamnus*.

TALLOW TREE.
See *Sapium*.

TAM.
See *Juniperus sabina*.

TAMARACK.
See *Larix*.

TAMARIND-OF-THE-INDIES.
See *Vangueria*.

Tamarindus indica. ✤ 2

TAMARIND. A large evergreen tree from the tropics, also grown in south Florida for its fine shape, attractive foliage, and sweet fruit, which is very popular in Mexico and Latin America. TAMARIND is entirely insect-pollinated and is not known to cause allergy.

Tamarix. 📷 7

SALT CEDAR, TAMARISK. Deciduous trees native to the deserts of Arizona and California, and also native to parts of Africa and the Mediterranean. They are used in landscaping in the western desert and in many coastal areas. TAMARISK trees occasionally become summer-dormant and regrow their leaves as the weather cools.

Extremely-drought resistant, TAMARISK have tiny leaves, green stems, and many tiny pinkish flowers. They are the cause of some allergy, especially in Arizona and California, where they have an extended blooming period. At least one species, *T. dioica*, is separate-sexed. This small tree, native to India, Pakistan, Afghan-istan, and Iran, but also cultivated in the United States, causes more allergy than other *Tamarix* species. It has an allergy rating of 9.

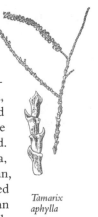

Tamarix aphylla

Tanacetum. 7

TANSY. A common, tall perennial with about 50 species native to the Northern Hemisphere. The leaves and flowers are highly aromatic and may cause allergy in perfume-sensitive individuals. TANSY also releases a large amount of airborne pollen and is the cause of allergy in areas where it is most common. All parts of TANSY are poisonous if eaten in quantity.

Tanakaea. *males 6, females* ✤ 1

A separate-sexed evergreen herb used in landscapes in China and Japan. The male plants produce airborne pollen.

TANBARK OAK.
See *Lithocarpus densiflorus*.

TANGERINE.
See *Citrus*.

TANNER'S SUMAC.
See *Rhus*.

TANNER'S TREE.
See *Coriaria japonica*.

TANSY.
See *Tanacetum*.

TANSY RAGWORT.
See *Senecio*.

TAPE GRASS.
See *Vallisneria*.

TAPE WORM.
See *Senecio*.

Taraxacum officinale. 6

DANDELION. A common European weed that has naturalized over much of the Northern Hemisphere. DANDELION sheds airborne pollen and causes limited allergy, but the weed killing lawn chemicals applied to eradicate it cause more allergy. These chemicals can cause not only allergy, but also leukemia in dogs and cats using the lawn. Avoid these chemicals. DANDELIONS can be held in check by applying high-nitrogen lawn fertilizer frequently, mowing regularly, and if necessary, pricking them out with a "dandelion digger."

TARO.
See *Colocasia esculenta*.

TARRAGON.
See *Artemisia*.

TASMANIAN TREE FERN.
See *Dicksonia*.

TATARIAN MAPLE.
See *Acer tataricum*.

Taxodium.   8
BALD CYPRESS, MONTEZUMA CYPRESS, POND CYPRESS. Two species of coniferous trees hardy in zones 7–10. BALD CYPRESS, which grows in swamps and shallow lakes of the southern United States, produces a buttressed lower trunk. MONTEZUMA CYPRESS is a tree of the Pacific Coast, growing southward into Mexico. Both species are well-known allergens, both produce copious amounts of airborne pollen, which is the cause of wintertime allergy. Occasionally used in landscapes in wet situations, *Taxodium* is best left in the swamps.

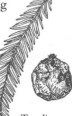
Taxodium distichum

Taxus. 📷   *males 7, females* ✳ *1*
YEWS. Eight species of evergreen coniferous trees and shrubs, all native to the Northern Hemisphere. Several species are native to the United States and some are imported from Japan and China. Most *Taxus* are separate-sexed. Young female *Taxus* species often make fine foundation shrubs, adding a luxurious look to the landscape. If there are male plants present, the female plants will often form red berries, which are highly poisonous. (All parts of the plant are poisonous.)

Taxus are slow growing, long lived, and shade tolerant, and they thrive only in moist, acid soils. The bark of *T. brevifolia*, the WESTERN YEW, is the source of the anti-cancer drug, Taxol. Although there is some disagreement about the prevalence of allergy from *Taxus*, YEW pollen is very similar to the well-known allergenic JUNIPER pollen, and likely shares its allergenic potential. Plant female YEWS only.

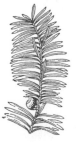
Taxus brevifolia

T. baccata, is the ENGLISH YEW. 'Fastigiata' is an upright, variegated female.

T. brevifolia, is the PACIFIC or WESTERN YEW. It is not sold sexed; look for the red berries that indicate a female plant.

T. cuspidata is the JAPANESE YEW, which is hardier than the ENGLISH YEW, into zone 3. Again, look for berries.

T. × *media* is a hybrid cross between the JAPANESE and ENGLISH YEWS, and nearly as hardy as JAPANESE YEW. 'Anthony Wayne' is a tall, vigorous female, despite its masculine name, as are 'Hicksii', 'Kelseyi', 'Pyramidalis', and 'Sentinalis'.

TEA.
See *Camellia; Thea sinensis*.

TEA TREE.
See *Leptospermum*.

TEABERRY.
See *Gaultheria; Viburnum*.

TEAK.
See *Tectona grandis*.

Tecoma (Stenolobium).   3
A group of TRUMPET VINE species for zones 9–10 that needs heat, sun, rich soil, and ample water to thrive.

Tecomaria capensis.   3
CAPE HONEYSUCKLE. A shrub or vine native to South Africa and common in zones 9–10. It grows best in full sun or partial shade, and can be clipped to form a hedge. *Tecomaria's* orange tubular flowers are attractive to hummingbirds. There is a yellow-flowering variety that needs more light and heat to thrive. *Tecomaria* is unrelated to COMMON or JAPANESE HONEYSUCKLE (*Lonicera*).

Tectona grandis.   ✳ *2*
TEAK. A very large (to 150 feet) deciduous tree native to India and Myanmar, and occasionally grown in zone 10. A fine landscape plant and an important timber tree.

TEDDY BEARS.
See *Cyanotis*.

Tellima grandiflora. ✤ 2
FRINGE CUP. Unusual perennial with spotted leaves and tall spikes of reddish flowers, hardy in zones 6–10. It thrives in the partial shade beneath large deciduous trees.

TENDER MAPLE.
See *Acer rubescens.*

Tephrosia. 4
CATGUT, FISH POISON PEA, RABBIT'S PEA. A group of over 300 species of the LEGUME or PEA family from the tropics and subtropics, some used in zones 5–10. Several species produce poisonous seeds that are used by native fishermen to kill fish and are also used to produce the organic insecticide *Rotenone.*

Ternstroemia gymnanthera. ✤ 2
A group of about 80 species of evergreen shrubs and trees from Japan and India, used in landscapes in the United States in zones 7–10. Related to the *Camellia,* they require well-drained, moist, acid soil to thrive. *Ternstroemia* grows in sun or shade, but leaves are reddish in full sun.

Tetraclinis. ✳9
ARAR TREE. A small coniferous evergreen tree from the dry areas of the Mediterranean regions, grown in zone 10. The ARAR TREE closely resembles its relatives, the CYPRESSES, and like them may also cause allergy.

Tetragonia. 5
Fifty species of herbs or small shrubs from Australia, New Zealand, Africa, Asia, and South America. *T. tetragonioides* or NEW ZEALAND SPINACH, is grown as a perennial vegetable. These are occasionally separate-sexed plants but the allergy potential is small.

Tetrapanax papyriferus. 6
CHINESE RICE PAPER PLANT. A tall, very large-leafed evergreen shrub for sun or shade in zones 8–10. It bears white flowers that are not implicated in allergy, but the leaves are coated in fine hairs that cause skin rash and serious irritation.

Tetrastigma. 6
JAVAN GRAPE. About 90 species of separate-sexed evergreen vines, natives of Southeast Asia and the Philippines, for zones 9–10. *T. voinieranum,* the LIZARD PLANT, LIZARD VINE, or CHESTNUT VINE, is used in landscaping in California and Florida. There is little evidence of allergy from the pollen-producing males, but because *Tetrastigma* is not sold sexed, it is wise to avoid its use.

Teucrium. ✤ 2
GERMANDER. Small shrub-like plants for hot, dry situations in all zones. The white flowers are attractive to bees.

TEXAS BLUEBELLS.
See *Eustoma grandiflorum.*

TEXAS BUCKEYE.
See *Ungnadia.*

TEXAS MOUNTAIN LAUREL.
See *Sophora.*

TEXAS PALM.
See *Sabal.*

TEXAS RANGER.
See *Leucophyllum frutescens.*

TEXAS UMBRELLA TREE
See *Melia.*

Thalictrum. ✳9
MEADOW RUE, BUTTERCUP. Perennials for all zones, but grow best in zones 2–8; they are common plants in the high latitudes of the Northern Hemisphere. MEADOW RUE usually grows 2 to 3 feet tall, but one species, *T. dipterocarpum,* the CHINESE MEADOW RUE, may grow to 6 feet. The yellow, violet, lavender, purple, or white flowers are often used in floral arrangements. All *Thalictrum* are heavy producers of airborne pollen that may cause allergy during their extended bloom period— March through August.

THATCH PALM.
See *Thrinax*.

THRIFT.
See *Armeria*.

Thea sinensis. ✳ 2
TEA. An evergreen shrub or tree, similar in many ways to its close relative, the *Camellia*. TEA is grown in India, Ceylon, Japan, Indonesia, Pakistan, Russia, Brazil, Chile, and Peru. Unpruned, a TEA tree can grow to 50 feet, but commercial plantation shrubs are usually kept clipped to about 6 feet. Like *Camellia*, *Thea* causes little or no allergy.

Thrinax. ✳ 2
FLORIDA THATCH PALM, KEY PALM, PALMETTO THATCH, THATCH PALM. Several species of medium-sized FAN PALMS, native to Mexico, Honduras, West Indies, and Florida. All are insect-pollinated and do not cause much allergy.

Theobroma cacao. ✳ 2
CACAO TREE. An evergreen tree, to 25 feet, from Central and South America, the seeds of which are used to produce cocoa and chocolate.

Thuja. 8
ARBORVITAE, THUYA, WESTERN RED CEDAR, WHITE CEDAR. Five species of evergreen coniferous trees native to North America and eastern Asia. Many of these trees are used as either trees or shrubs in all plant zones in the United States. Many cultivars of *Thuja* are sold as ARBORVITAE. Popular shrub forms of *Thuja* are sold as either "globe" or "pyramid" types. All species of *Thuja* release large amounts of airborne pollen over an extended period of time; those allergic to CYPRESS or JUNIPER have a good chance of cross-allergic reaction to ARBORVITAE.

Thuja plicata

Theophrasta. Not rated.
About 60 species of evergreen shrubs and trees from Hawaii and tropical America, many of them separate-sexed. In Florida a shrub called JACQUINIA is used in landscaping. Most of the *Theophrasta* family has not been rated yet, but may well contain numerous allergy plants.

Thevetia. 4
BE-STILL PLANT, LUCKY TREE, YELLOW OLEANDER. A fast-growing small tree or shrub from tropical America and Mexico, used in landscapes in zones 9–10. Its common name of BE-STILL PLANT derives from the fact that its long green leaves tremble in the slightest breeze. *Thevetia* tolerates a little light frost but does best in hot, frost-free areas. The sap has allergy potential and all parts of the plant are poisonous.

Thujopsis dolabrata. ✸ 9
BATTLE AX CEDAR, DEERHORN CEDAR, FALSE ARBORVITAE, HIBA ARBORVITAE, HIBA CEDAR. A large evergreen, coniferous tree native to Japan and growing to 100 feet in its native land. In the United States zones 7–10, the many named cultivars of *Thujopsis* are used as landscape plants.

Thunbergia. 📷 ✳ 2
BLACK-EYED SUSAN VINE, ORANGE CLOCK VINE, SKY FLOWER. Perennial vines for sunny areas of zones 9–10, and hanging basket annual plants elsewhere.

THORN APPLE.
See *Datura*.

THREAD PALM.
See *Washingtonia*.

THREADLEAF FALSE ARALIA.
See *Dizygotheca*.

THUYA.
See *Thuja*.

Thymus. 3

THYME. Perennial ground covers, small shrubs, or culinary herb for sunny areas of zones 4–10. The fragrance may affect perfume-sensitive individuals.

Thymophylla.

See *Dyssodia.*

TI.

See *Cordyline.*

Tibouchina urvilleana (Pleroma). 📷 ❊ 2

GLORY BUSH, PRINCESS FLOWER. A tall, loosely limbed, evergreen shrub with large, very soft, velvety leaves and large attractive purple flowers, hardy in the mildest areas of zones 9–10, and as a green houseplant elsewhere. Native to Brazil, *Tibouchina* is actually a large genus of plants with over 300 species, the best known of which is *T. urvilleana*, the PRINCESS FLOWER. Fast-growing under the right conditions, *Tibouchina* grows best with its roots in shade and its top in the sun, in mulched, well-drained, slightly acidic soil with adequate water.

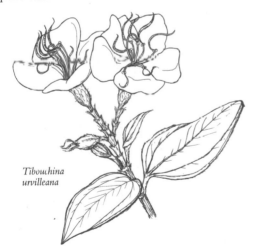

*Tibouchina
urvilleana*

TICKSEED.

See *Coreopsis.*

TIDYTIPS.

See *Layia platyglossa.*

Tigridia. 3

TIGER FLOWER. The brilliant orange, trumpet-shaped flowers, flecked with black, are held aloft on stiff, erect stems. *Tigridia* bulbs are hardy in zones 8–10.

Tilia. 📷 7

BASSWOOD, CRIMEAN LINDEN, FEMALE LINDEN, LIME TREE, LINDEN, LITTLELEAF LINDEN, MALE LINDEN, MONGOLIAN LINDEN, SILVER LINDEN, WHISTLEWOOD, WHITE LINDEN, WHITTLEWOOD. A group of about 30 species of fast-growing, spreading, deciduous trees, native to most of the Northern Hemisphere and popular as street trees and valuable lumber trees. They thrive only in areas of adequate moisture.

Despite some of their common names, no LINDEN is actually either a male- or female-only tree. They produce many small white flowers; although honeybees visit these flowers often, the trees are imperfectly insect-pollinated, and a good deal of pollen becomes airborne. *Tilia* pollen, although often allergenic, is fairly heavy and does not easily travel far from the tree. Exposure to LINDEN pollen is often caused by trees growing in the allergy sufferer's own yard or workplace.

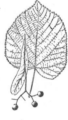

*Tilia
americana*

Tillandsia.

See *Bromelia.*

TIMOTHY.

See *Phleum.*

Tipuana tipu. 3

PRIDE-OF-BOLIVIA, ROSEWOOD TREE, TIPU TREE. An evergreen or deciduous tree native to South America, and used in the United States in zones 9–10 as an ornamental. *Tipuana* is hardy to about 20 degrees. It bears clusters of apricot-colored pea-like flowers in spring, and has long leaves divided into 11 or 12 leaflets.

Tithonia rotundifolia. 7

MEXICAN SUNFLOWER. Tall perennial with large bright orange flowers, used as an annual in sunny areas of most zones.

TITI.
See *Cyrilla racemiflora; Oxydendrum.*

TOADFLAX.
See *Linaria.*

TOBACCO, FLOWERING.
See *Nicotiana.*

Tobira.
See *Pittosporum.*

TODDY PALM.
See *Borassus.*

Tolmiea menziesii.   ✳ 1
PIGGY-BACK PLANT. Native to California's Coastal Range, the PIGGY-BACK PLANT is popular in gardens in zones 8–10 and as a houseplant elsewhere. It is tolerant of wet soil, grows well in the shade, and causes little or no allergy.

TOMATILLO.
See *Physalis.*

TOMATO.
See *Lycopersicon lycopersicum.*

TOONA TREE.
See *Cedrela toona.*

TOOTHACHE TREE.
See *Zanthoxylum.*

TORCH LILY.
See *Kniphofia uvaria.*

TORCHWOOD FAMILY.
See *Burseraceae.*

Torenia.   3
BLUEWINGS, WISHBONE FLOWER, WISHBONE PLANT. About 40 species of annuals and perennials, most used as summer annuals. The colorful flowers resemble those of *Gloxinias.*

TORNILLO.
See *Prosopis.*

Torreya. 📷   males 7, females ✳ 1
CALIFORNIA NUTMEG, FLORIDA TORREYA, JAPANESE NUTMEG TREE, NUTMEG TREE, STINKING CEDAR, STINKING YEW. Six species of evergreen coniferous trees native to California's cool canyons, Georgia and Florida, China and Japan, and used in zones 6–10. The very slow-growing JAPANESE NUTMEG produces edible seeds; it thrives only in moist, shady situations. *Torreya* is related to YEWS (*Taxus*) and like the YEWS some species of *Torreya* are separate-sexed. Because they are not sold sexed, it is best to avoid their use.

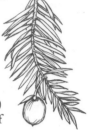

Torreya

TOTARA.
See *Podocarpus.*

TOUCH-ME-NOT.
See *Impatiens.*

TOWER OF JEWELS.
See *Echium.*

TOYON.
See *Heteromeles arbutifolia.*

Trachelospermum (Rhynchospermum). 📷 6
CONFEDERATE JASMINE, STAR JASMINE. A group of about a dozen species of shrubby, vining evergreen plants with bright star-shaped, highly fragrant white flowers. These very popular landscape plants are often used as ground covers in sun or shade, in zones 8–10. STAR JASMINE's milky sap can occasionally cause rash, and the heavy fragrance is allergenic to those who are perfume-sensitive. The fragrance is most intense on still, warm summer nights and it should not be planted near bedroom windows. Unrelated to true JASMINE (*Jasminum*), those who cannot tolerate the heavy fragrance of *Jasminum* may not be as affected by *Trachelospermum.*

Trachycarpus. 📷   *males* ✳ *9, females* ❉ *1*

WINDMILL PALMS. Several species of small- to medium-sized palm trees native to the Himalayan region of Asia. One species in particular, *T. fortunei*, the CHINESE WINDMILL or HEMP PALM, is among the hardiest of all palms, down to 7 or 8 degrees. Used in landscaping in zones 8–10, WINDMILL PALM is also commonly grown in all zones as a houseplant. Landscapers in zones 8–9 like these palms because of their ability to tolerate cold; in warm areas the trees grow quickly to 40 feet tall, but in colder, more borderline hardy areas they grow much more slowly.

Separate-sexed, they are not sold sexed. The females produce fruits that resemble large BLUEBERRIES. The male trees produce allergenic pollen. It has been erroneously stated that fan-leafed palms cause no allergy because they are perfect-flowered and pollinated only by insects. The WINDMILL PALM is not the only exception to the rule.

Trachymene coerulea (Didiscus).   *5*

BLUE LACE FLOWER. Two-foot tall annuals with clusters of lacy blue flowers on long stems; they grow best in cool weather.

Tradescantia (Zebrina).   *4*

CHAIN PLANT, SPIDERWORT, WANDERING JEW. Common houseplants or ground covers for shady areas with ample water in zones 9–10. WANDERING JEW has handsome multicolored leaves. It occasionally causes allergies—especially red, runny eyes—in dogs. In humans, allergy is uncommon.

TRAILING ARBUTUS.
See *Epigaea repens*.

TRANSVAAL DAISY.
See *Gerbera jamesonii*.

Treculia.   *males* ✳ *9, females* ❉ *1*

A dozen species of shrubs and trees from tropical Africa; one species, *T. africana*, the AFRICAN BREAD TREE, is grown in the United States in the mildest areas of zone 10. Separate-sexed plants related to MULBERRY, the female trees produce huge, seed-filled fruits (to 30 pounds) with many seeds. The male plants have high allergy potential; the females, none.

TREE FERN.
See *Blechnum*; *Cibotium*; *Dicksonia*; *Sphaeropteris*.

TREE FERN, TASMANIAN.
See *Dicksonia*.

TREE-OF-HEAVEN.
See *Ailanthus*.

TREE MALLOW.
See *Lavatera*.

TREE-OF-SADNESS.
See *Nyctanthes*.

TREFOIL.
See *Lotus*.

Trema.   ✳ *9*

About 20 species of trees or shrubs from the tropics and subtropics of both hemispheres. They are related to ELM, and some of these species have separate male-only flowers, which undoubtedly produce copious amounts of pollen. Unfortunately not much is known about individual species, so it is necessary to rate them all as a single group.

Trevesia.   *6*

SNOWFLAKE TREE. Houseplants grown for the large, snowflake-shaped leaves, held aloft on prickly, long stalks.

Trichosporum.

See *Aeschynanthus*.

Trichostema lanatum.   *3*

WOOLLY BLUE CURLS. An evergreen shrub native to California's Coastal Range, in zones 9–10; it is extremely drought-tolerant.

Tricuspidaria.

See *Crinodendron*.

TRIDENT MAPLE.
See *Acer buergeranum.*

Trifolium. 3

CLOVER. Allergy to fresh, growing CLOVER is uncommon, but adverse reaction to dried CLOVER hay is extensive and often severe. The cause of the reaction is not the CLOVER itself, but the MOLD spores that form when hay is baled while still wet. Dairy farmers, working in enclosed areas with this hay, are frequent sufferers of this allergy, known as "farmer's lung."

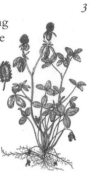

Trifolium pratense

Triglochin. ✹9

ARROW GRASS. A perennial grass-like plant common to marshy areas of much of the world, and used as a landscape plant around ponds and small pools.

Trigonella. ✽ 2

FENUGREEK. An annual grown for its aromatic seeds, which have both medicinal and culinary uses.

Trillium. ✽ 2

WAKE ROBIN. Hardy perennials for moist, shady areas in even the coldest zones. They bear attractive three-lobed white flowers in early spring.

Trillium

TRINIDAD FLAME BUSH.
See *Calliandra tweedii.*

TRIPLET LILY.
See *Triteleia.*

Tripleurospermum. 6

BRIDAL ROBE, TURFING DAISY. A group of spreading, ground cover perennials from Asia, Europe, Syria, and Lebanon, now naturalized in the eastern United States. They bear small daisy-like flowers.

Tripogandra multiflora. 5

BRIDAL VEIL. A houseplant very similar to WANDERING JEW, except that the leaves are much smaller and it produces numerous small white flowers. It is often sold as *Tradescantia multiflora.*

Tripsacum. ✹9

GAMMA GRASS. A common pasture or forage crop.

Tristania conferta. 5

BRISBANE BOX. An Australian evergreen tree with large leaves and interesting, molting bark, for zones 9–10. It is a popular landscape tree in Florida and California. BRISBANE BOX is related to *Eucalyptus* and sheds quantities of pollen, but little is known about its allergy potential. BRISBANE BOX leaves do not have the strong smell characteristic of *Eucalyptus* foliage.

Triteleia. 3

BRODIAEA, ITHURIEL'S SPEAR, TRIPLET LILIES. Native to California, *T. laxa,* ITHURIEL'S SPEAR, is grown from corms and bears large, trumpet-shaped blue flowers.

Trithrinax. 3

Small and medium-sized, spiny-trunked palm trees from South America, used in the United States in zones 9–10.

Triticum. 6

WHEAT. WHEAT is a type of grass and as such there are occasional cross-allergic reactions to its pollen, although the pollen usually does not travel far in the air. Because of this cross-allergic potential, many allergists suggest that people suffering from grass-pollen allergies refrain from eating foods made from WHEAT during peak grass pollen months. This avoidance technique often works quite well. Allergy to hay made from WHEAT is also common.

Tritoma.
See *Kniphofia uvaria.*

Tritonia.   *3*

FLAME FREESIA. Also known as *Montbretia*. Grown from corms in zones 9–10, *Tritonia* bears bright orange flowers on tall spikes.

Trollius.   *5*

GLOBE FLOWER. Large-flowered orange, yellow, or gold perennials, hardy in zones 3–10. GLOBE FLOWERS are long-lasting cut flowers.

Tropaeolum. 📷   *3*

NASTURTIUM. Two species of *Tropaeolum* are commonly used in landscaping. *T. majus*, the common garden NASTURTIUM, is a perennial that is used as a fast-growing annual. The large, round leaves and bright yellow or orange flowers are edible and piquant, and are occasionally added to salads. *T. peregrinum*, the CLIMBING NASTURTIUM, can reach 12 feet. It is yellow-flowered. Some individuals may be sensitive to its fragrance.

TRUMPET CREEPER.
See *Campsis*.

TRUMPET VINE.
See *Bignonia; Campsis; Distictis; Tecoma*.

TRUMPET VINE TREE.
See *Tabebuia*.

TRUMPET VINE, YELLOW.
See *Anemopaegma chamberlaynii; Macfadyena unguiscati*.

Tsuga.   ✳ *1*

HEMLOCK, HEMLOCK SPRUCE. A group of 10 species of tall evergreen coniferous trees, native to Canada, the United States, and Japan. The CANADA HEMLOCK is the most hardy, to zone 2, but the other species are all hardy to at least zone 6. HEMLOCKS are beautiful trees and can be used to good effect as clipped hedges or as bonsai specimens. They grow best in

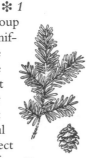

Tsuga canadensis

moist acid soil and do not do well in full sun or in spots with no protection from strong winds. *Tsuga* does not tolerate hot, dry conditions. Members of the PINE family, *Tsugas* shed abundant pollen, but because it has a waxy coating it is not irritating to mucous membranes.

TUBEROSE.
See *Polianthes tuberosa*.

TUCKEROO.
See *Cupaniopsis*.

Tulbaghia violacea.   *5*

SOCIETY GARLIC. A long-lived perennial with onion-like leaves and small lavender flowers. It has naturalized in some areas. The pollen is non-allergenic, but some find the smell of the crushed leaves objectionable; it may cause allergy in odor-sensitive individuals.

TULIP POPLAR, TULIP TREE.
See *Liriodendron*.

TULIP POPPY, MEXICAN.
See *Hunnemannia*.

Tulipa.   *4*

TULIP. A popular spring-blooming flower, grown from bulbs in all zones. TULIP pollen is rarely allergenic, but "tulip rash," caused by handling the bulbs, is not unusual and often severe.

TUNG OIL TREE.
See *Aleurites fordii*.

TUPELO.
See *Nyssa*.

Tupidanthus.   ✳ *2*

Tall plants that resemble *Schefflera*, for zone 10 or as houseplants elsewhere.

TURFING DAISY.
See *Tripleurospermum*.

TURKEY CORN.
See *Dicentra.*

TURKEY MULLEIN.
See *Eremocarpus setigerus; Verbascum.*

TURNIPS.
See *Brassica.*

Turraea obtusifolia. ✻ *2*
STAR BUSH. An evergreen shrub with large, bright-white, star-shaped flowers that thrives in light shade in the mildest parts of zone 10. It needs regular deep irrigation.

Tussilago. 6
COLTSFOOT. A common wildflower sometimes grown as a perennial for its very early spring bloom of yellow flowers. It may become invasive and is hard to eradicate where established. COLTSFOOT is used medicinally as a cough remedy.

TWINBERRY.
See *Lonicera.*

TWINFLOWER.
See *Linnaea borealis.*

TWINSPUR.
See *Diascia.*

Typha. 6
CATTAIL. A common wetland plant.

U

Allergy Index Scale: *1 is Best, 10 is Worst.*

✳ for *1* and *2*   ✸ for *9* and *10*

📷 See insert for photograph

Ugni molinae. *3*

CHILEAN GUAVA. Also known as *Myrtus ugni.* An evergreen shrub from Chile, hardy in zones 9–10. This handsome shrub has dark green leaves with a slight bronzy tint, rosy-white flowers, and small, fragrant, delicious dark purple fruit. *Ugni* grows best in slightly acid soil with ample water.

Ulmus. 📷 8

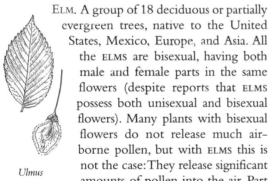

ELM. A group of 18 deciduous or partially evergreen trees, native to the United States, Mexico, Europe, and Asia. All the ELMS are bisexual, having both male and female parts in the same flowers (despite reports that ELMS possess both unisexual and bisexual flowers). Many plants with bisexual flowers do not release much airborne pollen, but with ELMS this is not the case: They release significant amounts of pollen into the air. Part of the confusion about the ELM flowering systems is probably caused by the fact that some close relatives—*Aphananthe, Hemiptelea, Holoptelea, Planera, Trema,* and *Zelkova*—produce unisexual (one-sex) flowers.

Ulmus

All ELMS produce allergenic pollen. DECIDUOUS ELMS produce their pollen in early spring, just before or at the same time as new leaves are appearing. An exception to this is *U. crassifolia*, the CEDAR ELM, which blooms in the fall. It is rated at 8 on the allergy-potential scale. The CHINESE ELM (*U. parvifolia*), which can be found growing throughout zones 6–10, is often evergreen in the warmest winter areas. CHINESE ELM releases its pollen from late summer into early winter. It is rated at 10 (📷).

There are also at least three cultivars of ELM that never bloom, making them fine allergy-free landscape trees: *U. americana* 'Ascendens', a large columnar tree; *U. glabra* 'Horizontalis', a weeping selection of SCOTCH ELM; and *U. minor* 'Gracilis', a cultivar of the EUROPEAN SMOOTHLEAF ELM. All three of these nonflowering ELMS are grown by cuttings or are budded onto seedling ELM rootstock. They are rated as excellent for the allergy-free landscape.

Because Dutch Elm Disease (DED) has killed off millions of ELM trees worldwide, the prevalence of ELM allergy has dropped considerably. In areas where ELMS have been replaced by disease-resistant look-alikes like the CHINESE ELM, however, the replacements may be more potent allergenic trees than the vanished ELMS. In fact, a strong argument can be made that the huge rise in urban allergy is directly linked to the millions of monoecious and dioecious male trees that were used to replace so many of the dead elms.

Umbellularia californica. 8

BAY LAUREL, CALIFORNIA BAY, CALIFORNIA LAUREL, MYRTLE, OREGON MYRTLE, PEPPERWOOD. A very large, spreading broadleaf evergreen tree, native to California and Oregon and hardy in zones 8–10. The leaves of this tree are occasionally used in cooking, in a similar fashion to its relative, *Laurus nobilis*, the BAY LAUREL or SWEET BAY TREE. However, unlike the pleasant odor of crushed *Laurus*

Umbellularia californica

nobilis leaves, the leaves of *Umbellularia* when crushed are malodorous. Inhaling this odor can cause immediate and severe (athough not long-lasting) head-ache. The fallen leaves also have this smell and odor-sensitive individuals should avoid it. The *Umbellularia* also produces numerous tiny white flowers with exposed stamens and plentiful pollen.

UMBRELLA PALM.
See *Hedyscepe canterburyana*.

UMBRELLA PINE.
See *Sciadopitys*.

UMBRELLA PLANT.
See *Cyperus*.

UMBRELLA TREE.
See *Brassaia; Melia*.

UMBRELLA TREE, QUEENSLAND.
See *Brassaia actinophylla*.

UMKOKOLO.
See *Dovyalis hebecarpa*.

Ungnadia.   6
FALSE BUCKEYE, MEXICAN BUCKEYE, TEXAS BUCKEYE. A small, shrubby deciduous tree native to Texas, New Mexico, and Mexico, and used in landscaping in zones 7–10. The 1-inch fragrant white flowers appear before the leaves, in early spring.

Ursinia.   7
A group of daisy-flowered annuals, perennials, and shrubs from South Africa, some used in all zones in the United States as ornamentals. Many are strong-smelling, and the pollen of all species may cause allergy.

Urtica.   ✺10
NETTLES. A large family of noxious weeds and allergy plants. *U. piluifera*, the ROMAN NETTLE, is a tall annual grown in greenhouses as an ornamental flower. It, like many others in this family, can cause allergy. STINGING NETTLES cause immediate con-tact rash. The plants produce abundant airborne pollen and have been implicated in allergy studies.

V

Allergy Index Scale: *1 is Best, 10 is Worst.*

✼ for *1* and *2*   ✳ for *9* and *10*

📷 See insert for photograph

Vaccinium.   ✼ *2*
BILBERRY, BLUEBERRY, CRANBERRY, CROWBERRY, FOXBERRY, HUCKLEBERRY. A genus of evergreen and deciduous shrubs, all with edible fruit, some hardy into zone 2. *Vaccinium* is an intriguing group of fruiting plants, most with small bell-shaped white flowers, that flourish only in very well-drained, moist, acid soil. They grow best when well mulched. BLUEBERRIES tolerate some shade but will not take drought. BILBERRY is said to be good for improving eyesight, and the juice of wild BLUE-BERRIES has long been an effective remedy for quickly curing diarrhea. CRANBERRIES and their juice are recognized as beneficial for curing or preventing bladder infections, and slowing or stopping gum disease. *Vaccinium* fruits and juices may also be useful in relieving severe lower back pain caused by liver disorder.

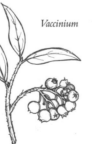

Vaccinium

VALERIAN.
See *Valeriana.*

VALERIAN, RED.
See *Centranthus ruber.*

Valeriana.   5
GARDEN HELIOTROPE, VALERIAN. Many species of ornamental and medicinal annuals and perennials, native to every continent except Australia and grown in all zones. The most commonly cultivated is *V. officinalis,* GARDEN VALERIAN, which has tall stems (to 4 feet) and clusters of tiny, fragrant, white, pink, red, or lavender flowers. The plants self-seed readily. The highly fragrant flowers may bother perfume-sensitive individuals. In *V. officinalis,* pollen is not a problem, but with some other species of this large group it may be.

Vallisneria.   7
EEL GRASS, TAPE GRASS, WATER CELERY, WILD CELERY. A small group of separate-sexed plants used in landscaping ponds and small pools. The males produce airborne pollen suspected of causing allergy.

Vallota.
See *Hippeastrum.*

Vancouveria.   3
INSIDE-OUT FLOWER. Deciduous and evergreen perennials native from California to Vancouver, Canada, and grown as a ground cover in shady areas of zones 7–9. They bear yellow, white, or white-and-lavender flowers.

Vanda.
See ORCHIDS.

Vangueria.   5
TAMARIND-OF-THE-INDIES. A group of shrubs and trees from the tropics, some with edible seeds or edible seed pods.

VAN HOUTTAN PALM.
See *Nephrosperma.*

VARIEGATED BOX ELDER.
See *Acer negundo* 'Variegatum'.

VARNISH TREE.
See *Firmiana simplex; Koelreuteria paniculata; Rhus; Semecarpus.*

VASE PLANT.
See *Billbergia.*

Vauquelinia californica. 3
ARIZONA ROSEWOOD. Drought-tolerant, evergreen shrub or small tree used in desert landscapes of zones 8–9. It bears single white flowers that resemble ROSES.

Veitchia. 7
CHRISTMAS PALM, MANILA PALM. A group of about 20 species of palm trees from the Fiji Islands, Vanuata, and the Philippines. Highly ornamental, these are widely used in tropical landscapes and in zone 10, especially in Florida.

VELVET GRASS.
See *Holcus.*

VELVET GROUNDSEL.
See *Senecio.*

VELVET PLANT.
See *Gynura.*

Venidium. 7
CAPE DAISY, NAMAQUALAND DAISY. A small group of perennial flowers from South Africa, the CAPE DAISY bears bright orange flowers and grows to 2–3 feet. It thrives in full sun.

Veratrum. 8
CORN LILY, EUROPEAN WHITE HELLEBORE, FALSE HELLEBORE, INDIAN POKE, ITCHWEED, SKUNK CABBAGE. A genus of about 45 species of perennial herbs native to North America, Europe, and Asia. *Veratrums* are usually wildflowers or weeds, but some species are used in the perennial garden. *Veratrums* thrive only in moist ground.

The FALSE HELLEBORES are an unusual group whose flowers may be white, green, brown, maroon, or purple, always borne in loose clusters on the ends of the stems. All parts are considered highly poisonous; sheep ingesting *Veratrum* give birth to lambs with fatal deformities. Even so, *Veratrum* species are used to make various forms of insecticides and are used also as medicinal plants. Avoid both products! *Veratrum* also causes skin rash, and is suspected of causing pollen-induced allergy.

Veratrum

Verbascum. 6
FLANNEL PLANT, MOTH MULLEIN, MULLEIN, PURPLE MULLEIN, TURKEY MULLEIN. A large genus of mostly hardy biennial herbs, native to Asia and Europe, but now common in most of the United States. Several species are used in flower gardens. Some species have leaves with a very disagreeable odor.

Verbena. 📷 5
BLUE VERVAIN, GARDEN VERBENA, VERVAIN, WHITE VERVAIN. A genus of about 200 species, annuals and perennials, some low-growing and others tall and almost shrub-like. *V. hybrida* is the common *Verbena* sold in most nurseries, and is grown as a short-lived perennial or ground cover in zones 9–10, and as an annual in other zones. *Verbenas* are heat-loving plants needing full sun and fast-draining soil for best results. Grown well, they flower profusely. Verbena is occasionally implicated in causing skin rash, and the scent of several species, especially when planted en masse, is unpleasant.

Verbesina. 7
BUTTER DAISY, CROWN-BEARD, WINGSTEM, YELLOW IRONWEED. A group of North and South American herbs, shrubs, and a few trees, rarely used in zones 5–10.

VERNAL GRASS.
See *Anthoxanthum.*

Vernonia. 7

IRONWEED. A very large group of herbs, shrubs, trees, and vines with almost worldwide distribution. Few, if any, are used in landscaping in the United States.

Veronica. ✲ *2*

BROOKLIME, SPEEDWELL. About 250 species of annuals and perennials from the North Temperate Zone, widely used in landscaping. (A New Zealand shrub called both *Veronica* and *Hebe*, and commonly used in most of California, is now placed in the genus *Hebe*.) Most garden *Veronicas* are hardy summer-flowering perennials, bearing white, rose, pink, or blue flowers on erect spikes. *Veronicas* grow best in full sun and need ample watering. Several prostrate varieties are used as ground covers.

Verschaffeltia splendida. *6*

A tall palm tree used in Florida.

VERVAIN.

See *Salvia; Verbena.*

Viburnum. *evergreens 5, deciduous 4*

ARROWWOOD, COWBERRY, CRANBERRY BUSH, CRANBERRY, GROUSEBERRY, GUELDER ROSE, LAURUSTINUS, LEATHERLEAF, MOOSEBERRY, NANNYBERRY, SNOWBALL BUSH, SQUAWBERRY, SUMMERBERRY, SWAMP HAW, SWEETBERRY, TEABERRY, WAYFARING TREE, WHITTEN TREE. Deciduous or evergreen shrubs or small trees, native to America, Asia, and Europe and hardy in all zones, depending on species. *Viburnums* are important long-lived landscape plants and are often used as foundation shrubs, hedges, solitary flowering shrubs, topiary, and as small trees. As relatives of the HONEYSUCKLES, most allergy occurs from close, direct inhaling of the pollen of the small, white, lightly fragrant flowers.

In California *V. tinus*, the LAURUSTINUS or EVERGREEN VIBURNUM, is commonly seen as a small tree or flowering hedge. *V. tinus* needs good air circulation and mildews in humid climates.

V. opulus, the CRANBERRY BUSH or SNOWBALL, is very popular in zones 3–10. Deciduous and hardy, it bears huge round clusters of small white flowers. Usually grown as a shrub, it makes a handsome little multitrunked tree. In some cultivars, the flowers are followed by bright red edible berries.

A very similar species, *V. carlcephalum*, produces more fragrant flowers and sets no fruit. *V. plicatum* 'Sterilis' is also similar and bears sterile flowers. (Sterility in flowers does not imply that there is no pollen; pollen is present, but the flowers don't set seed.)

Allergy to *Viburnum* pollen is uncommon; the pollen is heavy and rarely becomes airborne. Perfume-sensitive individuals may be affected by the scent of *Viburnum* flowers when in full bloom, and bees find them particularly attractive. Those with bee-sting allergies should limit the use of *Viburnums*. Evergreen species of *Viburnum* are often infested with aphids, scale, and spider mites, and these small insects may be potent allergens in themselves.

Vicia faba.

FABA BEANS. Large, robust upright growing annual broad beans. When some people eat FABA BEANS they develop a condition called favism, which makes them quite sick, or in some cases can be deadly. This reaction is most common in people from the Mediterranean area, Greeks, Italians, and Jews. In the population at large, 15 percent of blacks also cannot tolerate FABA BEANS. The pollen of FABA BEAN flowers can also set off favism in susceptible people. FABA is not allergy rated, but should be used with *caution*.

VICTORIAN BOX.

See *Pittosporum.*

Vigna. ✲ *2*

SNAIL VINE. A perennial vine for zones 9–10. SNAIL VINE and its flowers resemble those of a large BEAN vine. It dies back in winter and resprouts in spring.

Villebrunea. ✹*9*

A small group of shrubs and vining trees from Taiwan and Japan. *V. pedunculosa*, is used as a small landscape tree. Some of the species in this genus are separate-sexed and, as relatives of the NETTLES, all present distinct allergy potential.

Vinca.   ❋ 2

PERIWINKLE, MYRTLE. *V. minor* is a small-leafed, slow-growing, prostrate vine, hardy to zone 3, where it is used as a ground cover. *V. major* is a fast-growing, large-leafed version, not as hardy. Both vines bear five-petaled purple-blue flowers and have attractive dark, leathery leaves. Variegated forms of both species are available. *Vinca* grows well in full sun to full shade, but becomes tall and less compact in deep shade. Drought-tolerant once established, it performs better when provided with adequate water.

VINCA sap may cause allergic skin rash, and although this is uncommon, use care when shearing the vines. Because the flowers have almost no exposed pollen, *Vinca* makes a very good substitute for more allergenic ALGERIAN or ENGLISH IVY. The plant known as *V. rosea* or ANNUAL PERIWINKLE is a fine sun-loving annual flower properly named *Catharanthus roseus.*

VINE MAPLE.
See *Acer circinatum.*

VINEGAR TREE.
See *Rhus.*

Viola. 📷   ❋ 1

JOHNNY-JUMP-UP, PANSY, VIOLA, VIOLET. Common, cold-hardy, small perennials, usually grown as annuals and performing best in cool weather, *Violas* are planted in all zones. In zones 6–10, they grow well in spring, fall, and winter. In colder regions, *Violas* are best in spring. They thrive in full sun to partial shade and require ample water to thrive. The GARDEN VIOLAS bear medium-sized flowers. Those with very small flowers are known as JOHNNY-JUMP-UPS. Those bearing the largest and most colorful flowers are

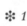

Viola

called PANSY. Long-lived and occasionally fragrant VIOLETS, *V. odorata,* are true perennials; this species is also quite poisonous. All *Violas* reseed with abandon and may become an invasive weed.

Violas produce little pollen and are entirely insect-pollinated. Perfume-sensitive individuals may have adverse reaction to the scent of fragrant VIOLETS.

VIOLET TREE.
See *Polygala.*

VIOLET TRUMPET VINE.
See *Clytostoma callistegioides.*

VIRGINIA BLUEBELLS.
See *Mertensia.*

VIRGINIA CREEPER.
See *Parthenocissus.*

VIRGINIAN STOCK.
See *Malcomia maritima.*

Viscaria.
See *Lychnis.*

Viscum cruciatum.   ✳ 9

EUROPEAN MISTLETOE. A dioecious, separate-sexed species; sprigs of berry-covered female plants are used as Christmas decoration. These do not cause allergy, although all parts of the plant are poisonous. The common AMERICAN MISTLETOE is *Phoradendron serotinum.*

Vitex. 📷   4

CHASTE TREE, HEMP TREE, MONK'S-PEPPER TREE. A large group of over 200 deciduous or evergreen shrubs or trees from the tropics and subtropics, hardy in zones 4–10. Some species have contact-allergy potential. The two most commonly seen *Vitex* are *V. agnus-castus,* the CHASTE TREE, and the less hardy *V. lucens,* or NEW ZEALAND CHASTE TREE, both of which bear spikes of blue or lavender flowers. They are used as large flowering shrubs or multitrunked small trees. *V. negundo* is a large shrub with clusters of blue flowers and is hardy to zone 4. CHASTE TREE needs good summer heat to produce the best flowers and has naturalized in some warm southern states.

Vitis. 3

GRAPE. All GRAPE flowers release pollen, but it is not a common allergen. More common is skin rash on those pruning or harvesting GRAPES: The undersides of the leaves are covered with fine hairs that may cause irritation, although not a classic allergic response. Dander from the small insects, especially aphids, that are common pests of GRAPES may cause inhalant allergy.

The MUSCADINE GRAPE is an exception, in that it is separate-sexed and produces airborne pollen, that has been implicated as causing allergy. It is not a good plant for the allergy-free garden.

Vittadinia australis. 6

A bushy subshrub used in Australia and New Zealand, the *Vittadinia* bears daisy-like white flowers on a low-growing fuzzy-leaved plant.

Vonitra. 6

Several species of slender palms from Madagascar, used to produce fiber.

Vriesea.

See *Bromelia*.

W

Allergy Index Scale: *1* is Best, *10* is Worst.

✻ for *1* and *2*　❋ for *9* and *10*

📷 See insert for photograph

WAFER ASH.
See *Ptelea*.

WAFFLE PLANT.
See *Hemigraphis*.

WAKE ROBIN.
See *Trillium*.

Waldsteinia fragarioides.　　　✻ *1*
STRAWBERRY GROUND COVER. A small, prostrate creeper for zones 6–10, bearing five-petaled yellow flowers that resemble those of STRAWBERRY.

Wallaceodendron celebicum.　　　*8*
A large and large-leafed tree from Celebes, used in tropical landscapes. Growing to 125 feet, this tree produces numerous, high pollen-producing flowers which have petals that are brown on the outside and white, yellow, and green inside.

WALLFLOWER.
See *Cheiranthus cheiri; Erysimum*.

Wallichia.　　　✻ *2*
Six species of small monocarpic palms that bloom once and die. They are used in zones 9–10. Because they flower only once, these plants produce copious amounts of pollen; they are, however, insect-pollinated and present little allergy threat. Some palms called *Wallichia* are actually *Arenga*.

WALLWORT.
See *Sambucus*.

WALNUT.
See *Juglans*.

WAND FLOWER.
See *Galax urceolata*.

WANDERING JEW.
See *Callisia; Tradescantia; Tripogandra*.

WARMINSTER BROOM.
See *Cytisus*.

Warszewiczella.　　　✻ *2*
A few species of trees from the tropics, occasionally seen in greenhouse collections in the United States.

WASHINGTON THORN.
See *Crataegus*.

Washingtonia. 📷　　　*3*
WASHINGTON PALMS. Two species native to dry areas of Mexico, California, and Arizona. *W. filifera*, the DESERT, CALIFORNIA FAN, or PETTICOAT PALM, is a thick-trunked, very stout palm tree that can eventually reach 80 feet. It is native to desert streams and springs, and is hardy to 18 degrees.

W. robusta, the MEXICAN FAN or THREAD PALM is a very tall tree with a slender trunk. It is the most common palm tree in California. It is hardy to about 20 degrees. Luckily for the many people living with these tall FAN PALMS towering overhead, both species are entirely insect-pollinated and shed very little pollen.

WATER CELERY.
See *Vallisneria*.

WATER ELM.
See *Planera aquatica*.

WATER HAWTHORN.
See *Aponogeton distachyus*.

WATER HYACINTH.
See *Eichhornia crassipes*.

WATER IVY.
See *Senecio*.

WATER LILY.
See *Aponogeton distachyus; Nelumbo; Nymphaea*.

WATER PINE.
See *Glyptostrobus lineatus*.

WATERCRESS.
See *Nasturtium*.

WATERMELON PEPEROMIA.
See *Peperomia*.

Watsonia. 3
BUGLE LILY. Easy-to-grow corms for zones 4–10, these tall, colorful plants often naturalize.

WATTLE.
See *Acacia*.

WAX APPLE.
See *Syzygium*.

WAX MYRTLE.
See *Myrica*.

WAX PALM.
See *Ceroxylon*.

WAX PLANT.
See *Hoya*.

WAX VINE.
See *Senecio*.

WAXBERRY.
See *Symphoricarpos*.

WAXFLOWER.
See *Chamelaucium uncinatum; Hoya; Stephanotis*.

WAYFARING TREE.
See *Viburnum*.

WEDDEL PALM.
See *Microcoelum*.

Wedelia triloba. 6
Tender ground cover perennial bearing small yellow flowers, for zone 10.

WEEPING WILLOW.
See *Salix*.

Weigela. 3
Deciduous shrubs that are widely used in zones 3–8, with many named cultivars. Because they flower on new wood, hard pruning after bloom encourages next season's blossoms. There are about a dozen different species of *Weigela*, usually bearing pink, purple, or carmine-colored flowers. All need ample water to thrive, but are otherwise easy to grow. Not often implicated in allergy, they are related to HONEYSUCKLE and those with allergy to HONEYSUCKLE should avoid inhaling the fragrance of *Weigela*.

Weinmannia. 7
A large genus of evergreen shrubs and trees from Africa and the Southern Hemisphere; several species are used around the world in landscapes for their large glossy leaves and pink or white flowers. Many species of *Weinmannia* are separate-sexed, and the group as a whole is closely related to several other important allergy plants.

Welwitschia mirabilis. Not rated.
A separate-sexed perennial from the deserts of Africa, occasionally found in the United States as a curiosity.

WEST INDIAN CEDAR.
See *Cedrela*.

WEST INDIAN CHERRY.
See *Malpighia glabra*.

WEST INDIAN SATINWOOD.
See *Zanthoxylum*.

WESTERN JUNE GRASS.
See *Koeleria*.

Westringia.   ✳ 2
A small group of shrubby Australian plants, similar in many ways to perennial *Salvia*. They are popular in zones 9–10, especially in California, where they are grown for their brown-spotted white flowers.

WHEAT.
See *Triticum*.

WHEATGRASS.
See *Agropyron*.

Whipplea modesta.   4
YERBA DE SALVA. A trailing sub shrub or ground cover for zones 7–10, *Whipplea* grows best in cool, shady woods where it bears clusters of white flowers.

WHISTLEWOOD.
See *Tilia*.

WHITE BLADDER FLOWER.
See *Araujia*.

WHITE CAMAS.
See *Zigadenus*.

WHITE CEDAR.
See *Cedrus; Chamaecyparis; Juniperus; Thuja*.

WHITE FORSYTHIA.
See *Abeliophyllum distichum*.

WHITE MULBERRY.
See *Morus*.

WHITE PEPPER.
See *Piper*.

WHITE VERVAIN.
See *Verbena*.

WHITETHORN.
See *Acacia*.

Whitfieldia.   ✳ 2
A small group of tropical African shrubs used in zone 10 for their white or red flowers.

WHITTEN TREE.
See *Viburnum*.

WHITTLEWOOD.
See *Tilia*.

WHYA TREE.
See *Robinia*.

Widdringtonia.
dioecious males ✹ *10, dioecious females* ✳ *2, monoecious species 8–*✹ *9*
AFRICAN CYPRESS, BERG CYPRESS, CLANWILLIAM CEDAR, MLANJE CEDAR, WILLOWMORE CEDAR. Evergreen, coniferous trees, some of which reach great height, native to Africa and Madagascar and used in the United States only in the mildest areas of zone 10. Some of the species are separate-sexed and, as close relatives of allergenic CYPRESS, they are a potent allergy threat.

WILD BUCKWHEAT.
See *Eriogonum*.

WILD CARROT.
See *Daucus*.

WILD CELERY.
See *Vallisneria*.

WILD CHINA TREE.
See *Sapindus*.

WILD CINNAMON.
See *Canella.*

WILD GINGER.
See *Asarum.*

WILD HELIOTROPE.
See *Phacelia distans.*

WILD HYACINTH.
See *Dichelostemma.*

WILD INDIGO.
See *Baptisia australis.*

WILD LILAC.
See *Ceanothus.*

WILD LIME.
See *Zanthoxylum.*

WILD MUSTARD.
See *Brassica.*

WILD OLIVE.
See *Nyssa.*

WILD RICE.
See *Zizania.*

WILD RYE.
See *Elymus canadensis.*

WILD SPINACH.
See *Chenopodium.*

WILD STRAWBERRY.
See *Fragaria.*

WILGA.
See *Geijera parviflora.*

WILLOW.
See *Salix.*

WILLOW SUMACH.
See *Rhus.*

WINDFLOWER.
See *Anemone.*

WINDMILL PALM.
See *Trachycarpus.*

WINE PALM.
See *Borassus; Caryota.*

WINGNUT TREE.
See *Pterocarya.*

WINGSTEM.
See *Verbesina.*

WINTER ACONITE.
See *Eranthis hyemalis.*

WINTER CREEPER.
See *Euonymus.*

WINTER DAPHNE.
See *Daphne odorata.*

WINTER HAZEL.
See *Corylopsis.*

WINTER SAVORY.
See *Satureja.*

Winteraceae.   Not rated.
WINTER'S BARK FAMILY. A group of about 8 genera and 70 species, mostly native to the Southern Hemisphere. They are related to *Magnolias* but have separate male flowers that produce airborne pollen. Only two kinds are used as ornamentals in the United States, *Drimys* and *Pseudowintera* (which see).

WINTERBLOOM.
See *Hamamelis.*

WINTERGREEN.
See *Gaultheria*.

WINTER'S BARK.
See *Drimys winteri; Pseudowintera*.

WINTERSWEET.
See *Chimonanthus praecox*.

WIRE VINE.
See *Muehlenbeckia*.

WISHBONE FLOWER, WISHBONE PLANT.
See *Torenia*.

Wisteria. 4

Less than a dozen species of woody vines native to Asia and the eastern United States. Two species, *W. floribunda* and *W. sinensis*, are commonly used worldwide. *W. floribunda*, the JAPANESE WISTERIA, is hardy in zones 4–10, long-lived, heavy-flowering, and may grow far up into trees or onto houses. Its fragrant flowers are white, purple, or lavender and are borne in long drooping clusters. The cultivar 'Plena' has fully double, deep blue-violet flowers. 'Plena' releases almost no pollen and is a fine choice for the allergy-free garden.

W. sinensis, the CHINESE WISTERIA, has shorter, faintly fragrant, purple flower clusters that open all at once, making them very showy in bloom. 'Alba' is a highly fragrant white cultivar. Hardiness is similar to *W. floribunda*.

W. macrostachya is a native species, found in wet areas of the Southeast, west to Arkansas. It has foot-long clusters of lilac-blue flowers and its pods are smooth. Another native is *W. frutescens*, also from the Southeast, west to Texas; it produces 5-inch-long lilac-colored flower clusters.

All species produce long pods filled with poisonous seeds which eject forcefully when ripe, often with a bang like a small firecracker. Frequently as one pod explodes, others quickly join in; it sometimes sounds like the yard has just come under gunfire! *Wisteria* is difficult to propagate from cuttings (as are most members of *Leguminosae* or PEA family) but it is easy from seed and good selections can be budded or grafted. Vines often take many years to bloom and occasionally, if the soil is too rich in nitrogen, the vines grow rampant but never bloom.

WISTERIA TREE.
See *Pterostyrax; Sesbania tripetii*.

WITCH HAZEL.
See *Hamamelis*.

WOLFBERRY.
See *Symphoricarpos*.

WONDER TREE.
See *Idesia polycarpa; Ricinus communis*.

WONDERBERRY.
See *Synsepalum dulcificum*.

WONGA-WONGA VINE.
See *Pandorea*.

WOOD FERN.
See *Dryopteris*.

WOOD SORREL.
See *Oxalis*.

WOODBINE.
See *Lonicera; Parthenocissus*.

Woodfordia. 5

Two species of shrubs from Africa, Madagascar, and Asia, occasionally used in Florida. *W. fruticosa*, a large shrub, is the most common; it bears clusters of red flowers.

WOODRUFF.
See *Galium*.

Woodwardia fimbriata. 7

GIANT CHAIN FERN. Easy to grow, very large fern for zones 7–10.

WOOLLY BLUE CURLS.
See *Trichostema lanatum*.

WOOLY SENNA.
See *Cassia.*

WORMSEED.
See *Chenopodium.*

WORMWOOD.
See *Artemisia.*

Wrightia. 6
Fifteen species of trees and shrubs from the tropics of the Old World, with poisonous seeds and a sap that causes contact allergy.

Wyethia. 6
A small genus of a dozen species of herbs native to the western United States and occasionally used as perennial plants for their yellow flowers.

X

Allergy Index Scale: *1* is Best, *10* is Worst.

❄ for *1* and *2*   ✹ for *9* and *10*

📷 See insert for photograph

Xantheranthemum.   ❄ *1*
A perennial herb from Peru, grown as a houseplant or greenhouse plant for its attractive dark green leaves with veins that are yellow above and purple below.

Xanthoceras.   6
Two species of shrubs or small trees from China, hardy in zones 6–10. They resemble HORSE CHESTNUT or BUCKEYE (*Aesculus*). The seeds are poisonous.

Xanthorrhoea.   5
BLACKBOY, GRASS TREE. A dozen species of palm-like perennials from Australia, occasionally used in landscapes in warm climates. The sap may cause skin rash.

Xeranthemum annuum.   6
IMMORTELLE. Six species of annual flowers from the Mediterranean region, grown in full sun; IMMORTELLE is a popular, long-lasting dried flower.

Xylococcus bicolor.   5
An evergreen shrub native to California and Baja California, and hardy in zones 7–10. It produces clusters of small white or pink flowers followed by small red fruit.

Xylosma. 📷   *males 6, females* ❄ *1*
About 100 species of spiny, glossy-leafed, separate-sexed evergreen shrubs or trees from the tropics and subtropics, increasingly used in landscaping in zones 8–10. The most common and cold-hardy is *X. congestum*, the SHINY XYLOSMA, a common landscape shrub often used as a tall hedge.

Because *Xylosma* does not have many commonly used close relatives, possible cross-allergic responses are sharply limited. Nonetheless, male shrubs shed airborne pollen and those living or working where a great deal of *Xylosma* grows may develop allergy. Female shrubs are identified by their small berries.

Xyris.   ❄ *2*
YELLOW-EYED GRASS. A perennial for zones 5–10. Not a true GRASS, several species of YELLOW-EYED GRASS are grown for the small, yellow, three-petaled flowers they produce. Not particular about soil, they grow best with ample water and tolerate wet soil.

Y

Allergy Index Scale: *1* is **Best,** *10* is **Worst.**

✳ for *1* and *2*   ✺ for *9* and *10*

📷 See insert for photograph

YARROW.
See *Achillea.*

YARROW GILIA.
See *Gilia.*

YATE.
See *Eucalyptus.*

YELLOW BACHELOR'S BUTTON.
See *Polygala.*

YELLOW-EYED GRASS.
See *Xyris.*

YELLOW FLAX.
See *Reinwardtia indica.*

YELLOW-FLOWERED DAISY.
See *Bidens ferulifolia.*

YELLOW IRONWEED.
See *Verbesina.*

YELLOW OLEANDER.
See *Thevetia.*

YELLOW PALM.
See *Chrysalidocarpus.*

YELLOW PARILLA.
See *Menispermum.*

YELLOW POPLAR.
See *Liriodendron.*

YELLOW POPOLO.
See *Solanum.*

YELLOW TRUMPET VINE.
See *Anemopaegma chamberlaynii; Macfadyena unguis-cati.*

YELLOWWOOD.
See *Cladrastis lutea; Rhodosphaera rhodanthema.*

YERBA BUENA.
See *Satureja.*

YERBA DE SALVA.
See *Whipplea modesta.*

YERBA MANSA.
See *Anemopsis californica.*

YESTERDAY-TODAY-AND-TOMORROW.
See *Brunfelsia pauciflora calycina.*

YEW.
See *Taxus.*

YEW, STINKING.
See *Torreya.*

YEW PINE.
See *Podocarpus.*

Yucca. 📷   ✳ *2*
ADAM'S NEEDLE, BANANA YUCCA, BLUE YUCCA, DAG-
GER PLANT, JOSHUA TREE, NEEDLE PALM, PALM LILY,
PALMA PITA, ROMAN CANDLE, SOAP TREE, SOAPWELL,
SPANISH BAYONET. A group of about 40 species of
sharp-spined plants native to the warm areas of

North America; some are hardy to zone 4, but few will flower north of zone 4. *Yucca* flowers are usually creamy white, tinged with pink or purple, and borne on tall, stiff stalks that rise well above the foliage. The flowers are entirely insect-pollinated and do not shed pollen.

The long, daggerlike leaves are dangerous, however, especially to small children, and placement of these vigorous plants requires good judgment. One species from Florida, *Y. recurvifolia*, lacks the sharp-tipped leaves and makes a better garden plant than most *Yuccas*. Another species, *Y. elephantipes*, the GIANT YUCCA, grows far too large for most gardens and is difficult to remove.

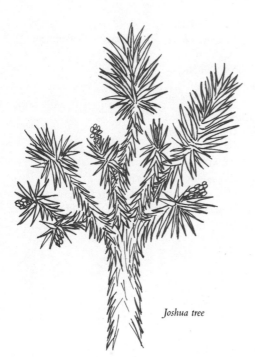

Joshua tree

Z

Allergy Index Scale: *1 is Best, 10 is Worst.*

❇ for *1* and *2*　　❋ for *9* and *10*

📷 See insert for photograph

ZABEL LAUREL.
See *Prunus.*

Zaluzianskya capensis.　　5

NIGHT PHLOX. A shrubby tender perennial for zone 10, grown for its fragrant tubular flowers that are white on the outside and purple inside. The scent may affect perfume-sensitive individuals, and the sap of these plants is poisonous and may occasionally cause skin rash.

Zamia.　　5

ARROW ROOT, COMPTIE, COONTIE, FLORIDA ARROW-WOOD, SAGO CYCAS, SEMINOLE BREAD. Small, separate-sexed, palm-like plants often used as houseplants, and sometimes as garden plants in zone 10. An occasional plant should pose little allergy potential, but because they are separate-sexed, the males may trigger allergic response. Female *Zamia* are identified by their central cone, which is considerably larger than that of the male. Viable seeds may be produced on the female plants.

Zantedeschia.　　4

CALLA, CALLA LILY. Tall perennials, with unusually prominent calyxes in white, yellow, pink, or red; they are easy to grow and hardy in zones 8–10. In cooler climates, the roots must be lifted and over-wintered indoors. They thrive in shade or sun, but require ample water.

The sap of CALLA LILIES has properties similar to that of DUMB CANE (*Dieffenbachia*), and it may cause contact rash. The pollen, which is prominently displayed on the stiff stamens, may cause allergy if inhaled. All parts of the plant are poisonous if eaten.

Zanthoxylum.　　6

HERCULES' CLUB, JAPAN PEPPER, PEPPERWOOD, PRICKLY ASH, SEA ASH, TOOTHACHE TREE, WEST INDIAN SATINWOOD, WILD LIME. Several hundred species of prickly, evergreen or deciduous shrubs and trees native to North and South America, Africa, Asia, and Australia. In California *Z. piperitum,* JAPAN PEPPER, a small evergreen tree, hardy in zones 8–10, is common. *Z. clava-herculis,* the SOUTHERN PRICKLY ASH, PEPPERWOOD, or HERCULE'S CLUB is common from Florida to

Zanthoxylum

Oklahoma, and hardy to zone 7. *Z. fagara,* the WILD LIME, is used in Florida and southern Texas into Mexico.

Several species of deciduous *Zanthoxylum* trees are used in Japan and China. *Z. americanum,* the TOOTHACHE TREE, is used for medicinal purposes and is hardy in zones 5–10.

Some members of this large genus produce airborne pollen, but allergy is uncommon. As *Citrus* relatives, some species may cause contact skin rash, and in fragrant varieties negative odor challenges are possible.

Zauschneria.　　4

CALIFORNIA FUCHSIA. Four species of woody perennials. *Z. californica* 'latifolia' is the hardiest, growing well in zones 6–10. It is a small shrubby plant with small tubular red flowers that resemble those of *Fuchsia.* Easy to grow in full sun, the flowers are attractive to hummingbirds. *Z. californica* has been reclassified in the *Epilobium* (FIREWEED) genus.

Zea mays. 6

CORN. Annual. The tassels at the top of the CORN plant are male flowers; the ears of corn themselves are actually female flowers. The pollen only goes airborne early in the mornng.

ZEBRA PLANT.
See *Calathea*.

Zebrina.

See *Tradescantia*.

Zelkova. 📷 ✳10

JAPANESE ZELKOVA, SAWLEAF ZELKOVA. Five species of ELM-like and ELM-related trees native to Japan and China and used throughout most of the United States. The most commonly used is *Z. serrata*, a hardy deciduous tree for zones 3–10. Also common is *Z. carpinifolia*, occasionally sold as *Z. ulmoides*, which is hardy to zone 4. Either of these two trees can grow to 50 feet; *Z. serrata* has a slightly wider growth habit and *Z. carpinifolia* forms a classic ELM-like vase shape.

Zelkova was little used in the past but has now become popular as a replacement tree for ELMS killed by Dutch Elm Disease — *Zelkova* is resistant to the disease. Little research has been done on allergy caused by *Zelkova*, but many have recently been planted and are only now starting to mature.

Zelkova is a direct ELM relative and, unlike the ELMS, which have bisexual flowers that do not shed much pollen, *Zelkova* has separate male flowers. When large and mature, *Zelkova* is able to put even more pollen into the air than an ELM of the same size. ELM pollen is the cause of some allergy, and reactions are often severe. *Pollinosis* (a big word for asthma and hay fever) to *Zelkova* will likely grow rapidly in importance in the future as these newly planted trees grow and mature.

Zenobia pulverulenta. 5

A deciduous shrub native to the southeastern United States and used in landscaping for its clus-

ters of fragrant white flowers. It needs moist, acid soil and grows well in partial shade. (Also known as *Andromeda speciosa*).

Zephyranthes. 3

FAIRY LILY, RAIN LILY, ZEPHYR FLOWER. A small hardy bulb, related to *Amaryllis*, for full sun or light shade in zones 4–10. It must be winter mulched heavily in zones 4–8.

Zigadenus. 7

ALKALI GRASS, DEATH CAMAS, STAR LILY, WHITE CAMAS. A bulbous perennial growing wild in fields from Minnesota to California and north to Alaska. It is sometimes used in perennial gardens for its white flowers. All parts are highly poisonous. Contact with the sap or roots may cause skin rash. This plant is sometimes confused with wild onions, with deadly results.

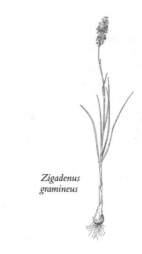

*Zigadenus
gramineus*

Zingiber officinale. 3

TRUE GINGER. An easy-to-grow tall perennial with greenish yellow flowers, for zones 8–10. Tubers of ginger root can be bought at the grocery store and planted in spring. Plants die back with the first frost and regrow in spring. In colder regions, a heavy mulch may carry the tender roots through the winter.

Zinnia. 📷 3

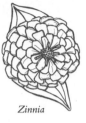

Popular garden annuals for full
sun, in many different sizes,
shapes, and colors. *Zinnias* are
related to the RAGWEEDS and as
such, may cause allergy. *Zinnia*
flowers, however, shed very little

Zinnia

pollen and in many tests, reaction to *Zinnia* was
neither common nor severe.

ZINNIA, CREEPING.

See *Sanvitalia procumbens.*

Zizania. 4

WILD RICE. Rarely implicated in allergy; the pollen
has low allergenicity.

Ziziphus. 7

CHINESE DATE, CHINESE JUJUBE, JUJUBE. Over 40
species of deciduous and evergreen shrubs or trees,
often with many sharp spines, and most producing
small edible, date-like fruits, hardy in zones 5–10,
although the fruits require high summer heat to
ripen fully. The fruits have a crunchy texture and a
flavor resembling PEAR and APPLE; these fruits are
sometimes dried and used like dates.

JUJUBE is related to the BUCKTHORNS and its
heavy pollen may cause allergy to those in the immediate vicinity of the trees.

The COMMON JUJUBE TREE, *Z. jujuba*, may reach
40 feet, although half that size is more common.
The cultivar 'Inermis' is thornless. 'Lang' and 'Li'
are two common fruiting cultivars; the fruit of 'Li'
are slightly larger (to 2 inches long), but 'Lang' is
faster to bear after planting.

Zombia antillarum. ❋ 1

ZOMBI PALM. A 10-foot FAN PALM from Haiti, the
ZOMBI PALM has a stout trunk sheathed in long
fibers. Completely insect-pollinated, it causes no
allergy.

Zoysia. 6

Three species of common lawn grass for milder
areas of the United States. *Z. japonica* is KOREAN
GRASS; *Z. matrella* is JAPANESE CARPET or MANILA

GRASS; and *Z. tenuifolia* is MASCARENE or KOREAN
VELVET GRASS. All three are propagated from plugs
or by stolons. *Zoysia* lawns are popular in parts of
zones 9 and 10. The lawns are coarse, thick, and
spongy and tend to produce a great deal of thatch.
Unlike BERMUDA GRASS, *Zoysia* does not often
flower while it is short, so regular mowing elimi-
nates most pollen producing potential. *Zoysia*
sometimes escapes cultivation to become a problem weed in vacant lots. In these circumstances, it
will produce pollen that, while allergenic, is not
nearly as potent as that of other lawn grasses. For a
similar but superior lawn grass for mild winter areas, see *Stenotaphrum secundatum*, ST. AUGUSTINE
GRASS, or a female clone of SALTGRASS or BUFFALO
GRASS.

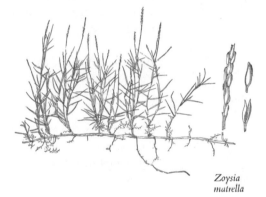

*Zoysia
matrella*

Glossary of Horticultural Terms

Annual. A plant that lives, flowers, produces seed, and dies within one year or less. Examples of annuals are corn, beans, and marigolds.

Asexual. No sex; not grown from seed. *Asexual propagation* (see *propagation*) is growing new plants from cuttings, divisions, runners, budding, grafting, layering, or tissue cultures. An asexually grown plant is essentially a clone; nonetheless there are sometimes slight variations even among these clones.

Biennial. A plant that lives for more than one year but not more than two years. Biennials usually flower in their second year. Examples of biennials are carrots, cabbage, and many, but not all, foxgloves.

Bisexual. A flowering system where both male and female functional parts are found in the same flower. Other names for bisexual are *perfect* and *complete*. Bisexual flowers are found in roses, apples, plums, and snapdragons.

Bract. A highly colored leaf that resembles a flower petal. Common plants with colorful bracts are *Bougainvillea* and poinsettia.

Complete flower. *A perfect* or *bisexual* flower, having both male and female functional parts in the same flower. A complete flower also has a full set of petals and sepals.

Conifer. A cone-bearing plant, usually evergreen, often with slender leaves or needles, belonging to the large plant order *Coniferales*. Examples of conifers are pines, spruce, yew, juniper, cedar, and cypress.

Coniferous. Belonging to the group of conifers.

Cross-allergic reactions. Also called *cross-reactive allergy*. When a person becomes highly allergic to one particular plant, they may easily become allergic to close relatives of that plant. For example, if you are highly allergic to pollen of the black walnut, it may not take long before you develop a cross-allergic response to the pollen of English walnut. In time you may also become allergic to pollen from butternuts, pecans, and hickories, all relatives of walnut. Likewise, after some time it is quite possible that you will also become allergic to eating these nuts, and to using the oil from them. Sometimes there are cross-allergic responses between plant groups that are not closely related, although this is not as common.

People who are already highly allergic to ragweed pollen often can develop cross-allergic reactions to daisy, coyote bush, marigold, calendula, aster, and sunflower, all of which are in the same large family of plants. Likewise, a person already allergic to poison ivy or poison oak will be at additional risk to develop cross-allergic reactions to their relatives, plants such as lemonade berry, smoke bush, and pepper trees.

Crown. A cluster of vegetative buds. Most hardy perennial plants form crowns at or just under the soil line. If the top part of the plant is killed off by frost, the plant usually resprouts from this crown. Crowns are protected by mulching. In certain plants, like strawberries, it is essential at planting to set the crowns in the soil at just the right depth. Buried too deeply, they rot, and not planted deep enough, they dry out and die.

Cultivar. A cultivated variety. Using the maple tree *Acer rubrum* 'Red Sunset' as an example, the cultivar is 'Red Sunset'. Cultivar implies that it is a cultivated plant, not just a variation of some species that only grows in the wild. A cultivar can only be duplicated asexually. They will not come true from seed.

Deciduous. A tree, shrub, or vine that loses its leaves, usually in the fall, and then grows new leaves in the spring. Common deciduous plants are maples, elms, willows, and apples. The opposite of deciduous is *evergreen*.

Dicot. Dicotyledon. Dicot seeds sprout and emerge from the soil with two first leaves. Examples of dicots are beans, tomatoes, maple trees, marigolds, petunias, junipers, and pines. Dicots typically have their flower parts in sets or multiples of five. Plum flowers, for example, usually have five petals, five sepals, and fifteen stamens. All flowering plants in the world are either dicots or *monocots*.

Dioecious. A separate-sexed plant, having only male flowers on one plant and only female flowers on another. Many of the most allergenic plants are dioecious males. Examples of dioecious plants are most willows, all box elders, some junipers, all yews, most of the ash and poplars, many palm trees, and all ginkgos, pepper trees, and hollies.

Dormant. Alive but not actively growing. Deciduous plants are dormant during the winter, as are many perennials. Many hardy plants go through a dormant period.

Evergreen. A tree, shrub, or vine that holds its leaves all year long. Common evergreens are pines, most hollies, lemons, and oranges.

Exserted stamens. In some flowers the male parts, the *stamens*, stick out from the flower, or are *exserted*. On the tips of the stamens are the *anthers*, and the anthers contain all the pollen. If a flower type has exserted stamens, the pollen is more easily contacted. Not all flowers with exserted stamens cause allergies; it is, however, always one of many factors considered in rating.

Family. A large group of related genera. In the beech family are found all the tan oaks, beechnuts, chestnuts, and oaks. Family members share common traits. For example, in the beech family, all the members are monoecious. In the study of allergy, we often find that someone who is allergic to a particular plant later may become allergic to different plants, which are in the same family. For example, someone allergic to the pollen of arborvitae may well become allergic to pollen from junipers. Both juniper and arborvitae are in the larger family, *Cupressaceae*, the cypress family.

Foundation shrubs. Permanent bushes planted around a building, often to hide the foundation lines. A good foundation plant is bushy, attractive, does not grow too large or too fast, is generally evergreen, and is easy to grow, pest-free, long-lived, and reliable. A well-landscaped house will always have a good selection of foundation shrubs.

Genus. Usually the first part of a plant's scientific name. Using the red maple as an example, the correct name is *Acer rubrum*. *Acer* is the *genus*. This system of giving all plants two names, called *binomial nomenclature*, was created by the great Swedish botanist, Carl Linnaeus. It was his intention that *genus* meant *group*, and that the next word, the *species*, meant *kind*. *Genera* is plural for *genus*.

Hardy, hardiness. The measure of a plant's ability to withstand frost and cold. This term is confused perhaps more than any other in horticulture. Hardy does not mean that a plant is strong, easy to grow, or tough. A hardy plant is one that can take frost and cold and not suffer. A tomato plant is not hardy, it is *tender*. A hard frost will quickly kill a tomato plant. A cabbage plant is hardy. Kale is hardier than cabbage, and a sugar maple tree is considerably hardier than either.

Herb, herbaceous. A plant without woody stems. A pepper plant is herbaceous, as is a potato plant. A shrub or tree is not an herb because it has woody stems.

Monocot. Monocotyledon. Monocot seeds sprout and emerge from the soil with one first leaf only. Examples of monocots are all grasses, lilies, onions, corn, wheat, and palm trees. In monocots, the veins run parallel to each other and the flowering parts are usually in threes. All the flowering plants in the world are either *dicots* or monocots.

Monocots do not form growth rings and they grow altogether differently than dicots. For example, if a slash is made three feet from the ground on the trunk of a young palm tree, ten years later this slash mark might be ten feet up on the tree trunk. If a similar slash were made on the trunk of a young dicot tree, ten years later the tree would be taller and the trunk wider, but the slash mark would still be exactly three feet from the ground.

Monoecious. A flowering system where separate male and female flowers are found on the same plant. In the example of corn, the top of the plant, the tassels, are the male flowers. The actual ears of corn are clusters of female flowers. In the example of a common cattail, a similar system is at work. The tip of the cattail has the male (pollen) flowers and the thicker, fatter, round part is composed of individual female flowers. Monoecious flowering systems are very important in allergy study because often the pollen will be dispersed not by insects, but by the wind. Some examples of monoecious plants are cypress, many of the palms, redwoods, oaks, some of the junipers, hickory, boxwood, pecans, and walnuts.

Naturalize. Some domestic plants will naturally spread by runners, corms, or *rhizomes,* while others drop much viable seed that will quickly sprout and grow. Certain cultivated plants, like daffodils, narcissus, ajuga, Japanese honeysuckle, and Mexican evening primrose often spread far from their original plantings. Sometimes this spreading or *naturalizing* is welcomed and other times it isn't.

Perennial. A plant that lives longer than two years. Perennial is a term most often used for winter hardy plants like phlox, poppy, peony, lupine, foxglove, delphinium, and columbine. Trees and shrubs are *woody plants*, not perennials. The top parts of a perennial plant may die to the ground in late fall but the plant will resprout from the underground crown in the spring.

Petals. Most flowers have petals, although in some they are totally lacking. Most *dicot* flowers have five petals (or multiples of five), although some have four. *Monocots* usually have three petals or multiples of three. Large, colorful, attractive petals are always considered a plus in allergy studies. All of the petals collectively form the *corolla*.

Poisonous. In this text the word *poisonous* means that the plant, its seeds, leaves, flowers, roots, etc. are toxic if eaten. There are many kinds of poisons in plants, some deadly, but because a plant is poisonous does not mean it causes allergy.

Propagation. To start a new plant. There are many methods of propagation used, such as seed, cuttings, spores, grafting, etc. Propagation using seeds is considered *sexual propagation*. Methods not involving seed are *asexual propagation*. To propagate cultivars, which do not come true from seed, asexual methods must be used. It is not legal to asexually propagate patented plants unless permission has been granted from the license holder.

Rhizomes. Thick, spreading, underground roots that are capable of sprouting new plants. Rhizomes are similar to runners, except that runners spread along the top of the soil, and rhizomes usually spread just under the soil line.

Seedling grown. Many plants are grown from seeds, and often these do not come true from seed, meaning that they may not be exactly like the seed parent plant. For example, a female cultivar of a red maple will set seed if pollinated; however, these seeds will grow maple trees, which will be both male and female. If a female cultivar is desired, it cannot be exactly duplicated from seed. To get an identical plant, it must be grown asexually.

Sepals. Leaf-like appendages just below the flower petals. The sepals are usually considered part of the flower. Most dicots produce five sepals, although sometimes four are present in species like evening primrose and poppies. Colorful sepals sometimes take the place of petals as insect attractors for pollination. In allergy studies, the presence of attractive sepals is considered a plus. All of the sepals taken together form the *calyx*.

Species. The second part of a scientific name. With the common tall marigold, the scientific name is *Tagetes erecta*. The species is *erecta*. The general meaning of species is *kind*. For example, in the name *Juniperus horizontalis*, *horizontalis* is the species and tells us that this species is a low-growing, spreading (horizontal) kind of juniper.

Stamens. The male parts of a flower. On the tip of the stamen is the *anther*, which contains the pollen. A flower that is all male is called a *staminate flower*.

Sub shrub. A woody plant that may grow like a big perennial, and sometimes become shrub-like. A sub shrub is not usually considered as permanent a plant as most species described as either shrubs or bushes.

Unisexual. A flowering system where separate-sexed flowers are present. Any flowering plants that are *dioecious* or *monoecious* are unisexual. Examples are hickory, walnut, sweet gum, and currants.

Variety. A subdivision of a species. For example in the tree often called rubber tree, the name is stated as *Ficus elastica* 'Decora'. In this example, the variety is 'Decora'. The difference between a *cultivar* and a variety is that a cultivar is only a *variety* of a cultivated species.

Vegetative. Growth that consists of stems and leaves, but not flowers. Often shrubs that are frequently sheared hard grow vegetatively only and do not produce flowers.

Volatile organic compounds (VOCs). Air pollutants released by trees and shrubs. Trees and shrubs remove huge amounts of air pollutants daily; however a few trees, such as *Liquidambar*, oak, and sycamore, produce more VOCs than they absorb, thus adding to industrial-produced smog.

Recommended Reading

*Note: This list of references is in no way complete, but included are a few of the books and articles that I found especially useful in the writing of *Allergy-Free Gardening*.

Bailey, Liberty Hyde, Ethel Zoe Bailey, and Cornell University Editors, *Hortus Third*. London, New York: Collier Macmillan Publishers, 1976.

Cairns, Thomas, *Modern Roses 10*. Shreveport, Louisiana: The American Rose Society, 1995. For serious rose lovers, this is *the* book.

Clark, David and Elizabeth L. Hogan, Editors, *Sunset Western Garden Book*. Menlo Park, California: Lane Publishing Company, 1986. For the Pacific West Coast, this is one of the most useful general gardening books.

Flint, Harrison L., *Landscape Plants for Eastern North America*. New York: John Wiley & Sons, 1983.

Jacobson, Arthur Lee, *North American Landscape Trees*. Berkeley, California: Ten Speed Press, 1996. One of the very best books on hardy landscape trees. Jacobson understands sex systems in trees and always includes this information. Great attention to detail.

Jelks, Mary, M.D., *Allergy Plants*, and also Mary Jelks, M.D., *Aeroallergens of Florida*. Immunology and Allergy Clinics of Naples, 1889: 381–399.

Jury, S. L., Cutler Reynolds, and F. J. Evans, *The Eurphorbiales*. The Linnean Society of London. London: The Whitefriars Press, 1987.

Lewis, Walter, H. and Wayne E. Imber, "Aeroallergens in the Midwestern United States: Pollen and Spores Hazardous to Health." IV Int. Palynol. Conf., Lucknow (1976-77) 3: 466–474, 1981.

Lewis, Walter H., "Airborne Pollen of the Neotropics." *Grana* 25 (20 March 1986): 75-83.

Lewis, Walter H., Prathibha Vinay, and Vincent E. Zenger, *Airborne and Allergenic Pollen of North America*. Baltimore and London: Johns Hopkins University Press, 1983. From a purely scientific point of view, I consider this the best book ever written on the connections between plants and pollen allergy.

Lewis, Walter H., Anu Dixit, and Walter Ward, "Distribution and Incidence of North American Pollen Aeroallergens." *American Journal of Otolaryngology* 12 (1991): 205-226.

Lewis, Walter H. and Memory Elvin Lewis, *Medical Botany*. New York: John Wiley and Sons Publications, 1977. A fascinating book!

Lewis, Walter H. and Prathibha Vinay, "North American Pollinosis Due to Insect-Pollinated Plants." St. Louis, Missouri, Washington University Department of Biology, May 1979.

Lewis, Walter H., *Tropical to Warm Temperate Aerospora of Vascular Plants*. St. Louis, Missouri, Washington University, 1990. This is a very extensive bibliography of useful sites up to 1990. For the serious allergy researcher, this is a good place to start.

McMinn, Howard E. and Evelyn Maino, *Pacific Coast Trees*. Berkeley, California: University of California Press, 1981. A fine easy-to-use book for identifying West Coast trees.

Mortensen, Ernest and Ervin Bullard, *Handbook of Tropical and Sub-Tropical Horticulture*. Washington, DC: USDA, May 1964.

Munz, Philip A. and David D. Keck, *A California Flora and Supplement*. Berkeley, California: University of California Press, 1968. This is not light reading, but is nonetheless the "Bible" on native California species.

Nowak, David J., P. J. McHale, M. Ibarra, D. Crane, J. Stevens, and C. Luley, *Modeling the Effects of Urban Vegetation on Air Pollution*. New York: Plenum Press, 1998.

Peattie, Donald Culross, *A Natural History of Trees of Eastern and Central North America* and *A Natural History of Western Trees*. Boston: Houghton Mifflin Company, 1991. These are two of my favorite books about trees, extremely readable and packed full of interesting and important observations that other writers miss.

Rapp, Doris, M.D., *Is This Your Child?* New York: William Morrow and Company, Dover Publications, Inc., 1961. Doris Rapp is a true pioneer in allergy study.

Sargent, Charles Sprague, *Manual of the Trees of North America*. New York: Dover Publications, Inc., 1965. One of the very best.

Snyder, Leon C., *Gardening in the Upper Midwest*. Minneapolis: University of Minnesota Press, 1978.

Taylor, Norman, *Taylor's Encyclopedia of Gardening*. Cambridge, Massachusetts: Houghton Mifflin Co., 1948. This is an old but wonderful book. One of my all time favorites, this is a very useful general gardening book.

Utterback, Christine, *Reliable Roses*. New York: Clarkson Potter Publishers, 1997. Good book for picking out roses with extra disease resistance.

Van Gelderen, D. M., P. C. de Jong, and H. J. Oterdoom, *Maples of the World*. Portland, Oregon: Timber Press, 1994. The very best book I've ever read on maples.

Winter, Ruth, *The People's Handbook of Allergies and Allergens*. Chicago: Contemporary Books, Inc., 1984.

Wodehouse, R. P., *Pollen Grains*. New York: McGraw-Hill, 1935. Wodehouse was one of the first and one of the best. *Pollen Grains* is a classic in allergy literature.

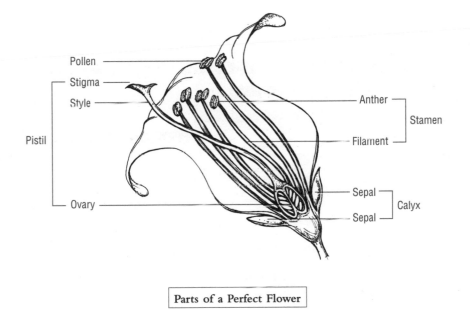

Pollen

Stigma

Style

Pistil

Ovary

Anther

Stamen

Filament

Sepal

Sepal

Calyx

Parts of a Perfect Flower

Pollen Calendar

Species	Jan	Feb	Mar	Apr	May	June	July	Aug	Sept	Oct	Nov	Dec
Acacia	■	■	■	■	■	■	■	■	■	■		
Acer		■	■	■	■							
Ailanthus			■	■	■	■						
Albizia							■	■	■	■		
Alder/Alnus		■	■	■								■
Almond		■	■	■								
Artemisia							■	■	■	■		
Baccharis									■	■	■	■
Bermuda Grass		■	■	■	■	■	■					
Betula			■	■						■		
Broussonetia		■	■	■	■							
Buxus		■	■	■	■	■						
Callistemon	■	■	■	■	■	■	■	■	■	■		
Calocedrus			■	■	■	■	■	■				
Carya		■	■	■	■							
Casurina	■	■	■								■	■
Catalpa					■	■	■					
Ceanothus			■	■	■	■						
Celtis			■	■	■							
Chionanthus					■	■	■	■				
Cinnamomum				■	■	■						

These are approximate dates of bloom periods of some of the most common allergenic trees, grasses, and shrubs. The actual blooming periods will be earlier in southern areas and later in northern climates. Poplars, for example, may start blooming in January in Florida, but in Washington state, they may not start until May. Some species of plants, for example cypress, may be in and out of bloom all year long in the areas furthest south.

Species	Jan	Feb	Mar	Apr	May	June	July	Aug	Sept	Oct	Nov	Dec
Cocculus				■	■	■	■					
Corylus			■	■	■							
Cryptomeria	■	■	■	■								
Cudrania		■	■									
Cunonia			■	■	■	■						
Cupaniopsis			■	■	■							
Cupressus	■	■	■	■	■	■	■	■	■	■	■	
Elaeagnus				■	■	■						
Eucommia		■	■	■	■	■						
Euonymus								■	■	■		
Festuca	■	■	■	■	■	■	■	■	■	■	■	■
Fraxinus	■	■	■	■								
Ginkgo		■	■	■	■							
Gymnocladus			■	■								
Hedera								■	■	■		
Hippophae		■	■	■	■							
Ilex		■	■	■	■							
Juglans				■	■	■						
Juniperus		■	■	■	■			■	■	■	■	
Laurus		■	■	■	■							
Ligustrum			■	■	■	■	■	■	■	■	■	

Species	Jan	Feb	Mar	Apr	May	June	July	Aug	Sept	Oct	Nov	Dec
Liquidambar				■	■	■	■					
Maclura			■	■								
Mallotus	■	■	■	■								
Maytenus		■	■	■	■							
Melaleuca			■	■	■	■						
Morus			■	■	■							
Myrica			■	■	■							
Myrsine			■	■	■	■	■					
Nyssa			■	■	■							
Olea				■	■	■	■					
Ostrya			■	■	■							
Palm Trees	■	■	■	■	■	■	■	■	■	■	■	
Pennisetum	■	■	■	■	■	■	■	■	■	■	■	■
Phellodendron			■	■	■	■						
Pistache			■	■	■							
Planera								■	■	■		
Platanus			■	■	■							
Platycarya				■	■	■						■
Platycladus			■	■	■	■						
Poa	■	■	■	■	■	■	■	■	■	■	■	
Podocarpus		■	■	■	■	■	■	■				
Populus			■	■	■	■	■					
Prosopis			■	■	■	■	■					
Quercus		■	■	■	■	■	■					
Ragweed								■	■	■	■	
Rhamnus		■	■	■	■	■	■					
Rhus			■	■	■	■	■					

Species	Jan	Feb	Mar	Apr	May	June	July	Aug	Sept	Oct	Nov	Dec
Ribes			███	███	███	███						
Ricinus					███	███	███	███	███	███		
Salix	███	███	███	███	███	███						
Sapium							███	███	███	███		
Sapindus							███	███	███	███		
Schinus					███	███	███	███	███	███		
Senecio								███	███	███	███	
Solidago								███	███	███		
Syringa				███	███	███						
Tamarix	███	███	███	███							███	███
Taxodium	███	███										███
Taxus			███	███	███							
Thujopsis	███	███	███	███								███
Tilia						███	███	███				
Ulmus	███	███	███	███								
Umbellularia		███	███	███	███							
Xylosma								███	███	███	███	███
Zanthoxylum	███	███	███	███	███	███						
Zelkova	███	███	███	███	███	███						███

Index

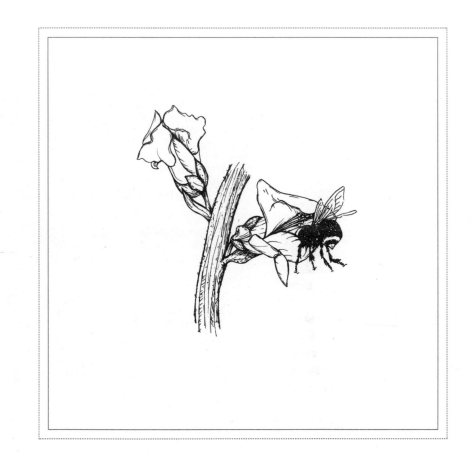